The Unofficial Guide to Getting into Medical School

EDITION
2

The Unofficial Guide to Getting into Medical School

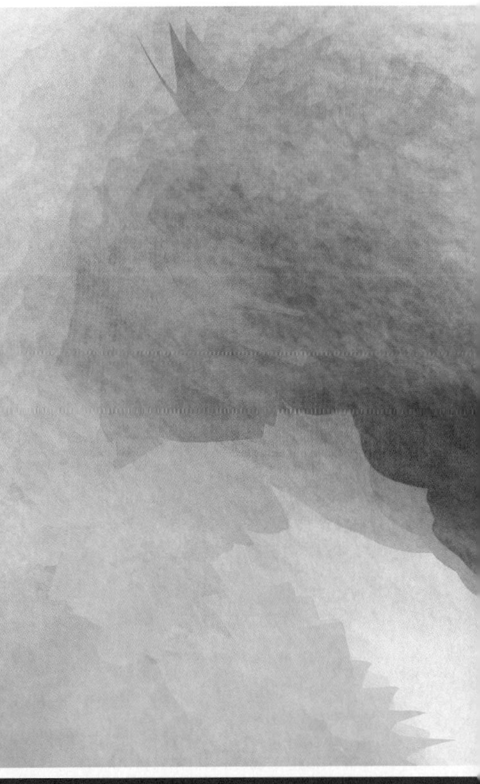

Bogdan Chiva Giurca BMBS, ClinEnt Fellow, DipIBLM
Specialty Doctor
London Deanery
United Kingdom
Council Member
College of Medicine
United Kingdom
Honorary Lecturer
University College London
United Kingdom

Series Editor
Zeshan Qureshi BM, BSc (Hons), MSc, MRCPCH FAcadMEd, MRCPS (Glasg)
Paediatric Registrar
London Deanery
United Kingdom

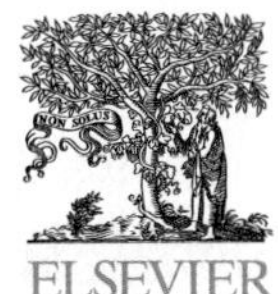

ELSEVIER

First edition 2019. Published by Zeshan Qureshi.

ISBN: 978-0-443-11338-3

Content Strategist: Trinity Hutton
Content Project Manager: Tapajyoti Chaudhuri
Cover Design: Miles Hitchen
Marketing Manager: Deborah J. Watkins

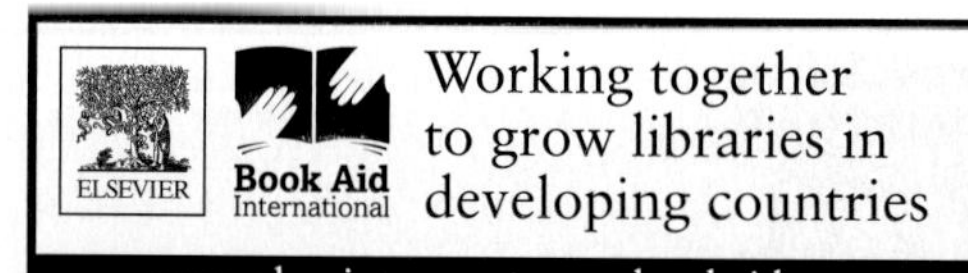

Printed in India.

Last digit is the print number: 9 8 7 6 5 4 3 2 1

This book is dedicated to the hundreds of medical students and medical school applicants who have shared their ideas and reflections to make this book possible. You have inspired us in ways you could never even imagine.

Bogdan Chiva Giurca

This extensive project would not have been possible without the guidance, inspiration and support of my dear mentors, mentees and colleagues, all of whom cannot be named, but I would particularly like to thank Dr Zeshan Qureshi for the opportunity to inspire the next generation of medical students and young doctors. To my mentors, thank you for your encouraging comments and feedback. To our dear applicants and current medical students who have reflected upon their current experiences with the medical school application process so passionately, I'd like to thank you wholeheartedly for sharing your journeys into medicine.

Contents

Series Editor Foreword

The Unofficial Guide to Medicine is not just about helping students study; it is also about allowing those that learn to take back control of their own education. Since its inception, it has been driven by the voices of students, and through this, democratised the process of medical education, blurring the line between learners and teachers.

Medical education is an evolving process, and the latest iteration of our titles has been rewritten to bring them up to date with modern curriculums, after extensive deliberation and consultation. We have kept the series up to date, incorporating new guidelines and perspectives from a wide range of students, junior, doctors and senior clinicians. There is greater consistency across the titles and more illustrations, and through these and other changes, I hope the books will now be even better study aids.

These books though are a process of continual improvement. By reading this book, I hope that you not only get through your exams but also consider contributing to a future edition. You may be a student now, but you are also the future of medical education.

I wish you all the best with your future career and any upcoming exams.

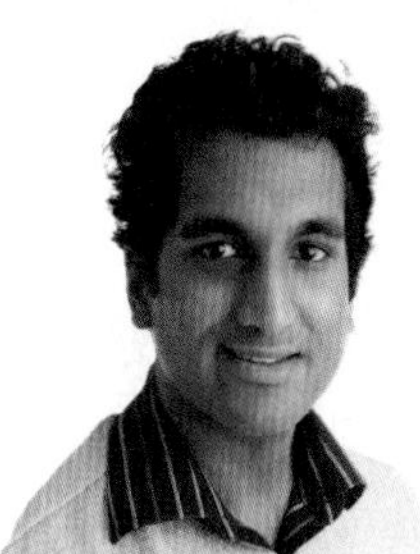

Zeshan Qureshi
November 2022

Foreword

Medicine is the most interesting and fulfilling career that you can choose. This also makes it one of the most competitive to enter. If you are someone who is caring, is compassionate, likes people and is socially aware, then you have made the right choice. If you have an enquiring mind, an interest in people and if you are prepared to lead, then you already have a head start. Nevertheless, every entry process has its hoops and processes, and 'The Unofficial Guide to Getting Into Medical School' is designed to help you navigate these and demonstrate why you are special and why you should be offered a medical school place. It is written by a distinguished group of medical students who have based their book on numerous surveys, discussions and personal experience. It may be the 'unofficial guide' but it is also the definitive guide for anyone wanting to maximise their chances of becoming a doctor.

Few jobs or professions have the potential of doing so much good for our fellow beings. We can help to prevent disease, detect it early, and cure it, and sometimes we have an important role in just being there for the patient who cannot be cured. No job in the world is so intellectually or emotionally stretching and also so important in the eyes of the public and media. Your future work will range from the biomedical to those much less specific and non-biomedical health-related aspects of the everyday lives of your patients. It is a job that constantly humanises us, putting us in permanent contact with joy and sadness, and allows us to make interventions and decisions that often change lives forever.

Now, more than ever, medicine requires fresh brains with new ideas. Medical science has played a major part in enabling longer life expectancy, but it has failed to stop an exponential increase in long-term disease including obesity, diabetes, stress, depression and cancer. As doctors of the future, you will need to enjoy and master the psychosocial as well as the biomedical and connect the body as a machine to the person as a self-healing individual. As all health systems become increasingly financially challenged, they will inevitably need to empower their patients as assets in their own healing, wherever possible, and also recognise the potential of local communities as assets in healing and health. They say that the only inevitability is change. A new young and enthusiastic generation of doctors is now required to face these new challenges and extend medicine's potential to benefit the physical and mental health of our individual patients and communities.

Being a doctor is not a job. It is a vocation. It is about becoming a healer and improving the health and resilience of the individuals and populations for which you are responsible. It inevitably affects your whole life and your relationships. If you are sufficiently passionate, determined, committed and resourceful, then you are likely to achieve becoming a doctor and, with it, the satisfaction at the end of every working day that you have made the world a better place.

Make this book your companion and your best friend. As you go through the application process, use it as a guide through the toughest storms until you finally succeed. Endurance lies behind the success of every great doctor and this book will help you to reach that starting point of the best career ever. Good luck and many congratulations for choosing to follow this path. It was certainly the best decision that I ever made.

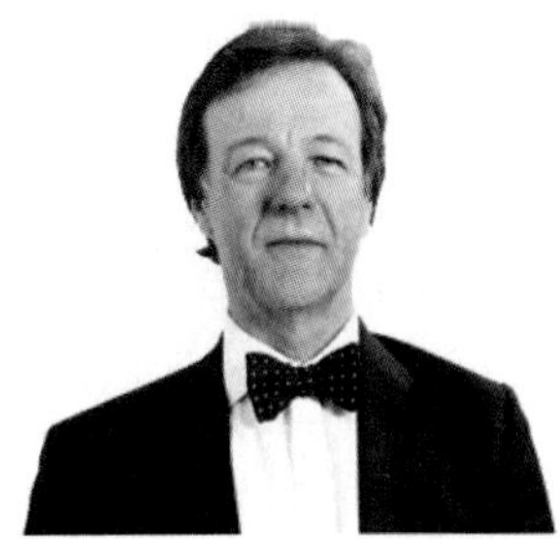

Professor Michael Dixon, LVO, OBE, FRCGP
Chair, College of Medicine and Integrated Health

About the Book

WHO ARE WE AND WHY ARE WE DOING THIS?

You are probably wondering why a bunch of medical students and doctors are writing this book instead of jogging around the hospital, or flipping through books and studying for exams day and night.

The truth is, a few years ago, we were all exactly where you are now, with a book in our hands, planning to apply to medical school, but fearing what at the time seemed like an impossible journey. Like yourself, we all had doubts, questions and worries regarding every single step of the application process. In fact, some of us didn't even know what the key application steps were!

Each and every author of this book has wondered why there aren't more resources written by the masters of the application process, by those who have been through the process themselves and can share their experiences retrospectively. We were also slightly frustrated that most resources available are reflections of senior academics and career advisers who, although experts in their fields, have not been through the new medical school application process themselves. The application process has changed and keeps changing significantly each year.

Fuelled by our constant passion to help others get into medicine, we set up a vast network of the most knowledgeable and experienced people: over 600 successful medical students from all the medical schools in the United Kingdom (UK). This book is the result of over 300 surveys and focus groups among successful medical students. A total of 67 current medical applicants, just like you, were also interviewed as part of our mentoring programme at Medefine Education (www.medefine.net). This book is a project based on your real needs, on the most commonly encountered uncertainties and difficulties as emphasised by YOU, the applicant.

For years now, we've been helping applicants like you to successfully secure a place in medical school. Most of them are now part of our growing team. You, too, can be part of our team and give something back to those who will be in the same situation such as yourself, so do get in touch!

WHAT ARE WE ATTEMPTING?

This is the first book of its kind that actually involved current medical school applicants in developing its content. With your help, we have understood what you want to see less of, and what you want to see more of.

You wanted less…

- Facts, contact details and information that are readily available on Google/university websites.
- Emphasis on General Certificate of Secondary Education (GCSEs), A-Levels and other grade requirements.
- Emphasis on Universities and Colleges Admissions Service (UCAS), student finance and costs.
- Emphasis on deciding to study medicine (since you have already made this decision).

You wanted more…

- Personal stories and real experiences of medical students written in an informal style.
- Use of analogies and interactive style.
- Emphasis on depth and requirements of background reading.
- Emphasis on effective strategies for the Personal Statement, UCAT, BMAT and interview.
- Further reading and preparatory materials upon completion of the book.

Essentially, we understand that you want fewer facts that are readily available elsewhere, and more real-life examples and insight that will make a difference to your medical school application.

The only assumption made in this book is that you are a massive geek and that you would do anything to get a place in medical school. Of course, this is not an easy decision. This decision should have been made over many years, as a result of all the activities and experiences of which you have been part.

Think really hard about this. It's not an easy choice; it's hard enough getting into medical school. It is a bit of a lottery at the moment. You need to get the grades, you need to work really hard, you need to present yourself well, and you need to be diligent.

You need to have a good personal statement, and it's very easy to start writing, 'I want to care about people…' and so on, but you really have to know that medicine is something you want to do, because there are so many other easier choices.

I do think it's completely worth doing, and if it is for you, then go for it. Don't let people put you off; don't let anyone dissuade you. The rewards are massive, not just for you personally, but more importantly for the patients that you're going to look after. It gives you a passport, you can work anywhere in the world with that passport, and it's a job for life.

So, don't worry about what's happening in politics or health economics—people are going to get ill, they're going get sick, and if you can help one person, it's going to make a massive difference, so stick with it!

Mr Vikram Devaraj, Consultant Plastic Reconstructive & Aesthetic Surgeon

To be completely honest with you, if you have the slightest doubt about going into medicine, then you may have to spend a bit more time exploring. Who in their right mind would go through 5 or 6 years of medical school to realise they don't actually love what they're doing? Think carefully, but if you're reading this, we will assume that this is your dream job and that you have put effort into exploring its positive and negative aspects.

CONTENTS AT A GLANCE

CHAPTER 1: INTRODUCTION

Before we dig deep into each section of the medical school application process, you and I need to have a quick chat about your personal reasons for doing medicine. Your siblings, your parents, your grandparents, your neighbour and even the lady who sat next to you on the bus will want to know, WHY medicine? Together, we'll set some goals to help you plan your journey through the application process. We finish the chapter by providing you with honest insight from successful medical students regarding their hosting medical schools within the UK.

CHAPTER 2: MEDICINE—PAST, PRESENT AND FUTURE

We continue with the first of four chapters aiming to equip you with the necessary theory before tackling each step of the application process. In this chapter, we learn by taking a time-travelling journey through the history of medicine. We discuss current affairs and set the vision for the future of medicine—all key aspects that should form part of your background knowledge before applying.

CHAPTER 3: UK MEDICAL PRACTICE AND CAREER PROGRESSION

How much do you already know about the medical school training programme in the UK? What about the National Health Service (NHS) and other important organisations? In this chapter, we lay out the inner workings of the UK healthcare system, explore the various teaching methods used by medical schools, and take a look at career progression beyond medical school. If you're going to study and work in the UK, you first need to be acquainted with its teaching methods, career prospects, and healthcare regulations.

CHAPTER 4: THE DIFFERENT ROLES OF A DOCTOR

Good awareness regarding the different masks worn by a doctor is key. Quite often, the general public associates the word 'doctor' with its clinical duties only. Chapter 4 uncovers a doctor's various roles as outlined by the General Medical Council (GMC). We also explore important terminology that will make you more knowledgeable during your medical school interview.

CHAPTER 5: MEDICAL ETHICS AND LAW

This chapter focuses on theory and background knowledge, and explores one of the most frequently discussed topics during medical school interviews: medical ethics and law. We begin by briefly outlining the essentials, including definitions and key differences. After equipping you with the necessary ethical principles and concepts, we put these into practice by exploring a few ethical dilemmas. We'll pass the stethoscope to you here—it's your turn to make decisions!

CHAPTER 6: WORK EXPERIENCE

When should I start? What counts as work experience? How do I boost my chances of getting work experience? These are some of the most common questions asked by applicants like you. Chapter 6 explores these and many other questions, such as how to make the most of your work experience placements. At your request, we have also included a ready-to-use reflective template that can be used after each placement.

CHAPTER 7: MASTERING ENTRANCE EXAMS

Perhaps the most dreadful and confusing subject of all: entrance exams. But not to worry, we start our chapter with top science-based studying hacks to help you gain confidence in learning everything and anything. This chapter outlines key strategies for tackling each section of the UCAT, including our successful 'twenty-hour rule for mastering the UCAT' through which we have significantly improved the scores of hundreds of applicants like you. We continue by outlining the BMAT's basic principles and structure. Using real examples, we provide general tips from high-scoring medical students before delving deeper in each individual section of the test. The bulk of the chapter is made of tips, tricks and strategies that you can apply when preparing for and sitting this exam.

CHAPTER 8: DISSECTING THE PERFECT MEDICAL SCHOOL PERSONAL STATEMENT

We next move into our own autopsy lab. Here we conduct a dissection of successful personal statements provided by medical students from all over the UK.

Furthermore, we begin the chapter by providing insight into the anatomy of a personal statement, and analyse its structure and components one by one.

CHAPTER 9: ACING THE MEDICAL SCHOOL INTERVIEW

Now that you have successfully prepared your passport for the interview (your personal statement), you are ready to explore the different types of interviews and most commonly encountered questions as suggested by medical students throughout the UK. In this chapter, we focus on preparatory tips, answering techniques and general tips to boost your chances of being selected following a medical school interview.

CHAPTER 10: A GUIDE FOR NONTRADITIONAL APPLICANTS

The final chapter of the book is dedicated to those of you who may have an extra thing or two to think about before applying. Graduates, internationals and gap-year students all need to tailor their applications slightly differently from their fellow undergraduate/Home-UK colleagues. We finish this chapter by providing hope and alternative ways for getting into medicine for those who may have not made it the first-time round.

BONUS Chapter: The Geeky Corner

This is a place where you can find recommendations and suggestions for some of the best medically related films, books, museums and other places to visit.

WHAT'S NOT INCLUDED?

Now that you know what's included, let us also be clear about what's not included. Based on your preferences, we won't bore you with irrelevant information. We will stick to the best advice that will boost your chances of getting into medical school.

Competition ratios, stats and numbers that differ throughout the UK and change from year to year have been left out. This book focuses on the aspects of the application process that YOU control. You've also told us that key contacts and details about individual medical schools can easily be located on the internet. Hence, we've focused only on personalised insights provided by successful medical students.

There's only so much that we can fit in one book. For this reason, you will see that our UCAT, BMAT and Interview sections represent comprehensive guides on HOW to master the strategies and skills required so you can practice correctly in your own time. To be completely honest, there isn't any secret to the previously mentioned topics—it's all about practice and hard work. HOWEVER, what truly matters is how you practice, and how you set and build on good habits from the start. Once you start, you are better off investing in online question databases, but according to the highest UCAT and BMAT scorers, developing key strategies to practice with from the beginning is crucial.

In essence, we want to teach you so that you start enjoying the preparation process, not dreading it.

HOW TO USE THIS BOOK

Make this book yours; make it your friend. Make this book your companion throughout both the stormy and sunny days of the medical school application process.

The number one rule of this book is that there aren't any rules. You should use this book as your notepad. Scribble ideas on its pages, highlight useful information and make the most of it. According to science, we tend to concentrate better and become more creative when we draw or scribble things down in books!

We suggest using colourful Post-it notes when encountering key points or when you want to jot down particular ideas—it's always useful to come back and reflect upon your thoughts, and you never know, it may save your life during the interview!

The following icons are used throughout the book. Here's what they all mean:

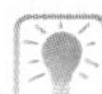

'Top Tip'—Look out for the light bulb as it represents some of the most important points throughout each chapter of this book.

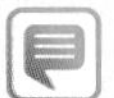

'An applicant's perspective'—This icon has been used to point out tips and opinions from medical school applicants, like you!

'A medical student's perspective'—As its name suggests, this icon includes tips from successful medical students.

'An academic's perspective'—The stethoscope icon marks tips provided by successful doctors, clinicians, academics and other healthcare professionals.

'Reflection time'—We've used this icon throughout the book to highlight times when you should pause and reflect. This allows you to reflect upon the newly acquired knowledge.

'Test yourself'—This icon will also appear towards the end of some chapters, giving you the opportunity to test your knowledge of what you've just learnt.

If you've got a burning question about getting into medical school, do get in touch with us—our army of medical students and junior doctors from all over the UK look forward to bringing you one step closer to your dream.

Bogdan Chiva Giurca

Acknowledgements

Thank you to the following contributors for their contribution to the first edition.

Medical student contributions
Winnie T.
Sarah M.
Roshni B.
Omowumi F. and Kusy S.
Joel C.
Kiyara F.
Katie K.
Alex S.
Tim W. and David L.
Tiffany L.
Joanna W. and Georgie L.
Krutika S.
Gladys L.
Dan H.
Waseem H.
Sandeep D.
Martina S.
Rumaysa A. Q.
Sarah P.
Akash M.
Dana T.
Jia C. C.
Elizabeth T.
Monica S.
Fady A.
Ryan H.
Pooja R.
Aisling B.
Keat K.
Lucia L.
Hanna W. P.
Jake R.
Rebecca F.
Kristie L.
Kushal K.
Laura P.
David H.
Tanya K.
Hannah B.
Taona N.
Marco F. N.
Connor J.
Cara J.
Amber P.
Andrel Y.
Daisy K.
Sashi G.
Eunice P.
Helena Q.

Medical school applicant contributions
Jasmine T.
Carice P.
Vincent K.
Minsu K.
Matthew L.
Jeremy C.
Nikki L.
Mark C.
Nick N.
Terence C.
Sharon K.
Jenny N.
Periklis G.
Hey-Gin K.
Benjamin T.
Ryan L.
Claudia Y.
Dan S.
Beatrice T. G.
Evita M.
Clarence C.

Doctor contributions
Professor Michael Dixon
Professor Peter Abrahams
Vikram Devaraj
Zeshan Qureshi
James Jarvie
Carwyn Watkins

Illustration contribution
Dominick Contreras

Abbreviations

A&E	Accident and emergency
ACT	American College Testing
AFC	Armed Forces Committee
AFCO	Armed Forces Careers Office
AR	Abstract reasoning
BC	Before Christ
BMA	British Medical Association
BMAT	BioMedical Admissions Test
BMJ	British Medical Journal
CBL	Case-based learning
CCG	Clinical commissioning groups
CCT	Certificate of Completion of Training
CMT	Core medical training
CQC	Care Quality Commission
CT	Computed tomography
CV	Curriculum vitae
DG	District general
DM	Decision making
DNACPR	Do not attempt cardiopulmonary resuscitation
DNAR	Do not attempt resuscitation
EBM	Evidence-based medicine
EPQ	Extended project qualification
FPAS	Foundation Programme Application System
FRCP	Fellow of the Royal College of Physicians
GAMSAT	Graduate Medical Schools Admissions Test
GCSE	General Certificate of Secondary Education
GEM	Graduate Entry Medicine
GMC	General Medical Council
GP	General practitioner
GPST	General Practice Speciality Training
GUM	Genitourinary medicine
IB	International baccalaureate
ICE	Ideas, concerns, expectations
IELTS	International English Language Testing System
IGCSE	International General Certificate of Secondary Education
IMCA	Independent Mental Capacity Advocate
MCQ	Multiple-choice question
MMI	Multiple mini interviews
MRCGP	Member of the Royal College of General Practitioners
MRCP	Member of the Royal College of Physicians
MSF	Medecins Sans Frontieres
NICE	National Institute for Health and Care Excellence
NGO	Nongovernmental organisation
NHS	National Health Service
OSCE	Obstructive Structured Clinical Examination
PBL	Problem-based learning
PCTs	Primary care trusts
PS	Personal statement
QR	Quantitative reasoning
SAT	Scholastic Assessment Test
SHA	Strategic Healthy Authority
SJ	Situational judgement
SJT	Situational Judgement Test
SMART	Specific, measurable, achievable, realistic, time-sensitive
SPIKES	Setting, perception, invitation, knowledge, empathetic response/silence, summary/strategy
STAR	Situation, task, action, results
TOEFL	Test of English as a Foreign Language
UCAS	Universities and Colleges Admissions Service
UCAT	University Clinical Aptitude Test
UK	United Kingdom
VR	Verbal reasoning

Contributors

SERIES EDITOR

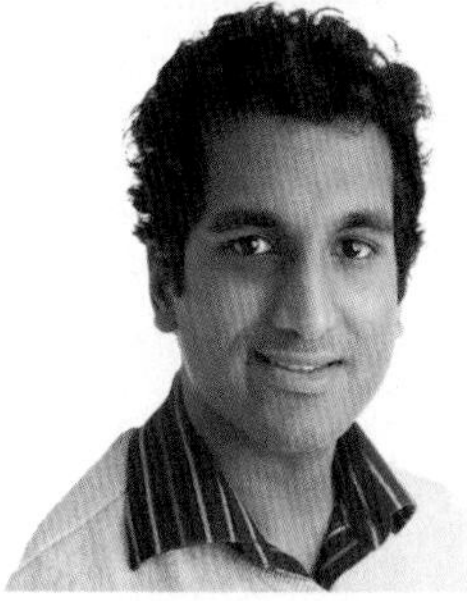

Zeshan Qureshi, BM, BSc (Hons), MSc, MRCPCH, FAcadMEd, MRCPS (Glasg)
Paediatric Registrar, London Deanery, United Kingdom

EDITOR

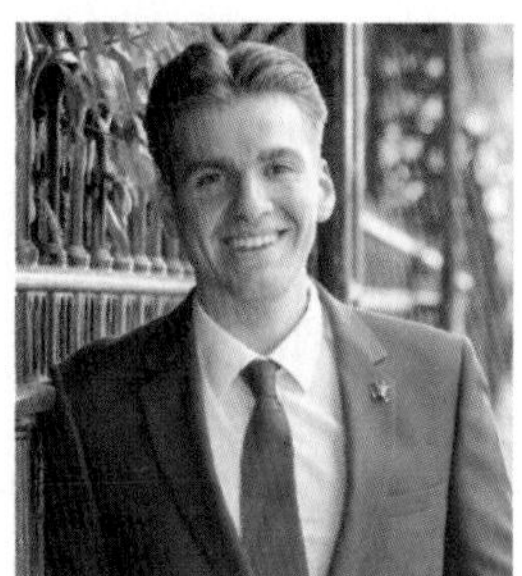

Bogdan Chiva Giurca, BMBS, ClinEnt Fellow, DipIBLM
Specialty Doctor, London Deanery, United Kingdom
Council Member, College of Medicine
Honorary Lecturer, University College London

AUTHORS

Polen Bareke
Medical Student, University College London

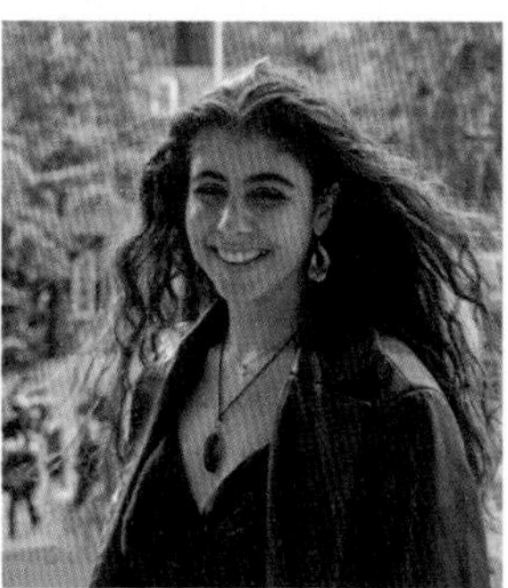

Jamie Christian Charlton
Graduate Entry Applicant, University of Exeter

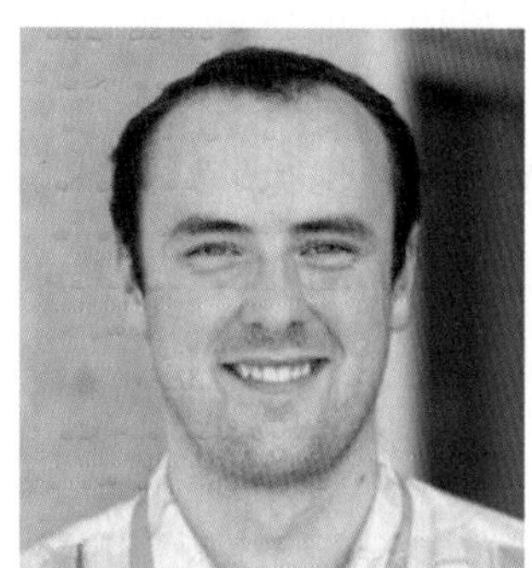

Kiyara Fernando
Junior Doctor, NHS England

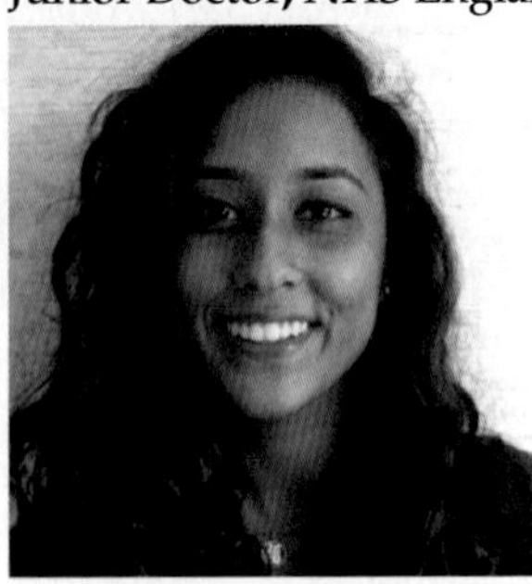

Gareth Lau
Junior Doctor, NHS England

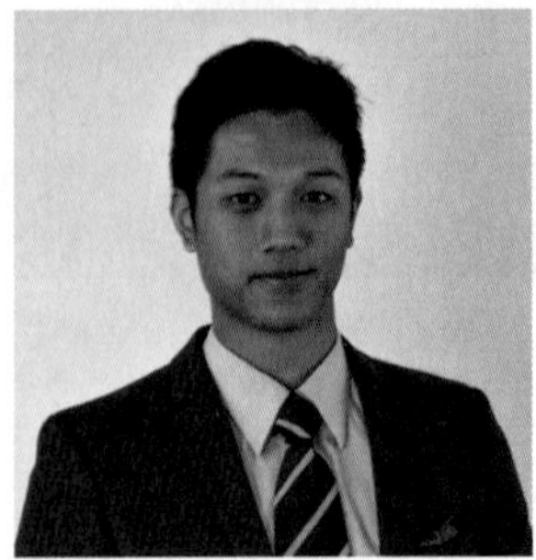

Caroline Gu
Medica Student, Exeter Medical School

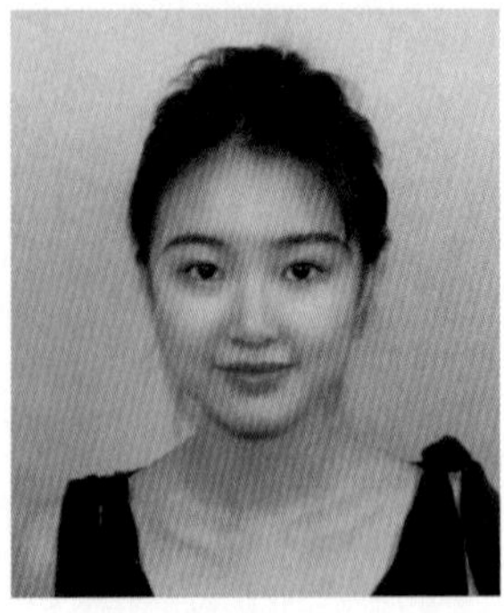

Matthew Lau
Medical Student, University College London

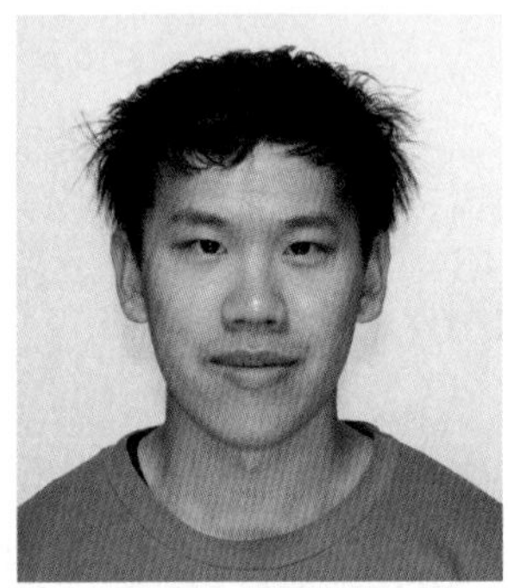

Rachel Howard
Junior Doctor, NHS England

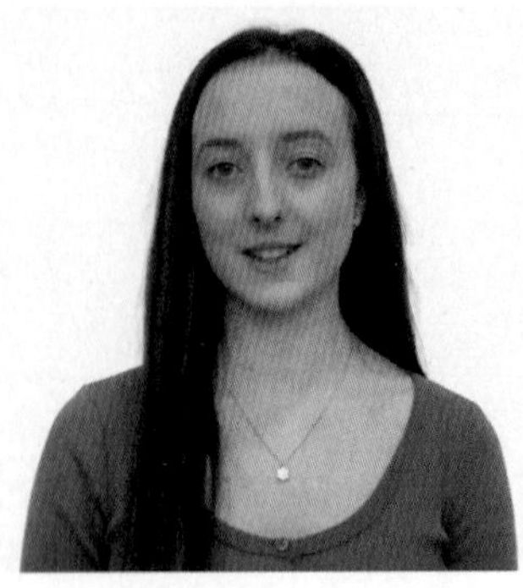

Navin Mukundu Nagesh
Specialty Doctor, NHS Wales

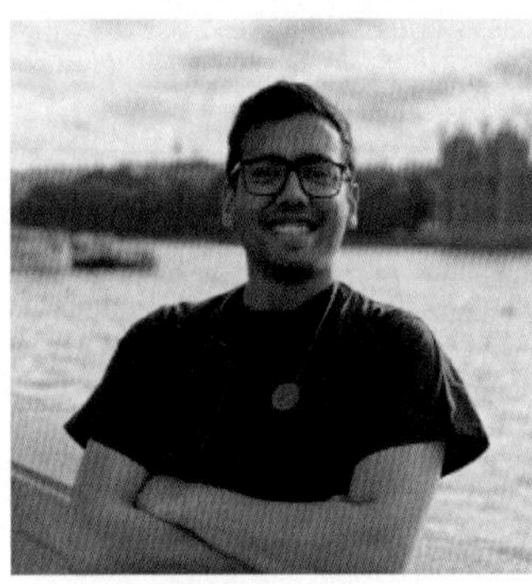

Hamaad Khan
Medical Student, Anglia Ruskin Medical School

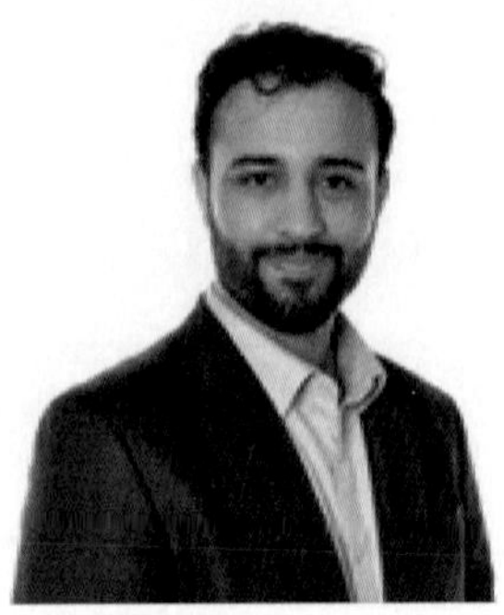

Teodora Popa
Reproductive Geneticist, University College London

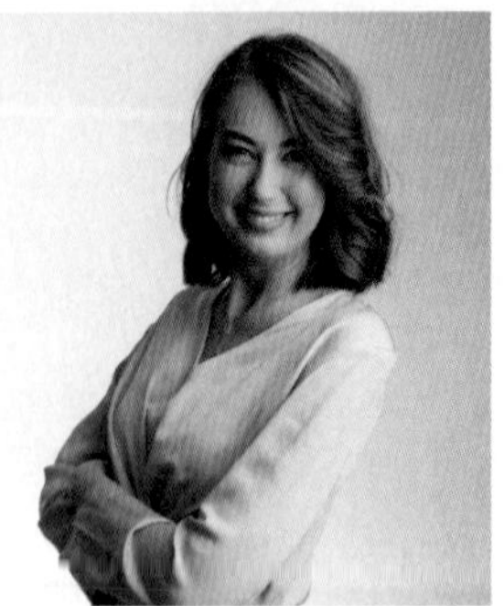

Dupinderjit Rye
Junior Doctor, NHS England

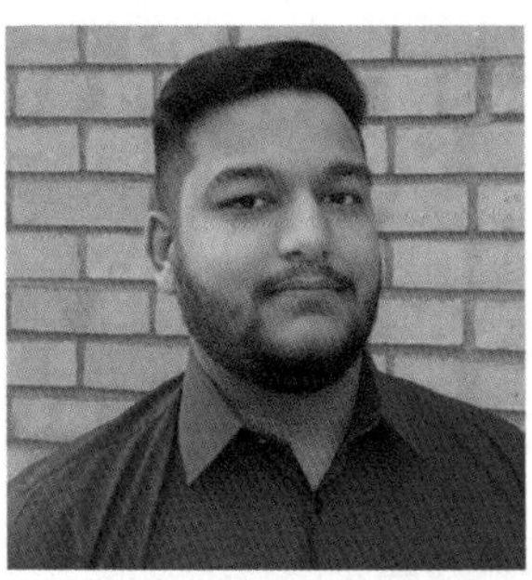

Alisha Sharif
Medical Student, Newcastle Medical School

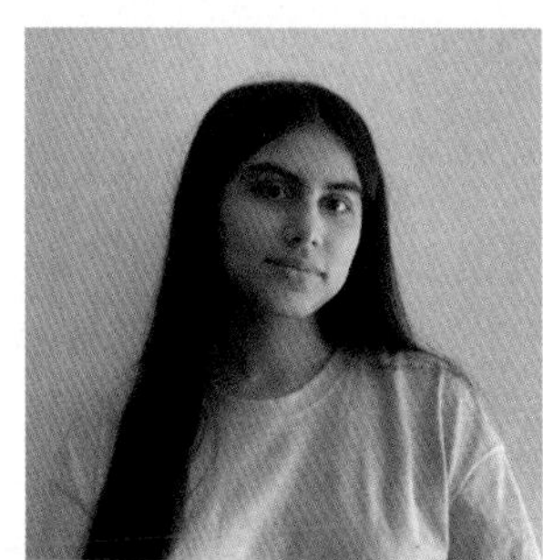

Ida Saidy
Medical Student, Manchester Medical School

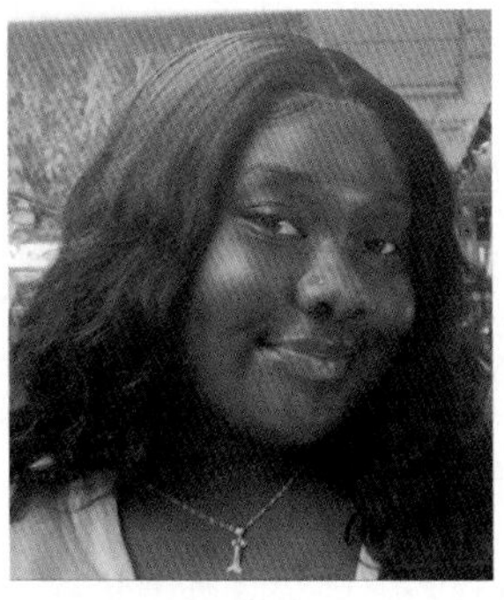

Charlotte Stoll
Medical Student, Leeds Medical School

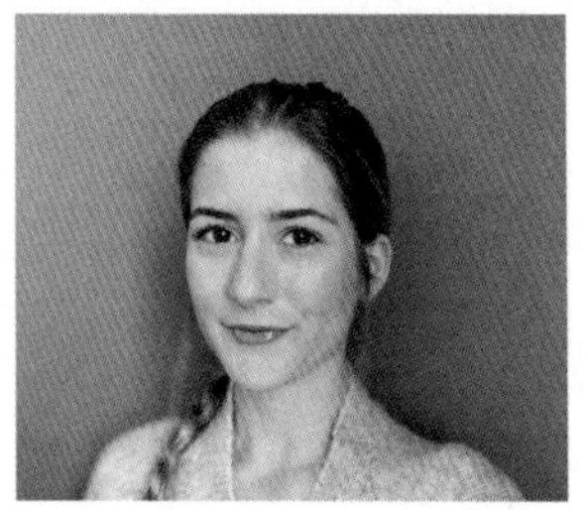

Aisha Sharif
Medical Student, University of East Anglia

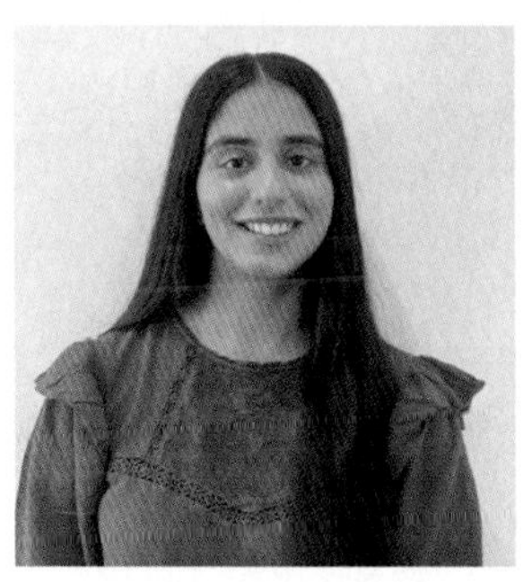

Akanksha Subramanian
Junior Doctor, NHS England

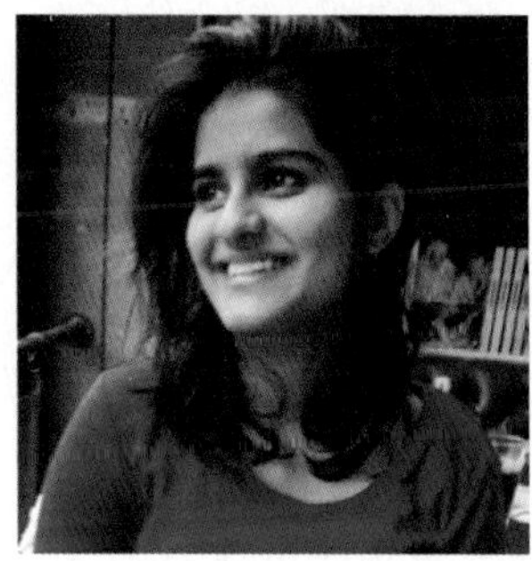

Introduction: Setting Up the Scene

1

Bogdan Chiva Giurca

Chapter Outline

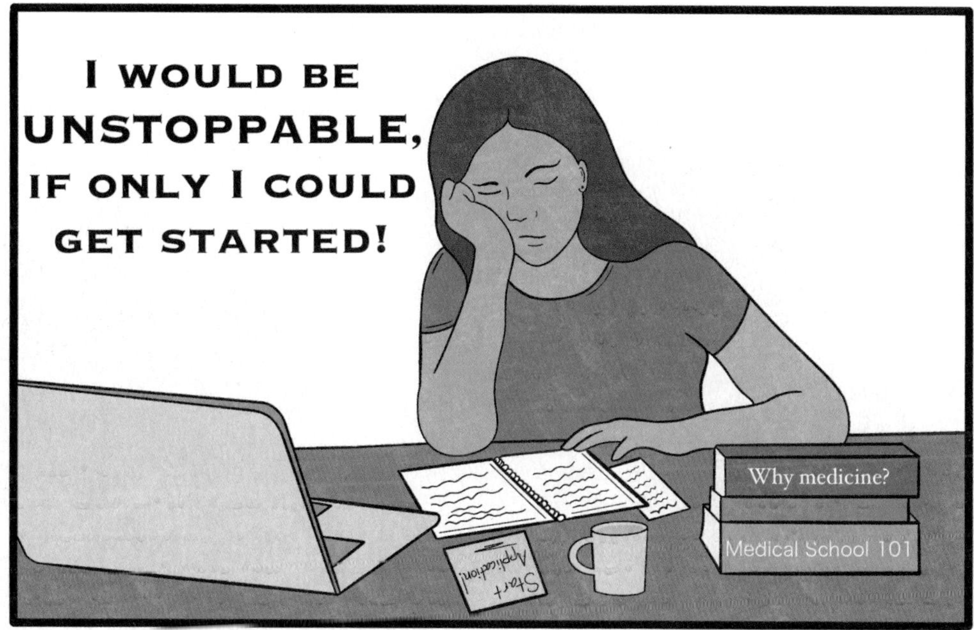
I WOULD BE UNSTOPPABLE, IF ONLY I COULD GET STARTED!
Why medicine?
Medical School 101
Start Application!

WHY MEDICINE?

Now is the time to arm yourself with a pen and spend some time on the most important question of your medical school application journey, your career as a doctor and quite possibly the rest of your life. Your family, teachers, school mates, potential employers and placement providers will all want to know this, but most importantly, YOU should know what fuels your passion for getting out of bed each day.

What makes you think you want to do medicine? What have you seen, done, felt and thought over the years to make you consider a career in medicine? How tempted are you to say that you love the sciences and that you want to help people?

Sure, you want to make a difference in someone's life and you certainly love the sciences, but can you make me believe this without stating the above word for word? What's your story? Can you think of a way to portray yourself as an empathetic person who wants to make a difference without actually saying it? Can you give me an example that convinces me you love the sciences?

Do you know why it is so hard to provide a good answer for this question? It's simple. You've spent most of your life in school, preparing for and answering questions that have a clear rationale that you can study for. 'Why medicine?', on the other hand, has no right or wrong answer. This question can only be answered using your life story and experiences. 'Why medicine?' is therefore the same as 'Who are you?' For some of the science geeks around, Carl Sagan once said, 'You have to know the past to understand the present' … or in your case, you have to know your past to understand your WHY.

I remember being asked this during my medical school interview. As much as I wanted to give a serious answer that I had thoroughly prepared in my free time, instead I started giggling and smiling because, at that point, I realised what a geek I am. Half-laughing, I told the interviewers that I was always that annoying child bombarding teachers with 'what, why, how' questions to the point of exhaustion. I told the interviewing panel that I could only focus for a few minutes when studying for other disciplines, but when it came to the sciences, I didn't even notice time flying by. I remember staying up until the middle of the night laughing at geeky medicine stuff, like how doctors used to taste a patient's urine (an 'accurate' test to see if a patient had diabetes or not). At this point, you may think the whole interviewing panel looked very confused, but they all laughed, agreeing that it sounded very geeky! This encouraged me to continue with my nonscripted answer, organically conveying my love for science and medicine.

Medicine is not just science, however. As a kid, my doctor explained how my airway swelled up due to certain allergens. I didn't care about the science behind this phenomenon; all I wanted to know was what was happening and why—I was only 12, after all! The doctor mimicked ingesting an allergen, spoke in a funny voice and used a balloon to explain what happens to my airway during an asthma attack. Whenever I went in for a vaccination, that same doctor would trick me into thinking the injection was pain-free, until I felt the needle and started crying. It made me laugh then, but looking back, there was more to it. That awesome doctor used skills beyond science—in fact, this is where medicine overlaps with art: the art of communication, the art of listening, choosing the perfect words and tailoring your practice to the patient in front of you. There are several examples that exemplify the 'art' of medicine, from breaking bad news to dealing with angry patients.

We are all unique in our own way, so our 'Why medicine?' is too. To inspire you, we have collected a couple of 'Why medicine?' examples from the authors of this book, all successful medical students with a passion for medicine.

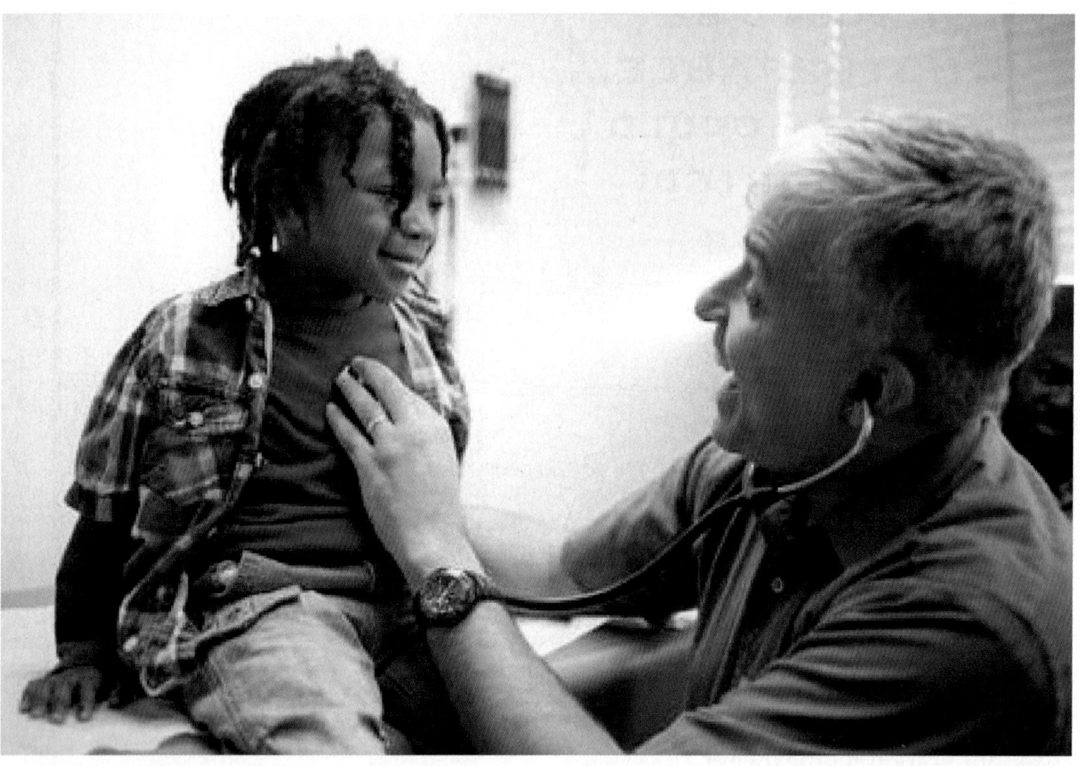

It gives me heartache to see people suffer and lose opportunities in their lives because of illnesses. Often, the suffering is augmented by a lack of healthcare, which is unfortunately inevitable in underdeveloped areas.

On a school service trip to Thailand, I was shaken by the poor living conditions in rural villages, where inadequate medical care left some bedridden and unattended. Apart from cooking and delivering food to them, I wished that I could have done more to ease their discomfort by attending to their medical needs.

I realised that by becoming a doctor, I could help bring back health and life opportunities to those stricken with illness. I will remain forever captivated by this vision.

Gareth, Medical Student, Exeter Medical School

'Why medicine?' is a question I couldn't answer for a long time. It was something I knew I wanted to do, deep down. It took a lot of reflection and soul searching to pick apart my motivations.

Primarily, it is the pure satisfaction of using one's skills and knowledge to pull people back from the edge of death and bring new life into the world. Being there for people in their best and worst moments, and being granted the privilege of doing something to help them, however small my contribution may be, means that I can give something back.

In today's world, we constantly hear about how humans are hurting one another or how bad things are. What is seldom mentioned is how people are also good and how people can help one another too. Medicine was the best way I felt I could express that.

It was also a vocation that would give me everything I wanted in life—a job where I look forward to going to work in the morning, that allows me to make new friends and meet fascinating people, teaches me something new every day and stretches my learning and abilities.

Jamie, Graduate Medical School Applicant

I believe the degree in medicine I am currently pursuing is only a gateway to the wonders of healing and helping people. It is the most sincere way I can give back to a community that has placed its trust in me during its most difficult times, both physically and emotionally.

Medicine also allows me to be the scholar that I have always aspired to be. I have sought the perfect mixture of knowledge and application. After a long couple of days in the hospital, I enjoy the clarity I get when I have the time to sit down and read something as simple as physiology or something as fascinating as a paper on the ethical use of social prescription in an age of allopathy.

Medicine opens so many windows into your personal interests by allowing you to develop insight into them; it helps you evaluate those skills or beliefs and integrate them into your practice. For instance, someone's passion in educational opportunities may translate into educational solutions for chronically ill children. This is a marriage between your interests and the knowledge that you gain on the ground.

I wanted to commit myself to something that would help me build real-life skills and make a real-life impact every time I interact with people. I wanted to maximise my ability to guide others towards feeling physically and mentally healthy. Now in my third year of medicine, I truly feel like I am as much medicine as medicine is me—it is a part of my day the same way that brushing my teeth is (although some Sundays I leave it till after brunch!).

Akanksha, Medical Student, Bristol Medical School

I was curious to read more, curious to find out more, curious to understand how and why things happen the way they happen. It was my avid interest in the sciences that sparked my interest in medicine. However, it was engaging in work and volunteer experience over the years that truly solidified my desire to be a doctor.

One experience that drew me to medicine was watching a junior doctor break the bad news to a cancer patient that his condition was now terminal. As a 15-year-old student, I observed how composed the doctor was when speaking to the patient. He showed expertise with empathy, and he ensured that the patient completely understood his diagnosis and had the support he needed.

As a member of the medical profession, you have responsibilities to care for patients, their families and members of your team. This is an aspect of the career that attracted me to medicine. There are several roles that a doctor plays; teacher, researcher, team player, listener and caregiver are just a few. These roles, and the dynamic nature of an ever-changing profession, drew me to the career at a young age, and my interest in medicine only grows with the years.

Kiyara, Medical Student, Bristol Medical School

Did you notice how everyone expressed their love for sciences, the human body, and for helping others, in an indirect and slightly different manner? We are all unique, which means we should all have an original, personal reason for doing medicine.

Your turn now—jot down a few parts of your own story. You may not know the full answer yet, but make a start and return to this section as you work your way through the book. If you are tempted to skip this without even trying, think again—I remember being tempted to do the same when I was in your position, but I promise that investing 5 minutes of mental effort will pay dividends in the end. Why medicine? My story, my reasons, my why....

HOW TO COPE WITH PEOPLE WHO THINK YOU'RE NOT GOOD ENOUGH TO GO TO MEDICAL SCHOOL IN THE UK

I just want to take this opportunity to clear some stuff out of the way. Have you ever been told by a teacher, relative or even a friend that you are not good enough to apply to medical school? We often receive questions from applicants who feel unmotivated to pursue their dream, purely because others don't believe in them.

The truth is, we've all been told this by someone at some point in our journey. People will always try to stop you from doing what they couldn't achieve themselves, by projecting their inner frustrations onto you. How would they know? They are not in your position; they have not put in the same amount of work that you are putting in.

What we want you to know is that we believe in you. Smile and carry on, because like us, you've got what it takes to succeed. Put in the hard work and all the rest will come. Put in the hard work and prove them wrong!

We hope Daisy's story will resonate with some of you and will keep you motivated to keep pushing, even when someone's trying to prevent you from applying just because they think that 'you are not good enough'.

My teachers said, 'If you were a horse, I wouldn't bet on you'. My story starts 3 years ago, when I was in my penultimate year of school. The careers lady told me that I would never get into medical school, that my grades weren't good enough and that I would embarrass myself by applying.

Looking in my eyes, she said, 'Let's put it this way, Daisy, out of all of the people applying, if you were a horse, I wouldn't bet on you'. Her words struck me like a knife in the chest. In a 45-minute appointment, this one woman shattered all of my dreams and ambitions. I barely made it out of the office before I started crying.

The following week, she sent me to a Biomedical Sciences UCAS convention and course information. It was the worst

(Continued)

humiliation possible. However, at the UCAS event, I discovered that there are other ways into medicine apart from the traditional A100 degree. I found out about different transfer schemes—'be in the top 10% of the cohort at Exeter and you can switch to medicine at the end of your first year'. With a lot of hard work, I managed to transfer, achieve my dream and prove my career advisor wrong.

I am now a medical student and will soon become a doctor. Do not let anyone tell you cannot achieve something. Dedication, passion and hard work will allow you to achieve your dream of studying medicine.

Daisy Kirtley, Medical Student, Exeter Medical School

TAKING AN OATH: A PROMISE TO YOUR FUTURE SELF

They say, 'If you can dream it, you can achieve it'. Quite often, imagination and dreams are one of our most powerful tools for success. Here, we'd like you to spend a couple of minutes envisaging yourself in the future. Can you draw your future?

Science tells us that in order to achieve a goal, you must first see it, then believe it and finally train your brain each day to execute your vision. Renowned TED-talk speaker Patti Dobrowolski refers to this as 'Drawing your dreams into reality'. However, it isn't as simple as just imagining yourself with a stethoscope dangling around your neck. Patti says that you must start by drawing your current state and, in as much detail as possible, outline the journey of getting to your desired new reality.

In simple terms, here's how this works. When you imagine something, your brain releases serotonin and other 'feel-good' neurotransmitters. Quite often, our brains are very good at guessing what will bring us closer to our desired goal; however, the big problem is getting started and taking that first step. The neurotransmitters mentioned earlier give you strength and empower you to take that uncomfortable, uncertain step. One of the most common mistakes is to dream of your desired goal without including difficult times into the equation. Your brain therefore gets a false sense of achievement, which will inevitably make you quit when you hit the tough steps of your journey.

Let's use getting into medical school as an example. Imagine how happy and fulfilled you'll be when you receive that letter saying, 'Dear applicant, we would like to formally offer you a place at our medical school…' Next, go step by step through each checkpoint of the application timeline and imagine what potential difficulties can arise, and how you will overcome them. By training your brain to think upfront that it's normal to encounter adversity, you will have the power to keep moving forward until you receive that coveted medical school acceptance.

? So, here's a question for you then: Where do you see yourself in 10 years? Feel free to draw and be as creative as possible. Can you map your biggest dreams and wishes? Will you be wearing a stethoscope, or will you have a scalpel in your hand?

Now that you have set a vivid image of yourself in the future, make a promise and take an oath to your future self.

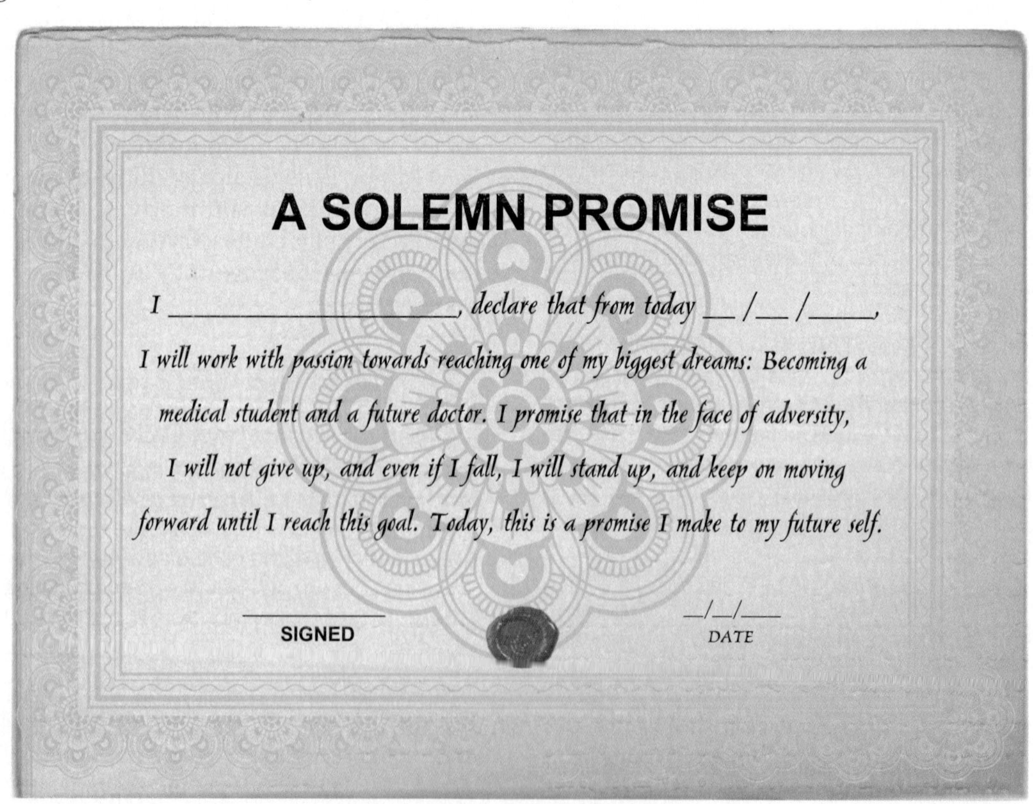

A SOLEMN PROMISE

I ____________________, declare that from today __ /__ /____,
I will work with passion towards reaching one of my biggest dreams: Becoming a medical student and a future doctor. I promise that in the face of adversity, I will not give up, and even if I fall, I will stand up, and keep on moving forward until I reach this goal. Today, this is a promise I make to my future self.

__________ SIGNED

__/__/__ DATE

APPLICATION TIMELINE AND KEY DATES

Fig. 1.1 shows the key dates of the application process. Please note we have only included the month and not specific days, since these change from year to year. You should check each specific date on the official websites and add these to your calendar to stay organised.

GOAL SETTING: STAYING ORGANISED

Some people might be intimidated by the complex application process, but not you. You don't expect this journey to be easy; otherwise, everybody would get a place in medical school, right? What you need to understand from the outset is that you have to take things one at a time. You want to build a wall, but you cannot do it in one day. What you can do, however, is start building the wall by adding one brick, day after day. Sure, it may not look like a wall in the beginning, but you already know what the outcome will be. In your head, it looks like a wall and it'll keep taking its shape after every single day.

High-performance athletes use this type of thinking to succeed. I'm sure many of you have heard of Michael Phelps, whose 28 medals make him the most decorated Olympian of all time. Want to know his secret? His coach said that Michael has a specific ritual, a number of steps that he takes before each training session and each race. Michael knows what's going to happen during the race, and in his mind, he has already won. However, his coach has mentioned several times during interviews that Phelps only focuses on one cycle of strokes and breaths at a time, short, specific, succinct goals that bring him closer to his victory.

Following his example, you can successfully march your way through the application process. You do, however, need to keep organised and set goals throughout.

HOW EARLY SHOULD YOU START?

This is by far the most common question from medical school applicants. The short answer is: the earlier, the better. It's never too early to start, but it may sometimes be too late. Although there isn't a specific answer giving you an exact number of days, our data suggest that most successful applicants started preparing approximately 2 years before the application deadline. By 'preparing', I mean getting involved in work experience, exploring medicine as a career, joining open days and talking to medical students, as well as building general knowledge and doing background reading around the subject. Of course, this can vary, and some may argue you can start later and still succeed, but statistically, the earlier, the better.

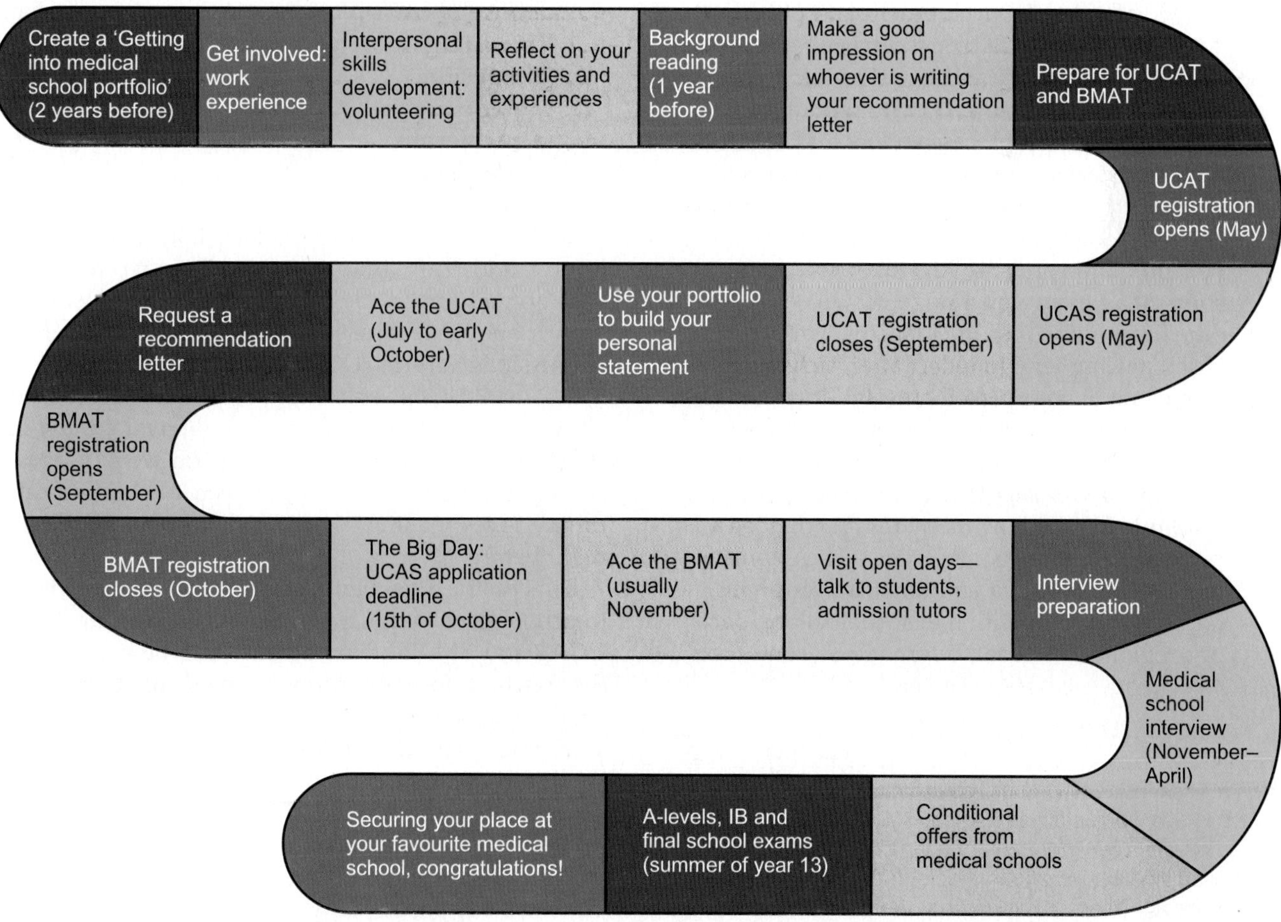

Fig. 1.1 Key dates for applications. *BMAT*, BioMedical Admissions Test; *UCAS*, Universities and Colleges Admissions Service; *UCAT*, University Clinical Aptitude Test.

The benefits of starting early include:

- Gaining a vast range of work experience
- Enough time to explore a career in medicine by talking to doctors and medical students
- Less stressful, some even begin to enjoy the application process (strange, right?!)
- Enough time to explore and prepare for University Clinical Aptitude Test (UCAT) and BioMedical Admissions Test (BMAT)

As for the benefits of starting late, well, there aren't any I'm afraid! I wish I could give you something, but instead, use the short time remaining to better your application as soon as possible.

WHERE TO START? CREATE A PORTFOLIO, FIND A MENTOR AND COME UP WITH A PLAN!

1. Getting into Medical School Portfolio

   Being organised and having your entire life in one place is key. Most successful applicants we have worked with in the past created a 'Getting into medical school portfolio'.

   Here's what you'll need:

   - An empty A4 binding portfolio
   - Subject dividers with the following sections
     - Work Experience
     - Prizes, Awards and Publications
     - Volunteering Projects
     - Professional Development and Others (e.g. CV, reference letters, work, etc.)

   Personalise your folder and make it yours. This folder will accompany you throughout the whole application process and increase in thickness as you grow through every experience to which you are being exposed. Don't be discouraged if you do not have anything to put inside yet, although I am sure several of you doing sports may have won a prize or two.

   For the first section, use the reflective template provided in Chapter 6 to reflect after each and every single one of your placements. Jot down the date and key points from each lesson and make a habit of documenting everything you've done.

   Many applicants struggle with the second section, until they realise how many things count as a prize or a publication. Winning a chess tournament, being part of a winning team, applying for an essay competition in school, taking part in a regional/national/international contest or Olympiad, the options are endless!

> I have created a portfolio that has all my high school deeds inside it: grades, certificates, work experience, prizes I have won so far, and so on…
>
> To me it is very important for a couple of reasons. Being organised and systematic is crucial for a smooth application process. When I'm asking my professors to write me a recommendation letter, I will give them this very folder so they have points of reference and can write with assurance that I'm worthy of their recommendation! Secondly, I document all my work experience placements with the exact date and things I have learnt. It's a great way to have everything in one place.
>
> I recommend this to any future medical school applicant since it is a quick strategy to organise personal documents needed for your application. Plus, you gain a sense of pride and productivity as your folder grows bigger.
>
> **Periklis, Medical School Applicant, Greece**

2. Find a Mentor

   Find someone who can motivate you when you don't feel like pushing yourself. Quite often, that's what parents are for. However, try to find someone more related to the field of medicine. Do you know any students who have already applied to medical school and have been through the process themselves? Do you know any teachers or doctors who may be willing to guide you in your journey? If the answer is no, then anyone can be your mentor as long as you feel motivated and inspired by their presence. Your school teacher, your friend, or even your neighbour can become your mentor.

3. Come Up With a Plan

   Have a clear idea of what your next step is by creating a SMART plan—not just any type of plan. It must be:

   - Specific
   - Measurable
   - Achievable
   - Realistic
   - Timely

If that sounds confusing, let's take two students, Jimmy and Tim. Jimmy loves planning his whole year out, adding in the calendar dates that he already knows about, such as the Universities and Colleges Admissions Service (UCAS) application deadline, the BMAT and UCAT, and when his holidays are—after all, who doesn't like Christmas holidays? Jimmy sets short-term goals that he can focus on weekly, as well as long-term goals that he can keep track of monthly. Jimmy loves making 'To-Do' lists to plan his day the night before.

Tim, on the other hand, goes with the flow. Tim goes to school each day, knows he has to sign up for the UCAT and BMAT at some point, and he is aware that the deadline for submitting his medical school application is at some point in October, but he's not really sure when. Tim does stuff as it comes into his head. He doesn't really have a plan, and he only knows that Christmas holidays are coming when his parents are asking him what he'd like from Santa this year.

Fig. 1.2 shows the difference between Jimmy's and Tim's weekly goals.

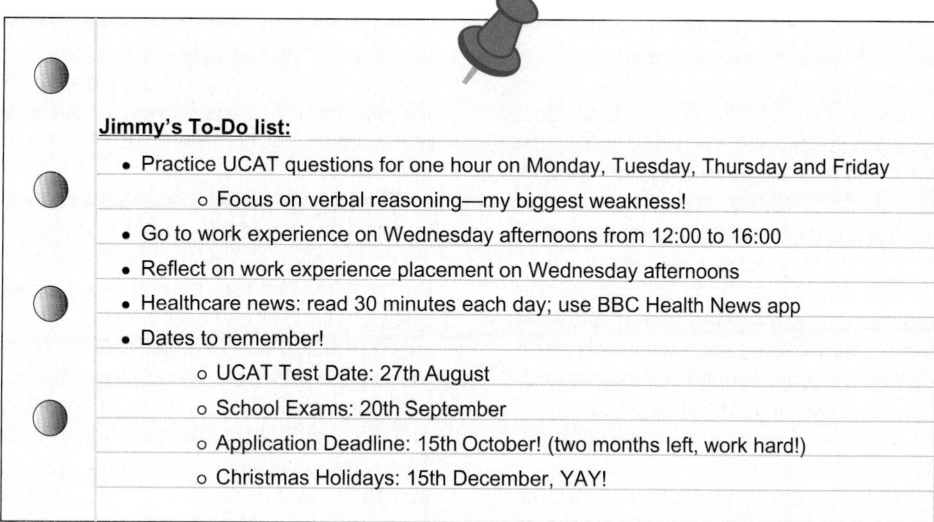

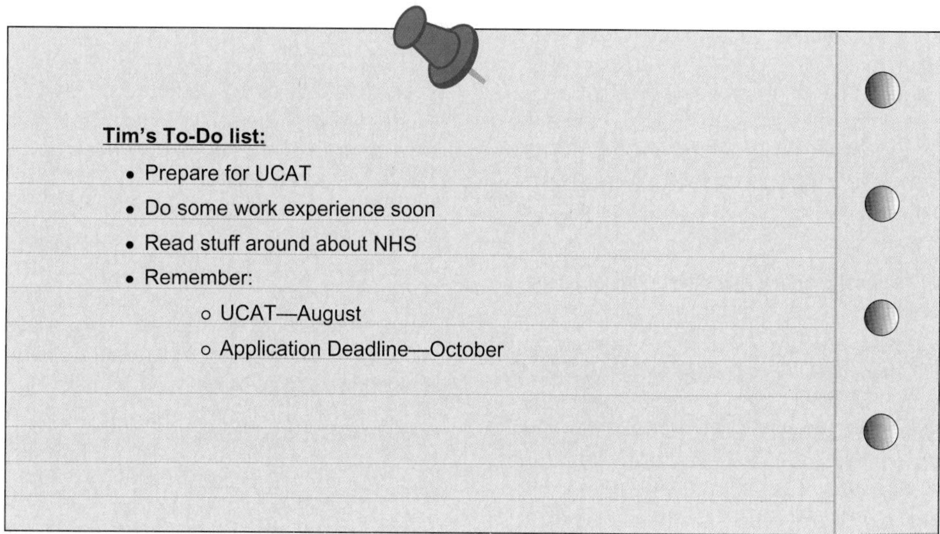

Fig. 1.2 Making a to-do list. *UCAT*, University Clinical Aptitude Test.

Your task now is to get a calendar and a blank piece of paper, and map out your medical school application journey. Put down all the important dates together with some short-term and long-term goals that you can refine as days go by. Place this sheet of paper above your desk and monitor your progress weekly.

A SHORT UNOFFICIAL GUIDE TO MEDICAL SCHOOLS IN THE UK

Finally, we'll finish this introduction chapter with an overview of UK medical schools. A bunch of amazing medical students (36, to be specific) have gathered to share their opinions about what makes their school unique. We've stayed away from advice and tips that you can readily find online, and selected personalised insights from current students.

Why are we showing you this? Firstly, you can use this as a map of existing medical schools in the UK. Highlight the medical schools that appeal to you most and use the power of the internet, open days, connections and so forth to find out more relevant information about the school you may be spending the next 5 to 6 years.

Secondly, we want you to get inspired. We want you to dream about your favourite place and write it down on your goals list. Imagine yourself being there, studying there, and one day your wish may come true. You too can be like Jake, who goes to St George's Medical School, where you can still find Edward Jenner's famous cow skin in the library (how geeky is that?), or like Ryan, who goes to Oxford, a medical school that has been involved in 16 Nobel Prizes for Medicine.

We hope you enjoy reading our guide. It is by no means a full list of everything you may want to know, but it certainly provides a taste of each medical school from those who study there—come back to it whenever you need a bit of motivation to get you through the tough study periods.

Aberdeen School of Medicine

Aberdeen puts a true emphasis on early exposure to clinical skills. The teaching methods are modern and allow you to translate all the theory you learn over the years into practice. Clinical cases stimulate you to correlate the medical knowledge you have learnt with practical management and counselling. You don't simply learn facts; you also get the chance to apply these in the community, and in the hospital, starting from year 1.

Besides exceptional clinical teaching and exposure to patients, Aberdeen offers a bit of everything. The remote and rural medicine component in year 4 offers a chance to see medicine practiced in the remote areas of Scotland. This is a very different setting than the more common large and modern hospital systems. The medical humanities block in year 3 provides students a chance to explore an entirely different side of medicine.

The hospital in Aberdeen is one of the biggest in Europe. Imagine the convenience of having a whole spectrum of medical specialities within 10 minutes of the medical school (and quite possibly your apartment). It is also a favourite argument of mine for 'my-med-school-is better-than-your-med-school' debates.

Apart from a wide range of extracurricular and medical societies that focus on different specialities, Aberdeen medical students have their own year club, which provides a sense of belonging and an opportunity to meet your peers through various activities like fundraising and hosting our own medical school ball.

Sarah M., Medical Student, Aberdeen Medical School

Barts and the London School of Medicine

Situated in the heart of London is St Bartholomew's Hospital, featured on the popular BBC drama 'Sherlock', including the iconic scene in which Benedict Cumberbatch falls from the hospital's roof. It's also where Sir Arthur Conan Doyle's characters Sherlock Holmes and Dr Watson meet. As a medical student at Barts, you will be enveloped in this institution's history and meet people who will become lifelong friends and colleagues.

Alongside the other main site, The Royal London Hospital in Whitechapel, you will enjoy clinical exposure to a unique patient population. From city bankers to new migrants, a variety of patients will educate you on diseases including tuberculosis, which you may not see elsewhere in the UK. We have placements in world-renowned specialist departments, so as students, you see both common and rare conditions.

The course itself includes clinical placements from the first semester of the first year. This early exposure to real patients is key in developing your communication skills, a highly valued component of clinical practice. Teaching is centred around problem-based learning (PBL), where groups of 8 to 10 students work to solve clinical scenario problems. It's great because you're always applying the knowledge you've learnt while being exposed to new things as well.

The Student's Union (BLSA) is excellent at mobilising the student body and arranging social events. You are part of Queen Mary University of London and, therefore, will have exposure to students from a variety of courses. At Bart's, all freshers are assigned a 'Mummy and Daddy' from the years above. This demonstrates the friendliness of the Barts community where there is always someone you can turn to for help on any matter.

Roshni B., Medical Student, Barts Medical School

Birmingham Medical School

Birmingham Medical School hosts one of the largest cohorts of medical students, and hence a very diverse group, with the opportunity to meet people from varying backgrounds and cultures, making the university experience all the more interesting.

Birmingham perhaps has an unfair reputation for being unconventional, but this is what makes it unique. It is an exciting combination of modern commerciality, but with the oasis-like calm and tradition of the campus at Selly Oak. It's not too quiet, but also not as hectic or expensive as other large cities.

The medical course is particularly engaging, with a strong focus on academics. The systems-based course structure integrates biochemistry, anatomy, histology, pharmacology, pathology and other aspects of each system into modules. This allows the student to better appreciate each system and their peculiar functionalities. There are two preclinical years and three clinical years, with a mixed learning style of traditional teaching by lectures and problem-based learning too. The course is supplemented by clinical cases at GP surgeries, which provide very useful clinical background to the biological science theory, as well as opportunities to develop your clinical skills by getting involved in GP consultations. All this helps students gain insight into illness and its effects based on the patients' experiences and perspectives. The cases provide useful clinical context that matches the biological sciences studied concurrently.

Living in Birmingham is absolutely wonderful! It is a very multicultural city that houses the second largest student population in the UK. As one of the largest cities in Europe, there is plenty to do to keep your stress level down. Galleries, music, restaurants and bars—you name it—they are all around the city.

Immediately after arriving, you'll feel welcome and a true sense of belonging. Whether you're an international student or not, nearly everybody is in the same boat. People are extremely supportive and kind, and you'll have the chance to form many friendships that will last a lifetime.

Omowumi F. and Kusy S., Medical Students, Birmingham Medical School

Brighton and Sussex Medical School

The uniqueness of BSMS can be put down to its ethos of 'quality not quantity' that is evident throughout all aspects of the school. Taking only 135 students a year ensures that from day one it is easy to build long-lasting friendships in this amazing part of the country. Teachings occur at both Brighton and Sussex University as well as the Royal Sussex County Hospital.

Teaching in small groups throughout the course ensures that key topics are not glossed over, and students are able to ask all their 'stupid' questions in judgement-free groups of usually eight or less students. This makes for excellent understanding and ultimately creates well-equipped and confident doctors of the future. What truly makes BSMS unique is the wealth of expertise available, and the school's drive to take student feedback on board and implement it swiftly to ensure the student body is always satisfied.

In the first 2 years, we are taught through systems-based learning of the human body. From year 3, we have the exciting opportunity to undertake ward-based attachments, offering extensive clinical experience.

Overall, there really is a community feeling—a feeling that the students matter to one another, to the teaching groups, and the overall institution. The medical school has a wide range of student societies, both medically and nonmedically related. Students have access to both the University of Sussex's and University of Brighton's student unions. As an added bonus, this is a wonderful and dynamic part of the country with the beach right next to you!

Joel C., Medical Student, Brighton and Sussex Medical School

 Bristol Medical School

If there were one word to describe Bristol, it would be 'supportive'. The *Sunday Times* named Bristol 'Britain's best city to live in' and I can definitely vouch for that! The street art, independent shops, theatre, outdoor activities, festivals and music make this a diverse city with character and culture. Bristol is very laid back and feels like home. Whether you're comfortable in the heart of a bustling city or prefer the serenity of the countryside, the University of Bristol caters to all preferences. I guarantee that whatever niche you fit into, there is a place for you in Bristol.

The University of Bristol has one of the best teaching faculties in the UK, with a teaching method that encourages self-directed learning augmented with an accomplished staff helping you along the way. The teaching style suited me perfectly, with a blend of lectures, practicals, case-based discussions, and in the future, assisting doctors and other healthcare professionals in the clinical setting. The medical course at Bristol trains you to be a doctor from day one, with patient contact starting in the first year. The transport network in Bristol makes travelling within the city and to neighbouring areas easy. I run for relaxation and since Bath is only 10 minutes away by train, I was able to run the half marathon in aid of breast cancer.

Bristol encourages its students to develop into global citizens, with internship opportunities ranging from final year electives in Angiers, France, and volunteering in first year to build water tanks in Uganda with Bristol Volunteers for Development Abroad. The degree emphasises early involvement with patients and focuses on developing clinical skills. During each year, the percentage of lectures, independent study and placements vary.

Bristol also offers a 6-year intercalated degree that provides an additional BSc qualification alongside the MBBS degree. Students have the option to research and explore their interests in fields like medical ethics, biochemistry and several other areas for a year. An intercalated degree at Bristol broadens your horizons and provides an additional qualification in a specific area external to the medical course syllabus.

A cardinal aspect of life as a Bristol medic is the easy accessibility to academics and academic resources. Our lectures are recorded online and can be viewed at any time. Our lecturers are medical pioneers, leaders of their fields, and top clinicians and researchers open to discussions and questions. Learning from them is a privilege. Each student is assigned an academic mentor who is a clinician in Bristol or a neighbouring area. They give advice and guide you for the duration of the course to help you make decisions beneficial to your career. Bristol has a state-of-the-art anatomy facility, including cadaveric prosections, to which we have access from year 1.

With outstanding medical teaching, a wide range of extracurricular activities and a focus on supporting one another, coming to Bristol was the best decision I ever made. I hope you will enjoy your time at Bristol as much as I am enjoying mine.

Kiyara F., Medical Student, Bristol Medical School

 Buckingham Medical School

There are several reasons I decided to attend this medical school. We have small group teaching, and each group is allocated a friendly personal tutor who is available at all times. This is a massive advantage because I can seek help whenever I need it, which is extremely important considering the fact that I am studying an intellectually demanding course.

The University of Buckingham was voted number one for teaching quality in 2015–2016, and this is clearly reflected in the school's innovative and modern teaching style. That we are a small cohort and have intimate group teaching ensures a coherent and supportive community.

Need another reason? Medicine at the University of Buckingham is 4 1/2 years as opposed to other universities where the course is 5 or even 6 years. There is also patient contact right from day one, allowing students to integrate the knowledge learnt in lecture into day-to-day clinical practice. You really get a feeling of what it's like to be a doctor, right from the start.

Another unique and interesting aspect of Buckingham Medical School is a core module that runs through the course called 'Narrative Medicine'. Each student is assigned a patient from the start of the course and follows up on the patient regularly throughout the year. This helps the student better understand the management of health conditions and its long-term impact, allowing students to think holistically right from the start.

The University of Buckingham is a private university located in a peaceful and serene countryside environment with fewer distractions than an urban campus, allowing students to focus on their work and studies. At the same time, London is only a 30-minute train journey away, which is very convenient for weekend getaways! Us medics study hard during the week and play hard on the weekends.

Katie K., Medical Student, Buckingham Medical School

 Cambridge Medical School

The unique course structure at Cambridge makes it suitable for a very particular type of medical student, with the preclinical/clinical divide being very marked. Years 1 to 3 are preclinical; students learn anatomy, physiology and the scientific basis of disease. Years 4 to 6 focus on clinical studies based in the hospital and community environment.

The inclusion of full-body dissection and the supervision system are two aspects rarely found at other medical schools, and they both offer fantastic opportunities for student-motivated learning. The college atmosphere is great for making friends and creating an inclusive community, and the formal dinners are a nice bonus too.

(*Continued*)

The inspirational environment, the unique collegiate system, and the outstanding teaching quality make studying at Cambridge a completely different experience compared to other universities.

Alex S., Cambridge Medical School

 Cardiff Medical School

Studying at Cardiff Medical School is a very stimulating experience, where students in small groups investigate a series of clinical cases, integrating physiological, anatomical, psychosocial and pharmacological teachings. Students learn through collective discussions, and supporting lectures and workshops.

The medical school offers a safe and stimulating learning environment, adopting a case-based teaching system that centres around a spiral curriculum, where aspects of medicine are built on year on year, rather than just being fed in isolated chunks. There is excellent early exposure to clinical and communication practices. Beyond lectures are a host of academic-related societies for paediatrics, emergency medicine, surgical societies, among others. Students can get involved in myriad activities, from being on the committee of the surgical society, to presenting posters at conferences, to competing for the healthcare basketball team. There's no shortage of opportunities for learning and socialising beyond the classroom.

Cardiff is a fantastic city to study and live in. It's student friendly, with a wide range of activities available, from nights out to outings at the Brecon Beacons. At the end of the day, it is the capital of Wales—there's no way you'll run out of things to do.

Tim W. and David L., Medical Students, Cardiff Medical School

 Dundee Medical School

For those of you who are thinking 'where even is Dundee?' the answer is simple—Dundee is the sunniest city in Scotland (proven by statistics!), located on the east coast. Our medical school is based in one of Europe's largest teaching hospitals, where the first ever laparoscopic surgery was performed in the UK.

Dundee Medical School is ranked first in Scotland and sixth in the UK for medicine in 2022. We have fantastic, passionate teaching staff that are active in both teaching and research in their specialities. Situated in Ninewells Hospital, medical students are given a lot of early patient contact, the earliest being within the first week of medical school, and clerking assessment submission within the first semester. It sounds daunting, but it is the best way to prepare you for being the best doctor you can be. Unlike some other medical schools, Dundee starts our clinical medicine teaching in the first year, giving you the most clinical exposure early on.

Medical students are encouraged to get involved in research projects, ranging from student-selected components within the curriculum to summer studentship schemes and even intercalated degrees.

With 195 societies to choose from, and a wide variety of entertainment and academic events, Dundee Student Association provides countless opportunities to make friends, learn new things and relax after a busy day in hospital.

Oh, and if that's not enough to convince you, did I mention that Dundee is one of the few medical schools that still teaches anatomy by doing full-body dissection on cadavers?

Tiffany L., Medical Student, Dundee Medical School

 Edinburgh Medical School

Edinburgh Medical School highly values personal development. Early patient exposure in the hospital setting and a wide variety of research options guaranteed by our university encourage students to face challenges with confidence and turn them into opportunities. Along with basic science courses and lectures, students constantly need to build their inner strength, stand up against their own weaknesses and overcome insecurities during their clinical rotations. The rationale behind this is to educate emotionally resilient doctors and inspire students' future development, since it is a lifelong task, no matter what career path you wish to pursue.

Founded in 1726, medicine at Edinburgh is an integrated, 6-year course with systems-based learning. The programme is broken down into 2 years of preclinical, 1 year of intercalation (from which you get a separate degree and graduate twice!), and then 3 years of clinical medicine. Anatomy is taught via prosection.

Students receive a lot of support through a personal tutoring system, where we all get assigned to an academic tutor from the medical school who is always there, ready to support you with any questions or concerns.

Edinburgh is a city university, not a campus, which I personally prefer as you have access to several opportunities. As the capital of Scotland, Edinburgh is an amazing city, beautiful and rich in history. Edinburgh has lots going on—why not get involved in ceilidhs and other traditional Scottish dancing events? The beach and a seaside town are just a 10-minute drive from the medical school. The Pentland Hills are great for long walks, and so is Arthur's seat (give it a Google).

Fun facts! JK Rowling lives in Edinburgh, just down the road, and you can visit the café where she wrote Harry Potter. Grave robbers and murderers Burke and Hare stole corpses to sell to the anatomy/dissections unit at the Edinburgh Medical School in the 1800s. They were arrested and executed, and Burke's skeleton still hangs in the old school's anatomy department—how cool (or creepy) is that?

Joanna W. and Georgie L., Medical Students, Edinburgh Medical School

 Exeter Medical School

A loud and intense banter ensues during every session, silent note-taking instantly forgotten. Each member speaks up, a forgotten anatomy term, an interesting research article, or even a helpful anecdote creating an atmosphere for discussion. This unique format for studying medicine has definitely helped me widen my medical knowledge, but more importantly, it has taught me to express this knowledge effectively to an audience. The University of Exeter Medical School has organised the course in an interesting manner that allows students the chance to interact with our colleagues and share information that fortifies our learning. There is a real community feeling as the course cohort is fairly small (~120 students). I love this because it means you get to know everyone very well.

Problem-based learning (PBL) is at the core of the course in Exeter. Learning in groups of six to seven students makes it easier for everyone to interact and build transferrable skills including, but not limited to, teamwork, leadership, communication, presentation and listening skills.

The curriculum is full of clinical skills sessions that give students the chance to put theory into action. A typical session would involve taking a history from a patient or an actor and practicing blood-taking or other skills. The Clinical Skills Resource Centre is open most of the time and you have a wide range of mannequins on which you can practice medical skills. From suturing to spirometry, there's always something to learn and to 'play' with. These sessions help students merge theoretical and clinical knowledge, making the heavy course load more relatable and easier to understand. You'll find it easier to visualise and remember the roles of the cranial nerves when identifying and testing their function on your peers.

Exeter is very receptive to student suggestions, especially since it's a relatively new course (Exeter and Plymouth used to be one medical school called 'Peninsula Medical School'). Student committees constantly give feedback and suggestions from each and every medical student. The professors actively modify their teaching styles to match the students' style and consistently ask for feedback, which makes them very approachable.

Exeter truly feels like home—there's always something to do, and the friendships you build here will last forever. By the way, fun fact for the Harry Potter fans out there: J.K. Rowling graduated from Exeter University and many of her sources of inspiration are dotted around the city and campus!

Krutika S., Medical Student, Exeter Medical School

 Glasgow Medical School

A typical week in the first 2 years of Glasgow Medical School consists of problem-based learning (PBL), vocational studies, clinical skills/visits, anatomy class, labs and lectures. From third year onwards, it is more focused on clinical placements. This combination helps students develop practical skills and professionalism alongside their scientific and clinical knowledge. One of the things I like most about the medical school is the spiral curriculum. By going over the same topics with increasing complexity each time, it consolidates one's knowledge and reinforces previous learning. In the first 12 weeks in first year, you will gain general knowledge of all body systems, which you will learn about in greater detail during each block in the coming years.

Having dissection class from first year onwards greatly facilitates students' learning of anatomy. The medical school library is open 24 hours a day with a large collection of books from all areas of medicine for references. The medical school also provides extensive student support through the peer support and medic family programmes, where you can talk to trained supporters or your seniors when problems arise.

Outside medical school, you will be able to enjoy a great student life on this big campus within a vibrant city. The school policy ensures that students have Wednesday afternoons off for extracurricular activities—that means there's no excuse for not enjoying your surroundings! The university has a huge variety of clubs and societies, both medically and nonmedically related. There are lots of volunteering opportunities, local or international, throughout the year and during summer.

The medical societies give students an opportunity to explore different specialties and start building up your CV from an early stage. They organise talks and study classes, which enhance your knowledge of specific areas and help you with your studies. The other societies and sport clubs help you relax and develop other interests. You can meet like-minded friends who study different subjects and are from different parts of the world.

Gladys L., Medical Student, Glasgow Medical School

 Hull York Medical School

Initially what attracted me to Hull York Medical School (HYMS) was the innovative teaching style, which combines a traditional lecture-based learning approach with PBL to deliver a modern and effective medical education.

In our first 2 years, we are randomly assigned to either the York or Hull campus. This means that unlike some other medical schools, our cohort sizes are relatively small (around 72 people on each site), making it easier to get to know the people on your course as well as the staff. This is a massive advantage, not only because you establish good relationships with your peers, who ultimately become your best friends, but also because you receive more support from those who are teaching you.

The HYMS curriculum is highly integrated and each week has its own unique theme. For example, if we are studying the respiratory system one week, then our lectures, PBL, anatomy sessions and clinical skills/placements will reflect this accordingly. Another unique aspect of the HYMS curriculum is the high level of clinical contact from term 1, in both primary and secondary healthcare settings. Here, we apply the same clinical skills taught earlier in the week, but to real patients under the supervision and guidance of a consultant or general practitioner. To me, this is what makes HYMS so strategic: You learn, you share learning with peers through PBL and then you put everything into action in the clinical world.

As for the area where you'll be spending your next few years, Hull was voted one of the UK's 'culture cities', while York is one of the most historical and most beautiful cities in the country. What could make studying better than this?

Danny D., Medical Student, Hull York Medical School

 Imperial College London

Initially, I was unsure which university to go to. Living overseas meant that I missed open days and lacked any geographical ties. Wanting my course to thoroughly cover the underlying mechanics of the body led me to narrow down my choices based on teaching ratios, rankings, reputation and research output. Imperial College London stood out in three ways. It's among the few medical schools that have full-body dissections, and it also has an integrated BSc year and course content with a strong biochemical focus.

(Continued)

These components make the university unique. Two elements that distinguish the medical course at Imperial College London are the people and the approach to medicine. Through lectures, labs and abundant opportunities to get involved in real research, I felt encouraged by the university to contribute as a clinician locally and as a scientist globally. The relevance of sociology and psychology in healthcare was highlighted through coursework that required drawing parallels between my regular encounters with patients and the theories I learnt in lectures. The wide spectrum of material also meant that lecturers include doctors, surgeons, non-governmental organisation (NGO) workers, psychologists and patients themselves. Most of them readily answered any questions after their presentations and in emails weeks after they had been held.

Imperial College London has challenged me to grow as an academic and a person, with the city enabling me to explore new places and cultures. With over 340 student societies, it was easy to find others who share my interests and hobbies.

I await the forthcoming years with restlessness, eager to further immerse myself in both this wonderful city and its world-leading medical school.

Waseem H., Medical Student, Imperial Medical School

Keele Medical School

Keele University Medical School is set within a rural landscape and will appeal to those looking for a relaxed environment compared to the hustle and bustle of a city. Despite this, both Manchester and Birmingham are less than an hour's train journey away. As it is a small medical school, staff and students get to know each other very well. Consequently, the support system is excellent, and staff will go out of their way to help students with any type of problem they may be experiencing, from academic to personal.

The course includes full cadaveric dissection (supplemented with prosection), which is an amazing way to learn anatomy, as it allows you to appreciate the body as a whole and I find details are easier to recall when I have dissected something myself. Clinical contact with patients starts early in year 1, and history taking and examination is taught in year 2. This provides a clinical context to the science and means that students can hit the ground running when the clinical phase of the course begins in year 3. Keele runs a PBL course, which personally I find much better than sitting through lectures, as you're in charge of your own learning and can tailor the course to your interests.

Keele's student union is also one of the best in the country, with over a hundred different societies and exciting line-up entertainment every year—this might be why Keele students have officially been known as the happiest in the country. Overall, the course is well designed, and I wouldn't hesitate recommending Keele Medical School to anyone.

Sandeep D., Medical Student, Keele Medical School

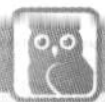

King's College London

The GKT School of Medicine at KCL has one of the largest cohorts in Europe, which means we have countless opportunities. During the early years, we perform full-body dissections as part of anatomy training, and during clinical years, we use simulation centre facilities with all sorts of tools and mannequins to practice on. It is almost guaranteed that you'll spend some time on a peripheral placement, i.e. outside of London, with accommodation provided for free. This means you'll experience training in both teaching and DG (District General) hospitals. The school just switched to a new curriculum with much more clinical exposure early on.

Having such a large student body, there are so many medical societies at KCL, ranging from specialty-focused, to volunteering, to sports, to anything in between—while maintaining access to the university-wide societies. You'll definitely find something suited to your taste, and if not, you can always gather some friends and start a new society. Being based in central London means higher rent, but it also means that you'll get to see the most exciting and novel things both in the hospital and outside. After all, you will be living in one of the largest, most dynamic and exciting cities in the world.

Martina S., Medical Student, King's College London

Lancaster Medical School

Lancaster University is one of the smallest public medical schools in the UK, admitting around 129 medical students per year. The teaching at Lancaster Medical School (LMS) offers a personalised and individual approach. Having fewer students in each group provides additional support as well as an effective and enjoyable student experience.

In year 1, teaching is mostly done at university, which allows you to consolidate knowledge learnt during lectures. In year 2, half your time is split between teaching on campus and clinical placements. Core patient examinations prepare students for practical hospital experience at Lancaster Royal Infirmary or Furness General Hospital in the second year. Early patient contact includes performing a full clerking on patients, taking histories and integrating clinical skills gained while conducting patient examinations to understand how pathology presents.

The course is well structured and balanced over 5 years, and includes weekly physiology and anatomy teaching sessions, but the particular focus on student/patient communication develops confidence and is a real added bonus. The academic staff at LMS are specialised professionals in their area of teaching and are approachable, helpful, and above all extremely supportive.

I believe that LMS provides a world-class education in a familial environment and generates outstanding doctors experienced in all aspects of medicine.

Rumaysa A.Q., Medical Student, Lancaster Medical School

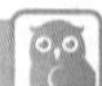

Leeds Medical School

Leeds is unique because we are one of the country's larger medical schools. I'm in my fourth year and my current year group has over 300 pupils. With such a large cohort, there are many societies that cater to different tastes, from sports clubs to life drawing, all within the medical school. As cliché as it sounds, there is something for everyone, and someone will always have similar interests and hobbies.

In terms of assessments, Leeds is great. We have one main exam (written exam and Objective Structured Clinical Examination (OSCE)) at the end of the year. While we get feedback for modules, which are useful for guiding further learning, this does not count towards a student's overall grade. This motivates you to study and improve because you want to, not because you have to!

Intercalation is not compulsory at Leeds; however, over half of the students choose to intercalate. Unlike some medical schools where there is a set time for intercalation, Leeds is flexible about when you can intercalate, with it being possible to intercalate any time between the end of fourth year and the start of fifth year.

Sarah P., Medical Student, Leeds Medical School

Leicester Medical School

My personal advice when applying to medical school is that the rankings should not be the sole motivator behind your university choices. Rankings always change, and most medical institutions are standardised across the board and provide high-quality education that prepares you for a career as a doctor. A more important factor to take into consideration is the teaching style and whether it matches your personality or not. Leicester University, for example, employs an integrated syllabus. This was ideal for me, as I found that learning in lectures and then applying this theoretical knowledge practically in group work is effective.

In addition to the academic factors, Leicester is a vibrant, multicultural city that has something for everyone. Another big plus is the affordability and comparatively low cost of living. Rent is quite reasonable for decent-sized houses.

Joining the course was a very straightforward experience, as we were all assigned a medic family. The 'medic parents' were senior medical students who volunteered to help out first years. They were very helpful and had a calming presence. I felt a lot more settled after speaking and spending time with my medic family as they shared their advice and experience.

The lectures were very well timed (approximately 2 hours/day), which meant we were not overloaded and retained a lot of the information. There was a strong emphasis on the practical side of medicine, including patient communication and clinical skills. Multiple patient simulations were organised to prepare us right from the beginning. Not long after the simulations, we were given the opportunity to visit a real patient on a regular basis. This was especially helpful, as you got to experience first-hand how it feels to have a patient and the responsibility that comes with it.

The availability of cadavers from the first day was another highlight that made anatomy so much more interesting. This ensured that each one of us got decent exposure to human anatomy and were able to practice dissection. As a result our learning has been very thorough, allowing us to retain the large curriculum, which can be assessed at any time (all topics from year 1 to year 5 may be assessed at any time).

In terms of infrastructure and facilities, including the top-class dissection room, the medical school has also built a new building complete with state-of-the-art technology.

I am wholeheartedly enjoying my time at Leicester University. I have gotten the work–life balance right. University hours are not particularly long, and this allows you to maintain hobbies and get involved with various societies, which is especially important in this field. Most importantly, the strong focus on practical skills has made me appreciate the course even more and will hopefully allow me to see the fruits of my labour in the near future.

Akash M., Medical Student, Leicester Medical School

Liverpool Medical School

Apart from the traditional method of learning through lectures, students at Liverpool School of Medicine actively discuss real-life scenarios via an interesting case-based learning approach. This equips us with the problem-solving and communication skills needed with our future colleagues.

To further improve our communication skills, we work with simulated patients throughout the year to prepare us for future professional interactions in clinical settings. Our medical school has a strong mentoring system that ensures we have sufficient support and guidance.

Outside the lectures, Liverpool is a city that has everything for everyone, from art, museums, and festivals to nightlife, theatre, and relaxing evenings. Sports, of course, are big in Liverpool as well, whether you're a football fan or not. The Liverpool Guild of Students provides a number of events that can help you relieve stress at the end of a busy day! By the way, did I mention that the Beatles are from Liverpool?

Dana T., Medical Student, Liverpool Medical School

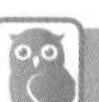

Manchester Medical School

My favourite aspect of Manchester? It has to be the teaching style: PBL. As some of you may already know, this means that there is A LOT of self-studying. First, a case study is given at the start of the week, including symptoms of a particular disease and names of drugs prescribed. We discuss these in a small group and set specific learning points. At the end of the week, we meet again to discuss what we have learnt and fill in any potential gaps in our knowledge. This unique system sometimes means we don't know how much to study, although the intended learning outcomes are still provided by the university. It takes a while to get used to PBL, but my colleagues and I love this style of teaching compared to the old traditional model filled with lectures from 9 a.m. until 5 p.m. PBL allows you to focus on your weaknesses and build on your strengths. Yes, it does require a bit of self-motivation on your side, but you'll get used to it. My top tip would be to visit the open days and experience a PBL taster session to see whether this teaching style fits your personality.

I chose the University of Manchester mainly because I had the impression that Manchester is 'the second London'. In other words, metropolitan and urban without the high-rise prices of a cutthroat financial hubbub. Cultural, urbane and diverse—these are the words that popped into my head when I first arrived in Manchester. This impression did not fail me. Besides, the University of Manchester ranks quite well in the university league tables.

Finally, the University of Manchester is the largest university by population in the country; it is a place that celebrates diversity, equality, and has the largest student union in the

(Continued)

UK. For those of you wishing to network further, it is very easy to meet new and interesting people. The university has all sorts of clubs and societies, and the location makes it easy to access various places inside and outside of the UK.

Jia C.C., Medical Student, Manchester Medical School

Newcastle Medical School

We gain clinical exposure early on in the course, with volunteers coming into our clinical skills sessions, as well as hospital and GP visits in the first 2 years. There are four hospital base units in the region, and in third and fifth year, we have the opportunity to be placed in different areas around the northeast.

Newcastle advocates case-based learning approach in years 1 and 2, which means students can integrate knowledge, skills, and professional communication across various subject areas. Students also have two 'Student-Select component' (SSC) placements. Essentially you get to choose an area that interests you and explore it during a given period of time. Intercalated study is also available for those who are interested.

Our Medical Society offers free drinks every Friday night and hosts annual events like the Winter Ball and Metroline, which involves touring Newcastle in scrubs!

Elizabeth T., Medical Student, Newcastle Medical School

Norwich (UEA) Medical School

In 2014, the GMC revealed results showing 97% of UEA graduates agree 'the skills I learn at medical school set me up well for working as a foundation doctor'. It's not difficult to see how UEA produces some of the best-prepared junior doctors in the country.

From year 1, we are introduced to patients in primary care 1 day a week throughout the year, followed by a block of secondary care placement, giving us the opportunity to understand health and disease holistically in a real-world context. This way, we are able to relate our learning back to patients we see every week, and, after all, we tend to remember things through connecting with people and their stories than the pages of a textbook. A strong emphasis on communication and clinical skills, as well as teamwork during PBL and IPL (interprofessional learning), are fundamental in producing well-rounded doctors capable of effectively managing patients and working alongside colleagues on the ward.

I've been told the gap from medical school to doctoring is steep, but the qualities and skills I develop at UEA will indeed set me up well for working as a foundation doctor and beyond!

Monica S., Medical Student, Norwich Medical School (UEA)

Nottingham Medical School

Initially wanting to go to a city-based university, I was pleasantly surprised by how much I loved the campus life at the University of Nottingham.

Here's what makes Nottingham's medical course stand out from other similar courses in the UK:

You get two degrees in 5 years (BMedSci and BMBS)—though the additional degree is no longer looked at by the FPAS application (foundation programme application system), it allows students to gain an extra qualification while taking time out of medicine—and the degree is always helpful in later applications!

University of Nottingham is one of the few universities that offer dissection when teaching anatomy (believe me, it makes life a lot easier).

There are many early opportunities to expose students to research and publication writing (which is an additional point on the FPAS application).

The medical course at Nottingham is a little more condensed because of the second BMedSci degree, which sometimes can be overwhelming. However, due to the many student-led societies like MedSoc Teaching and SCRUBS, you can rest assured there will always be someone to talk you through things if you are struggling.

As a medical student, you need the discipline to know when it's time to study and when it's time to have fun—nobody will force you to do either. There's a whole range of societies and clubs that you can get involved in, some medical, others nonmedical—it's completely up to you!

Fady A., Medical Student, University of Nottingham Medical School

Oxford Medical School

Oxford is a unique medical school and I am very grateful to be here. Students are more satisfied with their training here than at any other UK medical school (Complete University Guide). Beyond this, the overall quality of an Oxford medical education is considered by some to be the best in the world (Times Higher Education).

Oxford is split into 38 'Colleges' and every student is a member of one. They organise weekly 'tutorials' where you can discuss your favourite subjects with distinguished professors. I met a lot of my close friends living together in college, even though they study totally different subjects than medicine.

The city itself consists of beautiful architecture surrounded by lush green countryside. However, you are not isolated here: There are 24/7 transport links with London and nearby international airports.

Our university is the oldest in the English-speaking world, yet it stays incredibly modern. We are a world-leading research institution and have been involved in 16 Nobel Prizes for Medicine. Students here are encouraged to change our world for the better.

If you are excited about becoming the best doctor you can be, please consider Oxford—we would be delighted to welcome you here.

Ryan H., Medical Student, Oxford Medical School

Plymouth Medical School

Studying medicine at the Plymouth University Peninsula Schools of Medicine and Dentistry is stimulating, exciting, forward-thinking and patient centred. It is one of the largest medical schools in the southwest of England. The early clinical contact is one of the course's distinguishing features. There are also a wide variety of clinical placements available across multiple settings. In its initial years, the course adopts a problem-based learning (PBL) approach, moving on to placement-based learning in the latter years.

All the core scientific foundations of medicine are taught in a clinical context, which is unique to the school. Admittedly, I found this daunting in the first few weeks of the course. However, now I appreciate how beneficial this style of learning was, as I am much more confident in clinical settings than peers from other medical schools. It is often said that Peninsula produces some of the best foundation doctors and I believe that early clinical exposure contributes to this.

The setting in which this teaching is delivered is outstanding quality. Derriford Hospital, where most of our clinical placements occur, is one of the largest hospitals in Europe, as well as the only trauma centre in Devon and Cornwall.

As for the area, you're right by the sea and only 20 minutes away from Cornwall (one of the most beautiful areas in the UK—especially for the surfers out there). Words cannot describe how lovely it is!

Pooja R., Medical Student, Plymouth Medical School

Queen's University Belfast (QUB) Medical School

Choosing a university is one of the most important decisions you will ever make, and I couldn't be happier with mine. I am in my fourth year of study at Queen's University Belfast and I can honestly say I've loved every minute of it. Queen's is a university like no other in the UK, located in the North of Ireland where you get to experience the best of both worlds, with connections to both the UK and Ireland. Belfast is a thriving city with something for everyone; it has a great nightlife and shopping, and a rich culture unique to Northern Ireland. The Queen's quarter is a beautiful area of the city where most students live and study, creating a laid back and fun atmosphere.

Queen's is a Russel Group university, carrying out pioneering medical research in which students take part. Our facilities are state of the art and situated at the doorstep of Belfast City Hospital, a hospital that is world-leading in cancer care and renal transplant surgery. Your clinical placements are all over Northern Ireland, which allows you to travel, and the staff here are excellent, both in terms of teaching and pastoral support.

Aisling B., Medical Student, Queen's University Belfast

Sheffield Medical School

The University of Sheffield Medical School highly regards the need for each medical student to be competent and empathetic communicators straight from the first year of medical school.

University of Sheffield Medical School is also one of the few schools in the UK to still have dissection lessons of cadavers for anatomy. Sheffield is situated in a region where health inequalities are prevalent, with life expectancy varying up to 10 years just within different parts of Sheffield. This presents medical students with first-hand experience of health inequalities' social determinants and why such inequalities exist in the world today. This is perhaps something worth reading more about for your interview!

Well, one fun (or not-so-fun) fact is that the university library was voted the ugliest building in the UK, but apart from that, everything else here is beautiful. Peak district is close by and it is always nice to visit. The city is full of little cafes and vintage shops—it really feels like living in a town even though you are in a city.

Keat K., Medical Student, Sheffield Medical School

Southampton Medical School

If you like research, want early patient contact, like a busy city with a varied nightlife and are keen to join loads of sport/cultural/academic societies, then this is definitely the medical school for you. It has one of the largest medical student bodies of the country, with four different medical programmes, which means you get to meet tons of different people with various backgrounds and experiences, making your time at Southampton interesting and international.

Medicine is very demanding and has more contact hours than other degrees, so the medical school society, MedSoc, has set up around 15 societies dedicated to sport so that you can still do what you love around medical school commitments. They also organise social events and sponsor local, national, and student-led charities. Basically, anything you could think of that you want to do in your free time, chances are MedSoc has that on offer for you.

If you are interested in carrying out research part-time, Southampton has amazing research facilities and is a world-leading institution in many research areas such as cancer sciences, infection, population health and genomics. I honestly could not imagine myself studying medicine anywhere else, and I would recommend Southampton Medical School in a heartbeat.

Lucia L., Medical Student, Southampton Medical School

St Andrews Medical School

Founded in 1413, St Andrews was the first university established in Scotland. Perhaps one of the most noticeable buildings in the medical school is the recent £45 m building dedicated to medicine and life sciences. As you would imagine, this means A LOT of learning resources for students.

For many, the idea of a traditional medical course may be off-putting. However, this does not mean there is no patient contact. In fact, it is quite the opposite. Several clinical skills sessions a week, multiple opportunities to meet patients, and frequent visits to local general practitioner (GP) practices and hospitals ensure that we have plenty of opportunity to develop our clinical skills and patient communication, along with the fascinating opportunity to talk to real patients about their medical conditions. Our chance to spend more time in hospital comes after we graduate with our BSc (Hons) in medicine and transfer to our partner medical schools dotted all around the UK.

Perhaps what makes the medical school most unique are the integrated full-body dissection classes held every week to further expand our anatomy knowledge.

Although initially the prospect of such a small medical school (approximately 170 students per year) might be off-putting, in reality, it creates a very personal atmosphere

(Continued)

where all 3 years are integrated. This incredible community is bolstered by the medical school's Bute Medical Society (BMS). The BMS hosts many social events and informative talks, and raises money for charity every year. However, the BMS is not the only society available to join; from the Surgical Society to Médecins Sans Frontières (MSF) and a whole host of other university societies, you will never be bored!

Hanna W.P., Medical Student, St Andrew's Medical School

St George's University of London (SGUL)

SGUL is uniquely in tune with its history: From being the alma mater of Henry Gray (a book every science student owns) all the way down to the preserved skin of Edward Jenner's cow (from which his cowpox vaccine was created) in the library. Studying here, you feel connected to all the St George's doctors down through the centuries. It's also part of a major teaching hospital, and it's even on television! (In case you don't know, '24 Hours' on A&E is filmed in St George's hospital.) You get the chance to see incredible things you would be hard-pressed to find elsewhere, and the entire hospital and university is a tight-knit community you are instantly a part of from day one.

As for our course, some highlights include anatomy teaching via whole body dissections, patient-focused, case-based, and problem-based learning, as well as three choices of student-selected components in an area of your interest. SGUL is the only university in the country dedicated solely to healthcare education. Even so, the student union is not small at all and offers several extracurricular opportunities.

Jake R., Medical Student, St George's University of London

Swansea Medical School

'We're a small medical school', the admissions tutors like to tell new and prospective students. 'The good thing about that is everybody knows you; the bad thing about that is everybody knows you'.

This certainly rang true during my years at one of just two graduate-only medical schools in the UK. While my London friends were being left to their own devices in PBL groups, we had case-based learning weeks and were often taught in small groups by friendly tutors who made time for questions and feedback.

As was perhaps inevitable with its meteoric rise through the rankings (having gone from eleventh to third place in the league tables during my time here), the College of Medicine is slowly expanding. Despite this, Swansea has retained much of what made it appealing as a smaller school. Members of staff recognise you and say hello in the corridor and on the wards, and students are encouraged to email or stop by faculty members' offices with personal and academic issues.

Training in Wales also allows us to be part of a health system that is still recognisable from Nye Bevan's 1945 vision of an equal, nationalised service, free at the point of need.

As an older graduate with an interest in primary care, I'm glad to be at Swansea. As a human being who believes wholeheartedly in everything the NHS stands for, I'm delighted to be in Wales.

Rebecca F., Medical Student, Swansea University, Medical School

University College London Medical School

First of all, the student life is what makes UCL stand out. University College London (UCL) is right in the centre of London, offering an amazing choice and quality of food, nightlife, musicals, and shops.

There is a very well-structured welfare system in UCL. Apart from the welfare officer of the medical school student union—Royal Free, University College and Middlesex Medical Students Society (RUMS)—who offers individual advice on finance, health, etc., there are also other staff and students who are here and ready to help. From the day students come into the medical school, each student has a personal tutor who they meet regularly, a transition mentor who would meet weekly for the first term to support their transition into medical school, as well as RUMS Mums and Dads from the year above to pass on tips and tricks for surviving in medical school.

To improve our learning experiences, there are student representatives for each module from each year group, who take part in module, staff-led and student-led meetings each term to discuss issues raised by the students. The medical school staff and administrators listen to our suggestions and real changes happen.

On the academic side, in year 1, we get a diverse range of student-selected components (SSC) to learn more about other aspects of medicine, such as biomedical sciences, anthropology, and clinical application of knowledge. Dissections as opposed to prosections in many other medical schools make anatomy more real for us, along with early patient contact and community placements in year 1 as part of our clinical and professional practice module (CPP). The UCL medical degree includes a compulsory intercalated BSc in our third year, and we have a wide range of courses from which to choose. Ranging from anatomy to women's health, it is an invaluable experience for us to explore the field of medicine with a fresh perspective. Moreover, it is a plus that students in their first clinical year only rotate among the three UCL teaching hospitals (as summarised in the word RUMS) instead of around various hospitals all over London.

Apart from studying, there are many clubs and societies. RUMS has their own sports and music societies to accommodate the busy medic's schedule, but it's not exclusive and some societies have nonmedics on their team.

All in all, UCL offers an exciting and varied student life that's lots of fun!

Kristie L., Medical Student, University College London Medical School

Warwick University (Graduate Entry) Medical School

When pondering what makes Warwick Medical School unique, my first thought was of course the complete collection of Gunther von Hagen's plastinated specimens we have the privilege of using each week in anatomy teaching. Each specimen is so delicately preserved and perfect for our training. My next thought was the clinical exposure we get so early on in the course. With both clinical skills and bedside teaching introduced at the beginning of year 1, we get great opportunities to meet patients and put our learning into context from the start. However, what I think truly stands out at Warwick Medical School are my fellow students. As the largest graduate entry course in the UK, each student has a different background and range of experiences. Every student has a great story to tell, and many have had interesting first careers from being a paramedic to a firefighter and even a magician. Having a cohort of nearly 200 of some of the friendliest and most like-minded people I have had the pleasure of meeting is a brilliant support network, one that is invaluable in a career such as medicine.

Laura P., Medical Student, Warwick Medical School

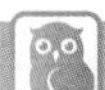 Anglia Ruskin Medical School

Anglia Ruskin is a relatively new medical school that opened in 2018; however, its curriculum, teaching, and student support is well established. The course is a 5-year MBChB degree with full-body dissections in anatomy from year 1 and clinical exposure throughout the 5 years. Each year, students take an SSC (student-selected component) which allows you to research a topic within medicine, expanding your academic knowledge and writing. I personally think it's an incredible opportunity that can lead you to getting summer research placements or even being published. Not many schools give students the opportunity to do SSCs every year, so it's definitely a privilege!

The campus itself is based in Chelmsford which is quiet enough to enjoy as a student, but there are also incredible opportunities and societies available for you to join. London is just about a 30-minute train journey away, and Cambridge is even closer—perfect for when you want to get away for the weekend!

Robert H., Medical Student, Anglia Ruskin Medical School

NEW MEDICAL SCHOOLS?

Since 2020, five brand new medical schools have been open to enthusiastic medical students such as yourself. This is part of the government's initiative to increase medical school places (and therefore future doctor positions) in England by 25%. Not only are there now more medical schools, but places at all other medical schools are also increasing. That's good news for you. While we are on the subject, it might be worth having a read around this topic as it often comes up in medical school interviews!

Many concerned parents and students have previously asked us about the quality of teaching at these medical schools. We have had the pleasure of speaking to numerous academics and clinicians who are part of the founding board of these new medical schools. As all medical schools do, new ones will also follow the same high-quality standards set by the UK General Medical Council. In fact, several (if not all) are using cutting-edge technology and state-of-the-art equipment for teaching, as well as focusing on modern topics of interest in medicine such as genetics, aging, and social determinants of health.

The following are the names of the newly founded medical schools:

- Anglia Ruskin School of Medicine, based in Chelmsford (Essex)
- Edge Hill University Medical School, based in Ormskirk (Lancashire)
- Kent and Medway Medical School, based in Canterbury (Kent) and as a partnership between the University of Kent and Canterbury Christ Church University
- Nottingham Lincoln Medical School, based in Lincoln (Lincolnshire) and in partnership with Nottingham University
- Sunderland Medical School, based in Sunderland (Tyne and Wear)

Up-to-date information can be found on their own individual websites and we urge you to check these websites often, especially when you're applying, as they are very likely to change during the first few years. As you'll notice, some of these new medical schools represent partnerships between universities and nearby medical schools, and therefore will also share similar teaching techniques and learning styles. The main aim (as set by the government) for establishing these new medical schools was to widen access to medical schools within the previously mentioned local regions.

SUMMARY, TEST YOURSELF AND REFLECTION

By now, I hope that we all agree that first you need to know your WHY. Write it down and stick it to the wall. Read it every day and use it as your motivation.

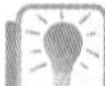

If You Want to Succeed, You Need To

- Start early and use it to your advantage.
- Come up with a 'SMART' plan and stick to it.
- Use your 'Getting into medical school' portfolio to track your progress.
- Find a mentor and surround yourself with people who share your passion.

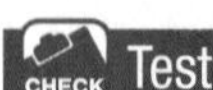

Test Yourself

- What does 'SMART' stand for and how can you use this to your advantage?
- What are the different sections of the getting into medical school portfolio?
- When is your UCAS application deadline?

Your homework, if you haven't already, is to follow the instructions outlined previously, get an empty folder and create your own 'getting into medical school' portfolio. Watch it grow as you add additional experiences to it and use it to track your progress. This folder will be invaluable when you start writing your personal statement or preparing for the interview.

How has this chapter influenced your perspective? How are you going to move forward? Do you have any plans or dates that you'd like to add to your calendar? What are your key application dates and what milestones can you use to keep track of your progress?

Reflection and Notes

RESOURCES

Cambridge Assessment, Admissions Testing. BioMedical Admissions test (BMAT). Available at http://www.admissionstesting.org/for-test-takers/bmat/. Accessed 20 September 2023.

Differences between medical schools. Available at https://www.medschools.ac.uk/media/2371/msc-infosheet-med-school-differences.pdf. Accessed 20 September 2023.

Universities and Colleges Admissions Service (UCAS). Available at https://www.ucas.com/. Accessed 20 September 2023.

University Clinical Aptitude Test. Available at https://www.ucat.ac.uk/

Medical school entrance requirements. Available at https://www.medschools.ac.uk/media/2357/msc-entry-requirements-for-uk-medical-schools.pdf. Accessed 20 September 2023.

Mind Tools Content Team. Setting SMART goals. MindTools website. Available at https://www.mindtools.com/pages/article/smart-goals.htm. Accessed 20 September 2023.

Medicine: Past, Present and Future

2

Bogdan Chiva Giurca, Hamaad Khan and Teodora Popa

Chapter Outline

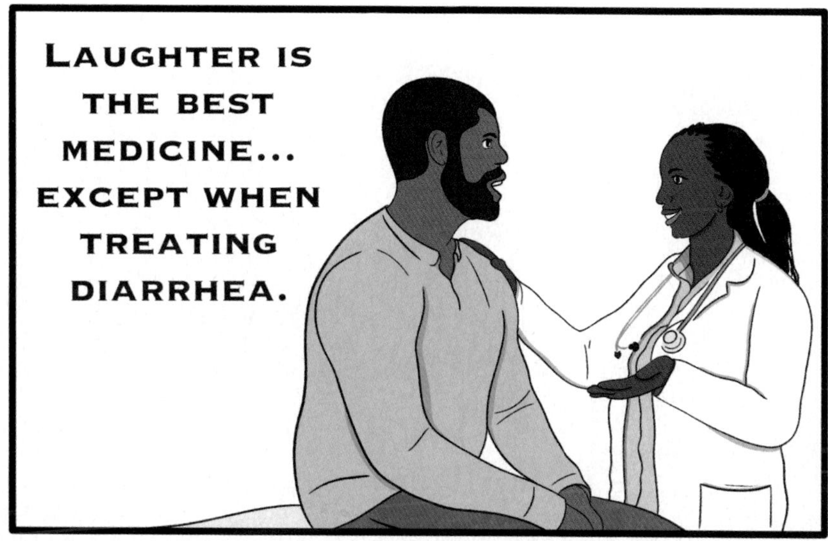

AN EXERCISE OF IMAGINATION: TIME TRAVELLING THROUGH THE KEY MOMENTS IN MEDICINE

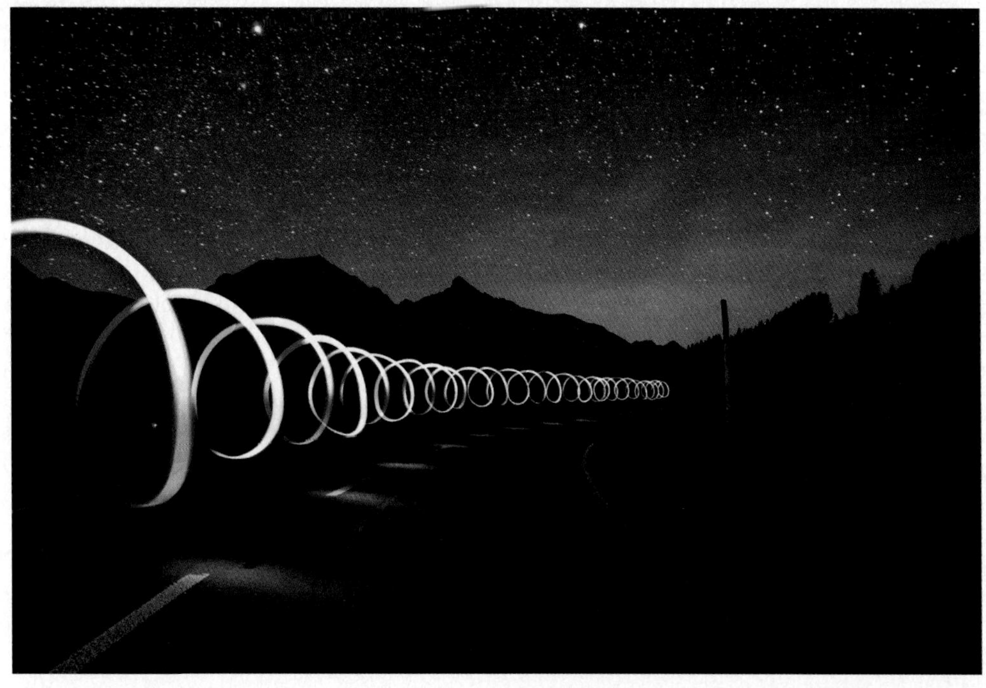

For this section, I need you to find a quiet place, sit back and relax. We are about to board the 'Time Express', taking us on a journey through the history of medicine. You're probably laughing now, thinking 'How can I relax when you've just mentioned the word 'history'?' No, no, no—not *that* kind of boring history that puts you and your desk-mate to sleep during school! I am talking about key discoveries and revolutionary breakthroughs in medicine that only happened by imagining the unimaginable. Revolutionary breakthroughs that have influenced the way doctors practice medicine and the way you will study once you get into medical school. Now, get a warm cup of tea and hold tight because we're about to start our journey.

PREHISTORIC MEDICINE AND SURGERY

Ah, here we are, thousands of years Before Christ (BC). Far away in the distance are two men with hunting bows… For some reason, they have stopped next to a tiny bush with red, fresh-looking berries. They seem to smell the berries, then touch them with their tongue. The texture is mushy, their taste is bitter. They look like raspberries, but their colour and texture are different. One of the men tries one, while the other man attentively watches him chewing and swallowing the wild fruit. They wait one minute, nothing happens, but suddenly the one who tried it drops down to the ground—he's having a seizure. Oh no, this cannot be good! His friend starts a very strange ritual, destroying the berry bush with his bow and singing in a high-pitched voice while looking towards the sky. After chanting, the almost naked man picks up a sharp arrow, places it on his friend's skull and drills a hole to release the 'evil spirits', making his friend seize. This early 'surgical procedure' was known as trephination. The precise cuts that can be seen on some skulls found by experts as well as evidence of bone regrowth point out that some 'patients' (if we may call them so) survived this type of 'surgery'.

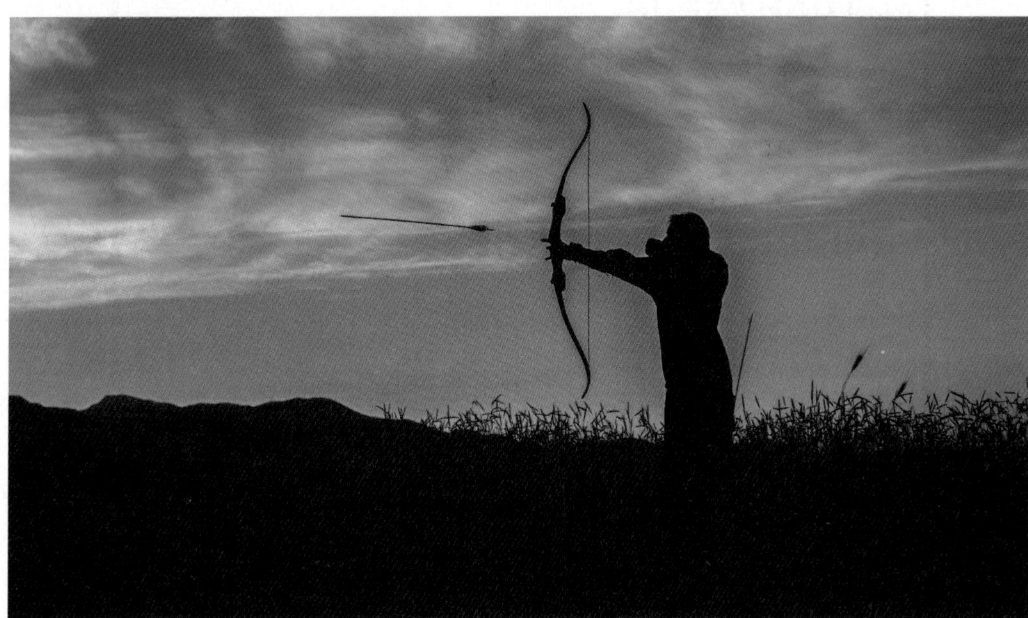

Will our friend be okay? We probably won't find out; but today, at least one of them learnt a very important lesson—never eat this type of berry again. This is pretty much how people living in prehistoric times remained healthy within their environment. The process of **trial and error** (observing what's poisonous and avoiding it in the future), as well as **natural selection** (survival of the fittest), ensured the survival of this generation, which was at the mercy of the 'elements within earth' and 'spirits of the sky'.

One small fact regarding our surviving friend before we move on: while running home from his productive hunting day, he fell through the floor of a cave and broke his leg, leading to an open fracture. He did, however, use his prehistoric orthopaedic skills. He used mud to fix the bone back into place before returning to his family—now, that's what I call creative!

EARLY CIVILISATIONS

Egypt (2600 BC)

As we approach our next stop, 2600 BC, you can already feel the hot sand under your feet and see a few pyramids in the distance. Be careful, there are plenty of scorpions around; I don't think you'd like to step on one. The interesting fact is that this place is known for having the first people to develop the profession of medicine.

One figure stands out during this time period in Egypt—Imhotep, also called the 'God of Medicine'. According to historians, he used plant extracts to treat over 200 diseases. Some say he was the real 'Father' of Medicine rather than Hippocrates, but we'll discuss this later. Imhotep took pulses, examined patients, asked questions and palpated the supposedly affected areas, similar to what modern doctors do.

Interestingly, Egyptians were the first to develop a type of 'evidence-based medicine' (using facts and observations) to cure disease, instead of simply seeking spiritual explanations. One interesting theory was the so-called 'Channel Theory'. While observing the old irrigation system, wise men found an analogy between the water channels and the human body. What they noticed was the damage caused to plants when the irrigation channels were blocked. Farmers easily solved the problem by unblocking the irrigation system so water could irrigate the plantation once again. This was a major breakthrough, allowing physicians at the time to 'unblock the channel' that may be causing disease. When someone complained of stomach pain, they tried unblocking the channel by vomiting or emptying bowels. They did the same with large cavities filled with blood or pus, draining the liquid and unblocking the channel. This analogy between water channels and the human body convinced doctors that the treatment used should be practical as well as spiritual.

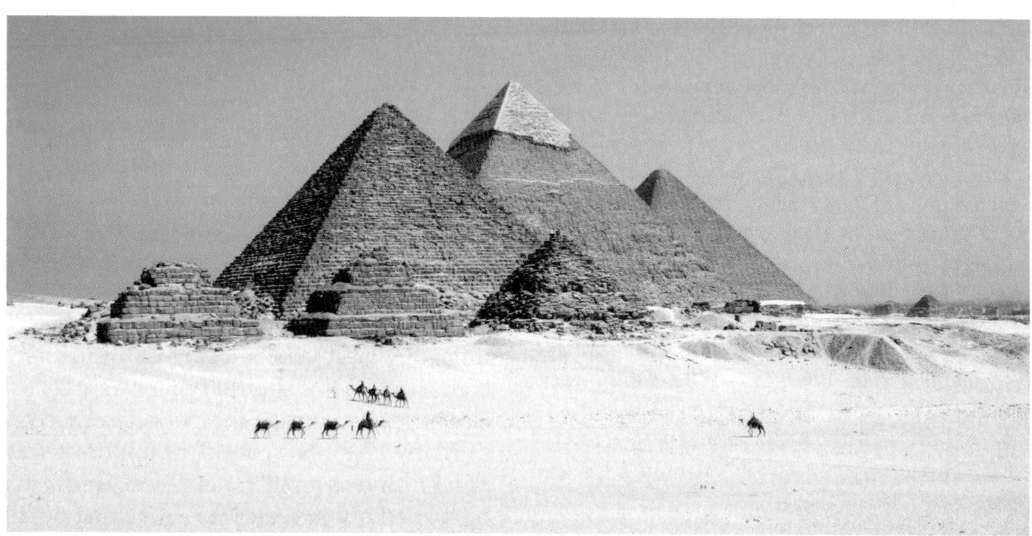

Here, smell this papyrus. This old paper allowed Egyptians to share ideas with colleagues and write textbooks about their experiences. Ultimately, they still insisted that disease was caused by gods. For this reason, every practical procedure was followed by a spell to intensify the treatment.

I know you're curious to hear one, so how about this: 'Oh Spirit, male or female, who lurks hidden in my flesh and in my limbs, get out of my flesh. Get out of my limbs!' This was the 'remedy' for pregnant women. Obviously, right?!

India (600 BC)

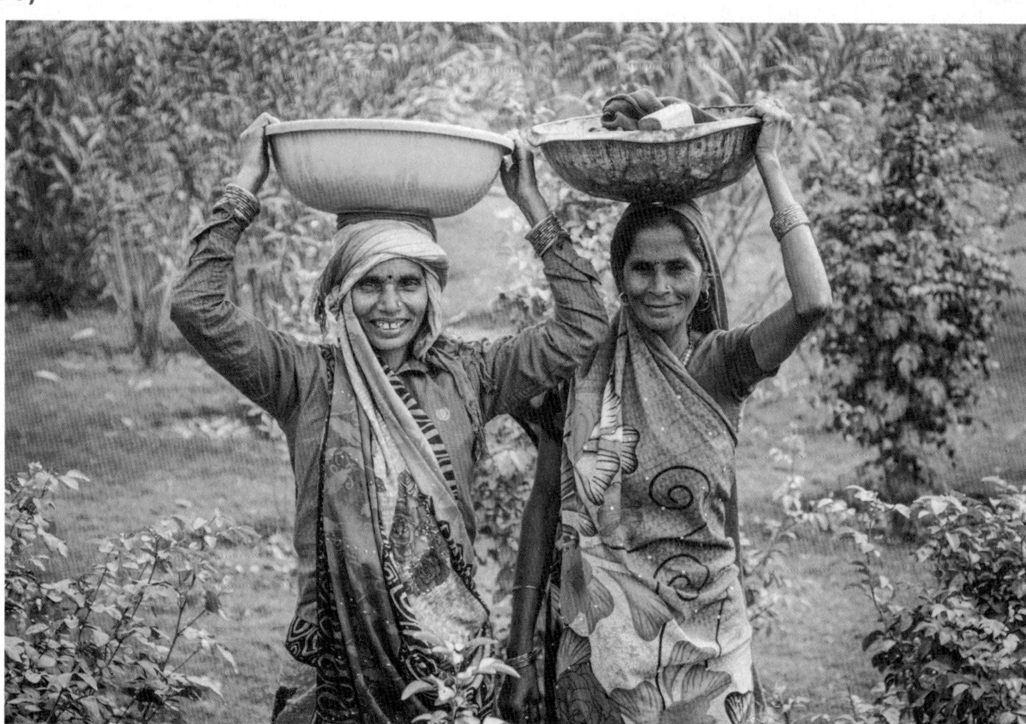

Are there any budding surgeons among you? Well, hold tight, because we're now travelling to India (600 BC), where the 'Founding Father of Surgery' was born. Strange things were happening during this period. One was punishing criminals and adulterers by chopping off their noses. There was one man, however, who saw the need to repair the external noses of those who were punished. His name was Sushruta, and he brought plastic and reconstructive surgery to life through his famous rhinoplasty procedure. Here's how he described it:

> *The portion of the nose to be covered should be first measured with a leaf. Then a piece of skin of the required size should be dissected from the living skin of the cheek, and turned back to cover the nose, keeping a small pedicle attached to the cheek. The part of the nose to which the skin is to be attached should be made raw by cutting the nasal stump with a knife. The physician then should place the skin on the nose and stitch the two parts swiftly, keeping the skin properly elevated by inserting two tubes of eranda (the castor-oil plant) in the position of the nostrils, so that the new nose gets proper shape. The skin thus properly adjusted, should then be sprinkled with a powder of liquorice, red sandal-wood and barberry plant. Finally, it should be covered with cotton, and clean sesame oil should be constantly applied. When the skin has united and granulated, if the nose is too short or too long, the middle of the flap should be divided and an endeavour made to enlarge or shorten it.*
>
> Bynum, 2008

Remember, this is a period when nobody had any clue what anaesthesia is. So how did Sushruta do it? Was it not unbearably painful? Sushruta specifically mentioned that 'wine should be used before operation to produce insensibility to pain'. He further remarks, 'The patient who has been fed, does not faint, and he who is rendered intoxicated, does not feel the pain of the operation'.

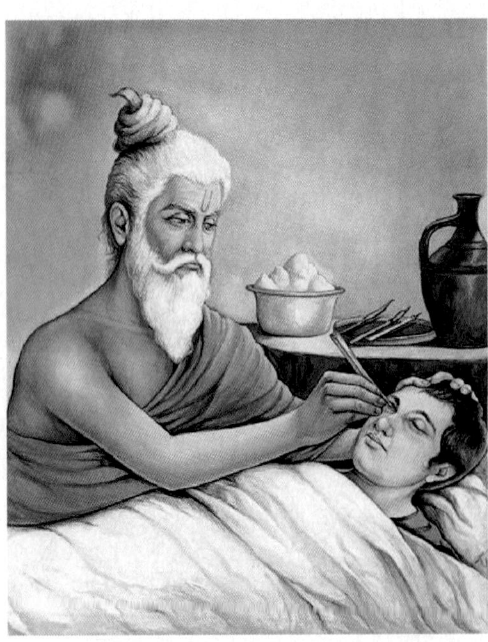

Sushruta later wrote the first surgical textbook, through which he described the detailed study of anatomy using a cadaver. His textbook also covered over 1000 diseases, various surgical procedures, medicinal plant uses and preparations from mineral or animal sources.

Greece (460 BC)

It looks like we've arrived right in the middle of some kind of ceremony. Why did all these people gather here? It sounds like an oath of some sort.

> *I swear by Apollo the Healer, by Asclepius, by Hygieia, by Panacea, and by all the gods and goddesses, making them my witnesses, that I will carry out, according to my ability and judgement, this oath and this indenture... I will use treatment to help the sick according to my ability and judgement, but never with a view to injury and wrongdoing. Neither will I administer a poison to anybody when asked to do so, nor will I suggest such a course. I will utterly reject harm and mischief....*
>
> Porter, 2004

Remember when we said that Imhotep was the 'real' father of medicine? Well, the more famous character who lived in Greece (approximately 460 BCE) was Hippocrates. Some of you may have already recognised the previous passage as part of the Hippocratic Oath. Every physician at the time had to take this oath before starting their career as a doctor. The Hippocratic Oath has been adapted over time, the latest version being published in 2017. We will come back to this shortly, but for now, let's find out what else happened during this period in Greece.

Many historians consider Hippocrates as the founder of medicine as a rational science. This is mainly because he carried out 'research' to prove that disease was a natural process, and that the doctor's role was to help the patient's body resist this natural process. Many of his treatments included medicinal plants, diets and other substances. This is further illustrated by his famous quote, 'Let food be thy medicine and medicine be thy food'.

Hippocrates was also a firm believer that natural matter was made of four elements: air, water, earth and fire. Similarly, philosophers at the time proposed the idea that the human body was made of four humours (blood, phlegm, black bile, yellow bile) that had to be kept in balance. If out of balance, these humours led to disease. Thus, Hippocrates urged doctors to look for a natural cause of disease instead of focusing on spiritual beliefs.

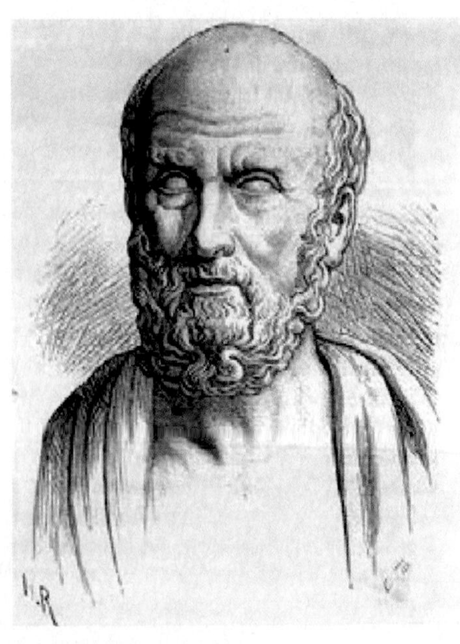

Contrary to the belief at the time that the body is made of separate, isolated parts, Hippocrates firmly believed that the patient should be considered as a whole, taking into consideration the mind, body and spirit altogether. This holistic approach (**holistic medicine**) is still being used today. Also important is the *'Hippocratic Corpus'*—a massive collection of books written by Hippocrates with other Greek doctors, encompassing several diseases and symptoms, as well as treatments and their effectiveness.

Ancient Greece also had the first 'Programme for Health', although this was only available to the rich. Hippocrates believed that in order to be healthy, people should keep themselves at a normal temperature, eat well, wash, clean their teeth and stay fit. However, Hippocrates acknowledged that the working class may not have the necessary time, or they might be too poor to engage in such activities and would therefore be less healthy than the rich. Even though this was thousands of years ago, it still holds true for most countries today. Although medicine has advanced, there still exists a huge health disparity between higher socioeconomic classes and lower socioeconomic classes.

A few centuries after Hippocrates, another Greek physician made a dramatic impact on medicine. Galen is known as one of the most successful researchers of the past—his work encompassed anatomy, pathology, pharmacology, physiology and logic, among others. His theories remained unchallenged and his books rated as 'bestsellers' (if Amazon existed back then) for 15 centuries!

But Galen's work wasn't all correct and accurate. You see, back then, people were afraid of performing dissections, as it would pretty much mean blowing your chances for getting into heaven. Galen's work was mostly based on animal dissection (dogs, apes and pigs in particular), which he accurately recorded in his notes. Although human anatomy is similar to some extent, this still led to Galen making several anatomical mistakes. For example, Galen said that the human jaw was made of two bones, like a dog's jaw.

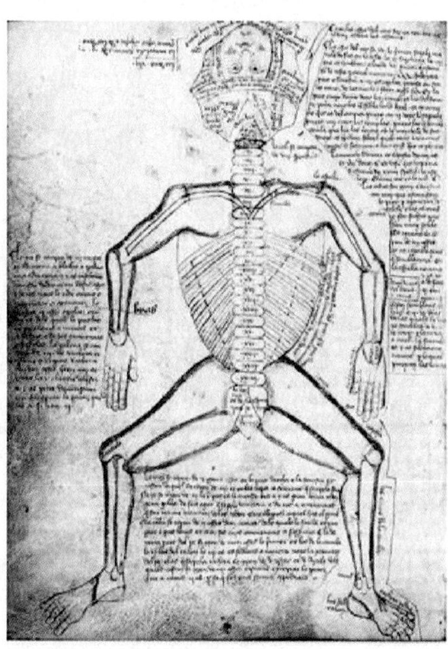

For the surgery enthusiasts among you, Galen described several procedures for breast cancer, including the excision of tumours. Although extremely painful and perhaps fatal at times, these procedures remained the sole treatment for cancer for many centuries to follow. Galen based most of his information about anatomy on what he saw when he dissected animals' bodies. This led him to make mistakes, including:

1. Thinking that muscles attach to the bone the same way in humans and dogs.
2. Thinking that blood was created in the liver. He realised that it flowed around the body, but said it was burned as fuel for the muscles.
3. Thinking that holes through the septum allowed the blood to flow from one side of the heart to the other.
4. Confusion about the blood vessels in the brain.
5. Thinking that the human jawbone was made up of two bones, like a dog's jaw.
6. Confusion about the shape of the human liver.

To summarise, here are a few important points about the Greeks back in the day:

- They knew about the inner workings of the body.
- They developed clinical observation.
- They studied the natural history of diseases.
- They realised that diseases had **natural** causes and cures.
- They developed the theory of the four humours and the 'use of opposites'.
- They wrote and used medical textbooks.
- They were professional and took the Hippocratic Oath.
- They were skilled at setting broken bones and slipped discs.
- They knew hundreds of herbal remedies.
- They had a reassuring 'bedside manner'.
- They developed a programme for health for personal health and hygiene.

MIDDLE AGES AND MEDIEVAL MEDICINE

As we continue our journey through the Middle Ages and experience a taste of medieval medicine, you'll soon realise that nothing much happened during this period in terms of medical breakthroughs. Wealthy kings invested money in wars, not health, leading to weak public health systems. Wars also disrupted learning and led to general social disorder, therefore promoting medical stagnation.

As always, religion played an important role. The church had forbidden dissection but encouraged superstition and prayer among the masses. The church insisted that people believe Galen's work was accurate, and disease was a punishment from God. If you were to ask people about what caused disease, they would pretty much give you one of the following answers:

- The result of God's will and a consequence of God and the Devil

- The result of bad smells (miasma) and an imbalance of the four humours
- The result of movement of the sun and planets

Things changed during the bubonic plague. The 'Black Death', as it was later named, made people lose faith in prayer. Regardless of religious beliefs and prayer, millions were dying.

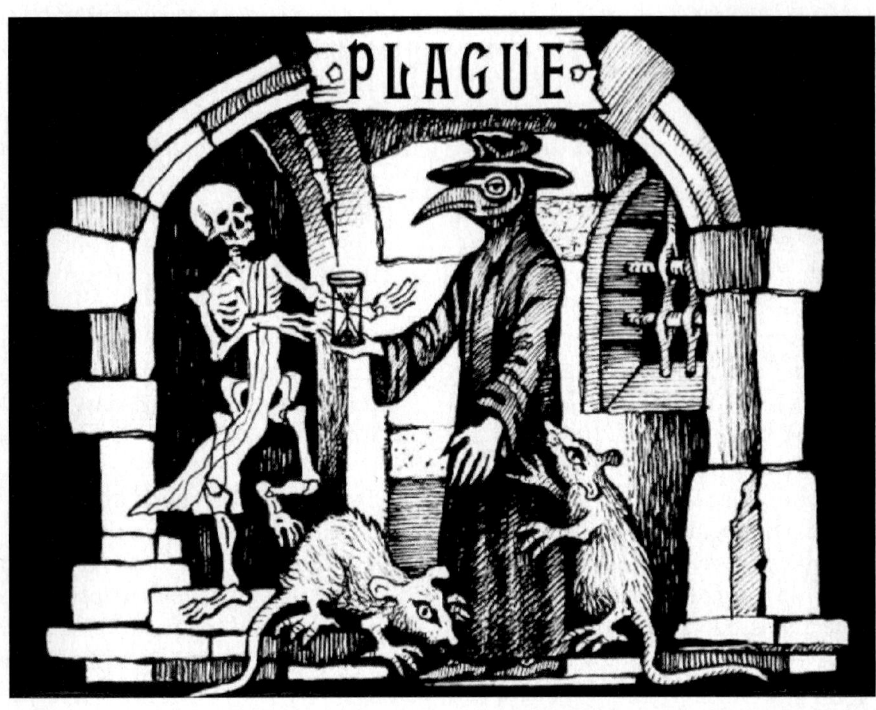

EARLY MODERN PERIOD (16TH–18TH CENTURY)

Pizza, pasta and football.... If this makes you think of Italy, you are correct! We are now standing in the world's first anatomical theatre in Padua, Italy. More than a hundred medical students are standing in a circle, hastily taking notes and listening to a young professor speak passionately while dissecting the human body. The theatre was purposefully built without chairs, so students could not fall asleep. We are now taking part in the first live anatomy demonstration. The professor? Andreas Vesalius (born in 1514), who is considered by many a hero of modern medicine. Vesalius was the first doctor to realise that human anatomy was different from apes and that Galen's work, which was praised for over 15 centuries, could be wrong.

Human dissection was still forbidden by the church during this period, so much of Vesalius's work was carried out illegally by digging corpses up from the cemetery during the night. Andreas Vesalius is known as the 'Father of Dissections and Anatomy' for publishing the first truly scientific anatomy textbook when he was only 28 years old. The book, entitled *De Humani Corporis Fabrica (on the Fabric of the Human Body)*, contained significant, and mostly correct, facts about most systems in the human body.

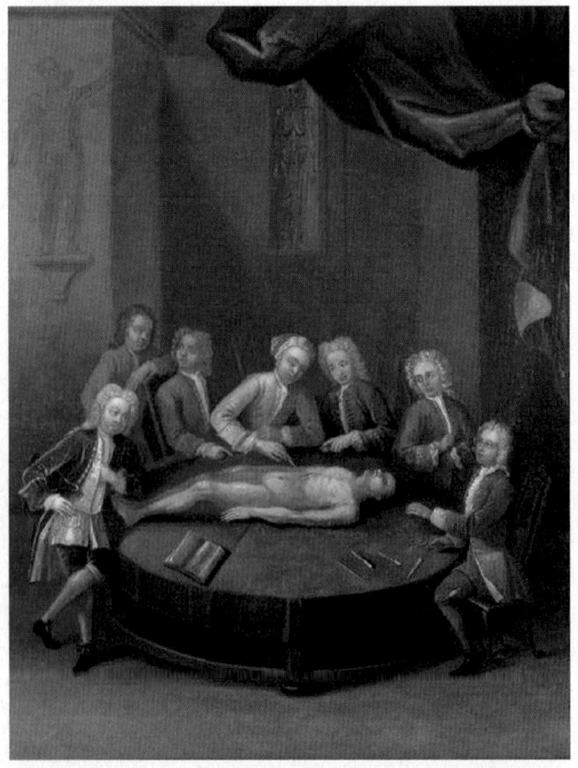

Vesalius also attempted to explore the heart and successfully portrayed the heart as a pump, but failed miserably by saying that blood flows directly through the walls of the heart's chambers.

The second person challenging Galen's theories was another young, curious and inquisitive British doctor named William Harvey. You see, because Galen was afraid of dissecting humans due to his religious beliefs, he could only base his theories on assumptions. Harvey proved that Galen's postulation that blood originated in the liver was wrong and explained the whole circuit, becoming the first person to correctly describe blood circulation.

Harvey was a well-known maverick at the time, ignoring all textbooks and preferring his own notes instead. He even ridiculed Galen's belief that there are two types of blood with two different colours—a theory unchanged for more than a thousand years. Harvey easily demonstrated that blood changed colour when exposed to oxygen.

His open-mindedness is encapsulated through his quote: 'I have often wondered and even laughed at those who fancied that everything had been so consummately and absolutely investigated by an Aristotle or a Galen or some other mighty name, that nothing could by any possibility be added to their knowledge'.

Did scientists at the time listen? Of course not—they all went medieval on Harvey by praising Galen's work. It was pretty much William Harvey versus everybody, including the church. Therefore, when he was asked about future plans and experiments, Harvey said, 'My previous research already caused a heavy storm. It is often better to grow wise in private at home than to publish what you have amassed with infinite labour, to stir up storms that may rob you of peace and quiet for the rest of your days'.

AGE OF ENLIGHTENMENT (18TH CENTURY)

We're now swiftly moving on to witness another fascinating moment in history. Ah, nothing better than fresh air, the mooing of the cows and organic milk. Sarah here is one of the many milkmaids working at this farm. Let's go say hi!

Oh no, can you see the small pustules on the cow's abdomen? I think that looks like cowpox. Let's warn Sarah before she starts milking the cow. 'Don't worry guys, I've had cowpox before and I don't seem to get it anymore', Sarah said. Did you hear that? Can we say that Sarah is 'immune' to cowpox? Well, that's certainly what a British physician, known as the 'Father of Immunology', thought.

Edward Jenner (1749–1823) observed that the milkmaids who were previously infected with cowpox not only didn't get infected with the disease anymore, but they were also immune to smallpox. As any curious researcher with no ethical regulations at the time would do, Jenner took a syringe and drew pus from a cow's pustule, which he later injected into his gardener's 8-year-old son—quite mad you'd think, right? The boy started sweating, developed a number of pustules and vomited for a couple of days, but then he got well.

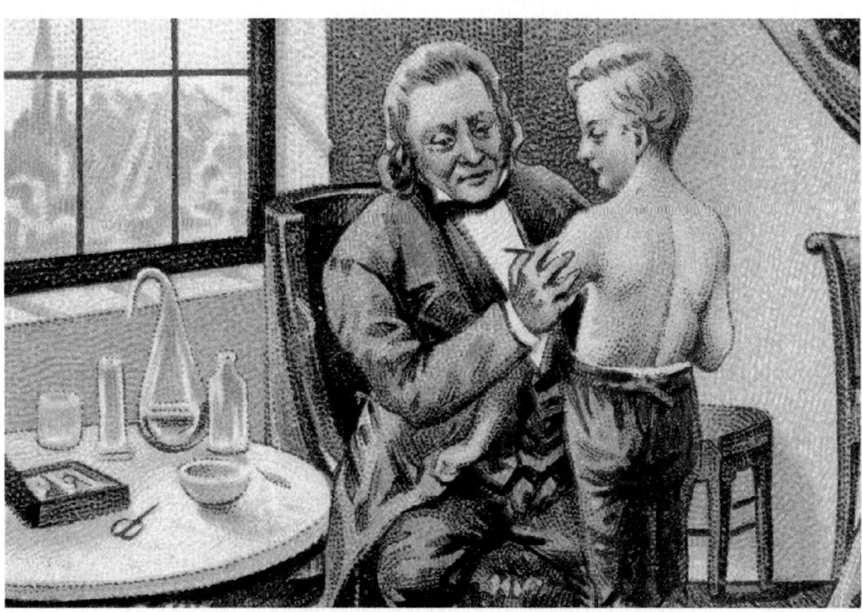

A few months later, Jenner injected the boy again. To our surprise, this time he used actual smallpox. The child was perfectly fit. Jenner's theory worked and led to the development of the first ever 'vaccine'. Vaccine? Why vaccine? 'Vacca' in Latin means 'cow'. The easy way to remember this is thinking that Jenner proposed 'cowinating' (vaccinating) people to prevent smallpox (that analogy doesn't make any sense, does it?).

How big was this discovery? Well, some say his work has saved more lives than the work of any other human throughout history. Now, we shouldn't forget to thank the milkmaids and poor 8-year-old James for being brave enough to be 'cowinated'. Sorry, I meant vaccinated. This is getting confusing now. After Jenner's death, the vaccine was made compulsory in England and Wales, leading to the eradication of smallpox.

Of a similar curiosity and enthusiasm was yet another British physician by the name of **John Snow**. I said John, not Jon. No, he's not the character from 'Game of Thrones', although he's quite cool too.

Cholera was a big public health issue in the 18th century. Everyone still believed that vapours in the air (otherwise known as 'miasma') caused disease. Snow firmly believed that something in the environment was causing cholera. Because people affected were vomiting and suffering from abdominal pain, Snow narrowed the cause down to something that people either drank or ingested. When challenging the idea that 'miasma' was the main cause of the sickness, the scientists simply said, 'YOU KNOW NOTHING, John Snow!' Yes, like in the series, for those 'Game of Thrones' fans.

Snow devoted his whole life to interviewing, surveying patients and investigating the cause of cholera. John Snow soon discovered the truth: faeces and waste had found their way into drinking water and those ingesting it later suffered from cholera. However, proving his theory took a long time. A very long time, in fact.

His first attempt to prove his theory was a case study of two different water fountains. Fountain A had waste flowing TOWARDS it, while fountain B had waste flowing AWAY from it (and was therefore not contaminated). All people drinking from fountain A were affected by cholera, while only one person drinking from fountain B had the disease. However, nobody believed him.

Frustrated, Snow took a break from cholera and spent time in academia. He pioneered several discoveries in the field of anaesthetics and was the first person to test dosages. He was so good at it, in fact, that he even performed it twice on the queen. At this point, the scientific community began to murmur, 'Well, you do know something, John Snow!'

Did he go back to his favourite topic? He did, but this time he managed to gather the evidence required to convince the whole scientific community of his initial hypothesis. As a result, he became the 'Father of Epidemiology' and founded an epidemiology society in London. Consequently, epidemiology has now become a well-known branch of medicine dedicated not only to investigating disease aetiology, but also studying the distribution and determinants of health. Hence, John Snow pioneered fundamental principles of public health control and subsequent prevention of disease.

Hand-washing Among Doctors

Hang on, let's take a brief diversion to Vienna to meet a moustachioed obstetrician known as the 'Saviour of Mothers'—you'll soon find out why.

Right, imagine two clinics running side by side. One was run by midwives and had a maternal mortality rate of 1 in 25. The other clinic was run by doctors who also taught medical students and had a mortality rate of 1 in 10 women, sometimes as high as 1 in 3. What was shocking for our moustachioed character, Ignaz Philipp Semmelweis, was that the mortality rate of women who insisted on giving birth anywhere outside the hospital was significantly lower than both of the clinics mentioned earlier.

He said, 'To me, it appeared logical that patients who experienced street births would become ill at least as frequently as those who delivered in the clinic. What protected those who delivered outside the clinic from these destructive unknown endemic influences?'

The main cause of this mortality was infection. What Ignaz observed was that very often, doctors came down with a fever after performing dissections and cutting themselves. The fever and disease were very similar to those experienced by mothers during childbirth ('childbed fever'). Ignaz believed there must be a difference in healthcare delivery between midwives and doctors too, since the mortality difference was so significant, but what was it?

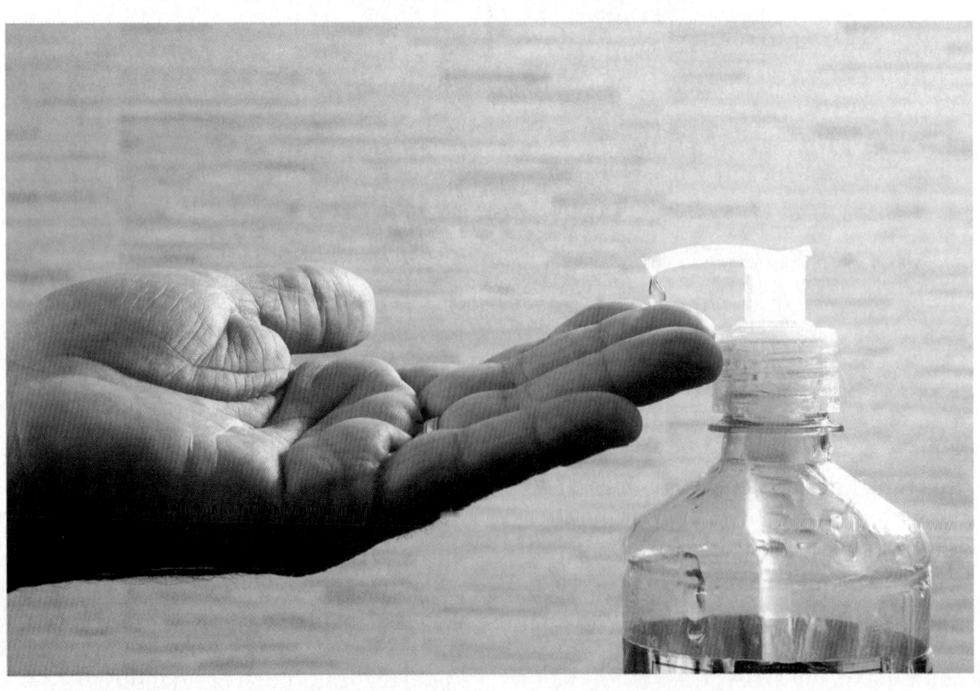

It may be obvious to you, but in those days, the medical society did not know about bacteria or infection. Ignaz made history. He was the first physician to make the connection between infection and the doctors who didn't wash their hands. After suggesting doctors hand wash before performing a clinical procedure, maternal mortality rates reduced dramatically. You'd think Ignaz would be praised for conquering childbed fever, right? Well, not really—as with many of our previous geniuses, nobody believed Ignaz. They thought he was crazy, and physicians kept dissecting—refusing to wash their hands for decades to come, before another hero scientifically proved the so-called 'Germ Theory of Disease'.

You see, this 'wandering clouds of poisonous miasma' theory was praised for hundreds if not thousands of years. However, around the 1840s, with the advent of microscopes and other fancy toys at the time, people grew sceptical. Robert Koch, another famous physician at the time, helped John Snow to prove the existence of cholera as an organism causing disease. Koch did so using his famous theories, nowadays called 'Koch's postulates'. For those of you who have not covered this in biology yet, why not go on YouTube and watch a short cartoon about it?

At the time, people still believed in a spontaneous cause of disease. Although it is obvious to you and me that in order to have life you need another organism first, people thought organisms and bacteria could just appear out of the blue. The man who eventually disproved this belief was **Louis Pasteur**. Pasteur was a French physician who designed the 'Swan-necked flask experiment' and contributed significantly to the Germ Theory of Disease.

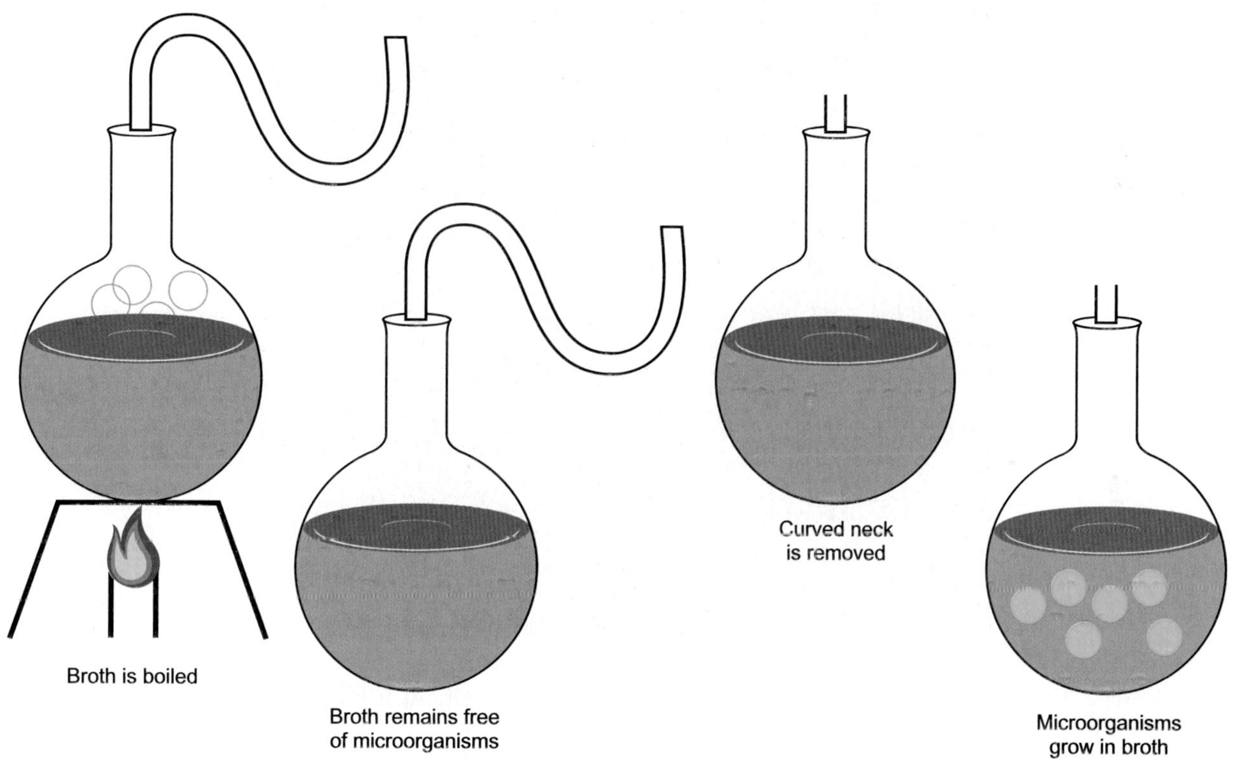
Broth is boiled
Broth remains free of microorganisms
Curved neck is removed
Microorganisms grow in broth

Essentially, Pasteur designed a bottle that allowed the air to go inside, but the twisted neck ('swan-necked flask') acted as a means of holding dust or bacteria, keeping the contents of the flask sterile. Pasteur filled the flask with broth, boiled it and let it sit. Even though the flask was exposed to outside particles, its contents did not get contaminated, disproving the theory that poisonous vapours in the air (miasma) caused disease once and for all.

The Use of Antiseptic

Inspired by Ignaz and Pasteur's work on hand-washing and bacteria, a British surgeon was determined to reduce mortality after surgery. This hero, **Joseph Lister**, a professor of surgery in both Glasgow and Edinburgh, firmly believed that carbolic acid had antiseptic properties and that it could be used to reduce infection rates postsurgery. Lister proposed treating all surgical instruments, bandages and operating environments with carbolic acid. He was right and his idea saved millions of lives and by 1879, his idea was accepted by almost all hospitals in Britain.

An Amazing Woman

As you may have already observed, most of the characters mentioned thus far are male. Some of you may know about the crazy laws that didn't allow women to go to university? There are, however, several heroines hiding behind the scenes whose stories must be told.

So where is our next stop? Warsaw, Poland. We're going to meet **Maria Sklodowska**—a curious woman from a poor family of five siblings. I know this name doesn't ring any bells just yet, but please bear with me. Let's explore her life and in no time, that 'AHA!' moment will hit you.

Maria loved school and was geeky and enthusiastic (quite like you, maybe?). She grew up and wanted to go to university, but guess what? At the time (1880), women were not allowed to study in Poland or many other countries around the world. However, Maria kept calm and carried on, or should I say 'Curie'd on'? You'll soon understand why. She joined a secret underground university designed for women, studied vigorously, then delivered lessons for years, saving enough money to move to Paris, where she earned degrees and masters in maths and physics.

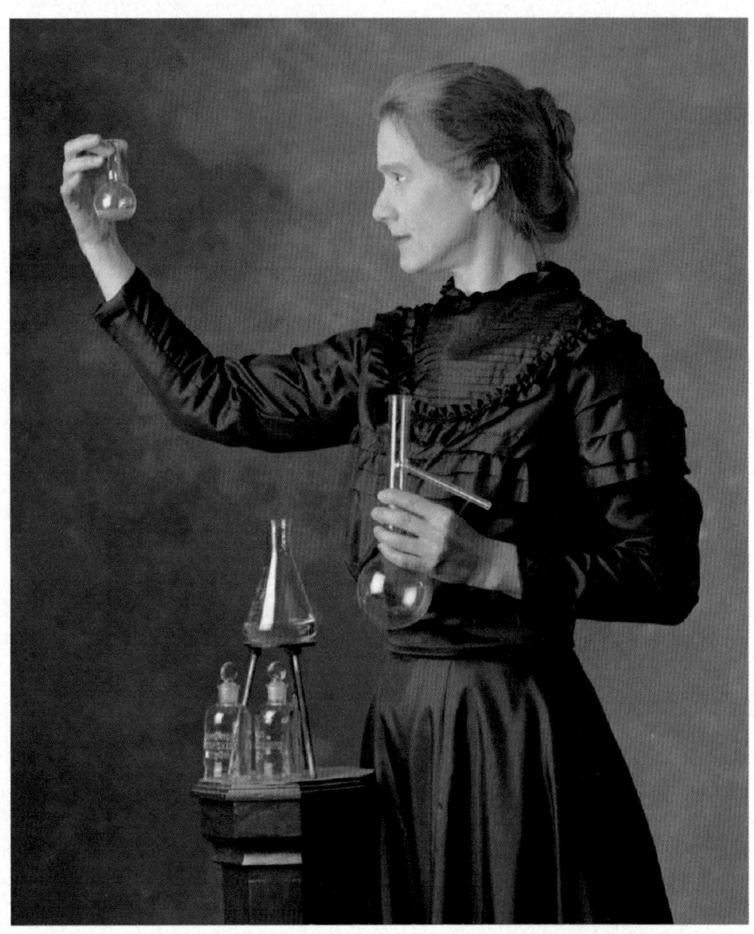

Maria, however, had a passion for research. When looking for a lab to continue her work, she met Pierre Curie, who happened to own a lab, and boy, did they work. Maria and Pierre fell in love, started working together and were soon married. Maria Sklodowska became **Marie Curie**.

So, what did Marie do? Well, firstly she coined the term 'radioactivity', discovering two new elements: radium and polonium (the latter named after her home country 'Polonia'). Marie also observed that radium could be used to treat cancer, leading to the development of the Radium Institute in Paris to treat cancer patients. In 1903, Marie was the first woman to receive the Nobel Prize, awarded to her and Pierre for their work on radioactivity. Her story doesn't stop there, however. Marie also became the first woman and only person ever to receive a second Nobel Prize, for a different category, chemistry. Curie used her scientific knowledge to build a fleet of X-ray wagons to be taken to the battlefield to diagnose soldiers. How's that for girl power?

What is noteworthy, however, is that this heroine never wore protection during her work. At the time, nobody knew about the dangerous effects of radioactive substances. She sacrificed her life in the name of science, dying from bone marrow disease in 1934. Her papers and corpse are still considered radioactive.

THE RISE OF MODERN MEDICINE (19TH–21ST CENTURY)

The Discovery of Penicillin

As we quickly travel in time towards the modern medicine of the 19th century, let me show you how accidents can lead to great discoveries. Many historians tell us that **Alexander Fleming** was a bright man who worked at St Mary's Hospital Medical School, in London. However, many historians also claim he was very unorganised and did not really maintain a clean working environment. One time, while researching influenza, Fleming went on a holiday and left all his culture dishes outside in the lab. Some say he just could not be bothered to clean, others claim this was a stroke of genius. Upon his return, Fleming noticed that mould had grown on a set of plates where he used to grow staphylococci germs. Much to Fleming's surprise, the mould cleared all the bacteria around itself, leaving behind a bacteria-free area.

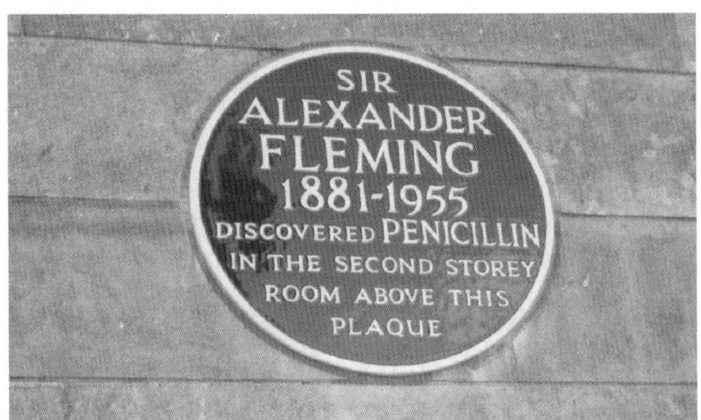
SIR
ALEXANDER
FLEMING
1881-1955
DISCOVERED PENICILLIN
IN THE SECOND STOREY
ROOM ABOVE THIS
PLAQUE

Fleming named the substance 'penicillin'. There were, however, two other people simultaneously working on the same research project with which he later shared the Nobel Prize that he received for this discovery (1945). So there you go, this is the only time when being unorganised and dirty probably paid off.

The Substance of Life: The True Heroine Behind the Scenes

Let us now meet another heroine whose work changed the course of history. Let me ask you a question first: How many of you have heard of Francis Crick and James Watson? Pretty sure most of you instantly thought of the discovery of the DNA, but how many of you have heard of Rosalind Franklin? Sadly, some books don't even mention her, although she contributed massively to the discovery of DNA. We've mostly talked about researchers who have been praised and rewarded for their discoveries. Well, this story is different.

Rosalind went to Cambridge, finished her degree in physics and chemistry, and became an expert in X-ray crystallography, a skill used in her later work at King's College. Here's where things get controversial. At the time, many research groups were trying to understand the structure of DNA and there was much debate as to whether it was a single, double or triple helix. Franklin worked in the same lab as Wilkins. Wilkins was another scientist, working on a different project, although his and Franklin's work often overlapped. Using her X-ray crystallography skills, Rosalind spent hundreds of hours trying to take pictures of crystallised DNA fibres. In 1952, one of her photos (labelled Photograph 51), which took 120 hours, clearly illustrated the first evidence of DNA being a double helix with multiple chains. Rosalind kept her work secret and kept working towards a model of DNA, without publishing or disseminating her recent discovery.

Meanwhile, in a laboratory in Cambridge, Watson and Crick were building their own models to uncover the structure of DNA, but they were UNABLE to confirm the helical structure. Are you ready for the biggest shock ever? Wilkins, who saw Rosalind's work, shared Photograph 51 with the competition, Watson and Crick, without Rosalind's knowledge or permission. A few months later, Watson and Crick announced the discovery of DNA's double helix structure. Their work was published, together with Rosalind's work, in Nature 1953, although Rosalind's work was added at the end, with readers and scientists implying that her work only confirmed Watson and Crick's data.

Two years later, Rosalind sadly died of ovarian cancer, probably because of carrying out her revolutionary X-ray work without wearing protection. In the meantime, Watson, Crick and Wilkins were awarded the Nobel Prize for their work on DNA.

To make matters worse, in 1968, Watson published a book about *The Double Helix*. Inside it, he describes Rosalind as 'belligerent, emotional, and unable to interpret her own data'. In his book, Watson also calls her 'Rosie', although she has never used this name, suggesting mockery.

Rosalind's lack of recognition is a transgression in history exposing the historical sexism within science and academia. Nevertheless, her legacy and devotion towards revolutionising the fields of biology, physics and medicine live on, and now you can also share her story. Rosalind Franklin, the unsung heroine or mother of the DNA helix, remains an inspiring example for women in science throughout the world.

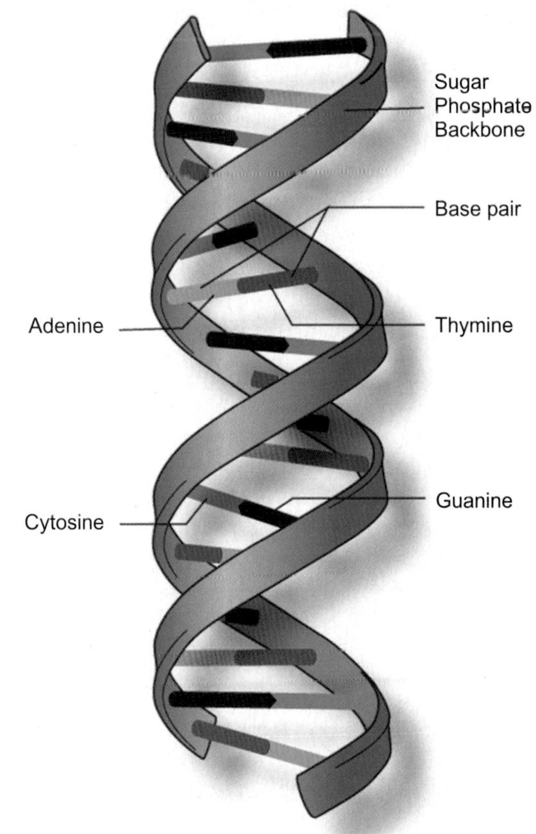

To further reinforce the contribution of women to science, I'd like to introduce you to Elizabeth Blackwell—the first woman to receive a medical degree. Her quote should be written on a Post-it on your desk:

> *It is not easy to be a pioneer—but oh, it is fascinating! I would not trade one moment, even the worst moment, for all the riches in the world.*

THE NATIONAL HEALTH SERVICE

Now we are approaching one of the most pivotal moments in recent medical history that established one of the most radical changes to healthcare.

July 5, 1948, represents the launch of a new health service in the United Kingdom, born out of the ideal that 'good healthcare should be available to all, regardless of wealth, race, or background'. This principle still remains at the core of the National Health Service (NHS). Throughout history, the NHS has been a constant battle full of compromises between politicians and doctors. However, the NHS is the world's biggest publicly funded health service. Furthermore, it is one of the most efficient, egalitarian and comprehensive health systems in the world.

Although the NHS has changed significantly since 1948, its three core principles have remained the same:

- Equality: meeting the needs of everyone
- Free of charge: free service at the point of delivery
- Based on clinical need and not on the ability to pay

You will get the chance to learn more about the newer principles and how the NHS is regulated in Chapter 3, as this is a common theme of discussion during the medical school interview process.

As we reach the end of this journey through the history of medicine and its biggest discoveries, you may be wondering, 'What about the discovery of insulin or computed tomography (CT) scans?' or the thousands of other breakthroughs that have contributed to medicine today. Well, this chapter was meant to provide you with a taste of medical research throughout history, to whet your appetite and make you hungry for more. Now it's your turn to investigate several other breakthroughs depending on your personal interest.

> This chapter goes to show how certain elements of medicine's past are still prominent and utilised in the medical world today. For example, the knowledge that bacteria and viruses cause disease is something we take for granted. However, the journey to discovering that microorganisms cause disease (Germ Theory) was a long maze that led us to many dead ends. For 1300 years since the Roman Empire, the predominant theory about what caused disease was Galen's miasma theory, which stated that diseases were caused by 'bad air'. A rather ridiculous notion of the time was that one could become obese by inhaling the smell of food. In 1546, a scientist called Fracastoro challenged this idea with a basic version of Germ Theory, but it took more than 300 years of further research by various other scientists, namely Louis Pasteur and Robert Koch, to eventually establish and prove the so-called Germ Theory.
>
> **Hamaad Khan, Medical Student**

THE PRESENT AND VISION FOR THE FUTURE

What a trip that was, right? Does it feel good to be home, or would you rather go back and help Andreas Vesalius dig out corpses and dissect them? Yeah, I thought so too.

Anyway, we need to consider what's being developed in the present as well. Previous breakthroughs have led to numerous advancements in the fields of medicine, surgery, public health and all other medical branches.

ARTIFICIAL INTELLIGENCE AND DIGITAL HEALTH

Let's fast forward to the current digital age and see how technology is changing medicine as we know it.

Only a few years ago, if you had trouble sleeping, experiencing some sharp chest pain or simply wanted to check your blood pressure, you would have to pay a visit to your doctor to do a check-up. Now, your phone can measure the quality of your sleep, and your digital wristwatch can perform an electrocardiogram, give an accurate reading of your blood pressure and even track a person's menstrual cycle! Digital health wearables are giving immediate in-depth insights into our health data and making us more aware of our own health without the need to always seek professional medical assistance.

Artificial intelligence (AI) is also making some startling advancements. AI has the potential to revolutionise the healthcare industry in the future. With the ability to analyse vast amounts of data and make predictions with a high degree of accuracy, AI can help doctors and researchers make more informed decisions about patient care.

One of the most significant ways in which AI is being used in healthcare is in the area of diagnostics. AI algorithms can be trained to identify patterns and anomalies in medical images, such as X-rays and CT scans, that may be difficult for human radiologists to detect. This can help to improve the accuracy and speed of diagnosis, leading to better patient outcomes.

Another area where AI is being used in healthcare is in the development of personalised medicine. By analysing a patient's genetic data, AI algorithms can help to identify the specific treatment that is most likely to be effective for that individual. This can lead to more targeted and effective treatments, with fewer side effects. In 2020, researchers from the Massachusetts Institute of Technology (MIT) used machine-learning algorithms to find a new and powerful antibiotic compound. At a time when we are increasingly faced with antibiotic resistance, AI is making vital breakthroughs advancing medical care. Most recently, AI-powered robots were used in Wuhan hospitals in China at the outbreak of COVID-19. These robots were able to autonomously move around the hospital, clean the wards and even deliver food and drugs to the patients.

In addition to these specific applications, AI can also be used to improve the overall efficiency of healthcare systems. By analysing patient data, AI algorithms can help to identify areas where resources are being wasted and suggest ways to optimise the use of those resources. This can lead to cost savings for healthcare providers and patients alike.

Intelligent machines and powerful algorithms are increasingly being used in healthcare, and it's important to consider how it might change medicine in the long-term. For example, digital health wearables and AI are increasing the rate and speed of diagnoses. This may be beneficial overall, but it might also burden health services with patients worried, for example, about why their blood pressure is a little higher than normal. Another effect could be that patients become more 'health-literate', gaining more insight into their health with data. The average patient in the future might already know quite a bit about their body, shifting the doctor–patient relationship from one where the doctor has to explain simple concepts to one where the doctor is informed by the patient!

Here's a list of other present discoveries that you can research on your own, be it on Google or YouTube, and reflect upon their implications at the end of this chapter. This represents an inexhaustible list.

- Robotic surgery (da Vinci Robot): minimally invasive surgery used in several branches of medicine, including urology, bowel, heart and others. Significantly more accurate, but what are the ethical implications?
- First HPV (human papillomavirus—correlated with cancer) vaccine—reducing the infection by 56%, thus saving countless lives
- Increased HIV survival rates
- Full face transplant achieved in 2010, taking 20 hours and involving more than 30 doctors
- Targeted cancer therapies and more precise drugs
- Tele-Surgery: performing robotic bladder surgery on a patient from Strasbourg, while the surgeon (Jacques Marescaux) was in New York
- Holistic care, social care and integration medicine
- The Human Genome Project

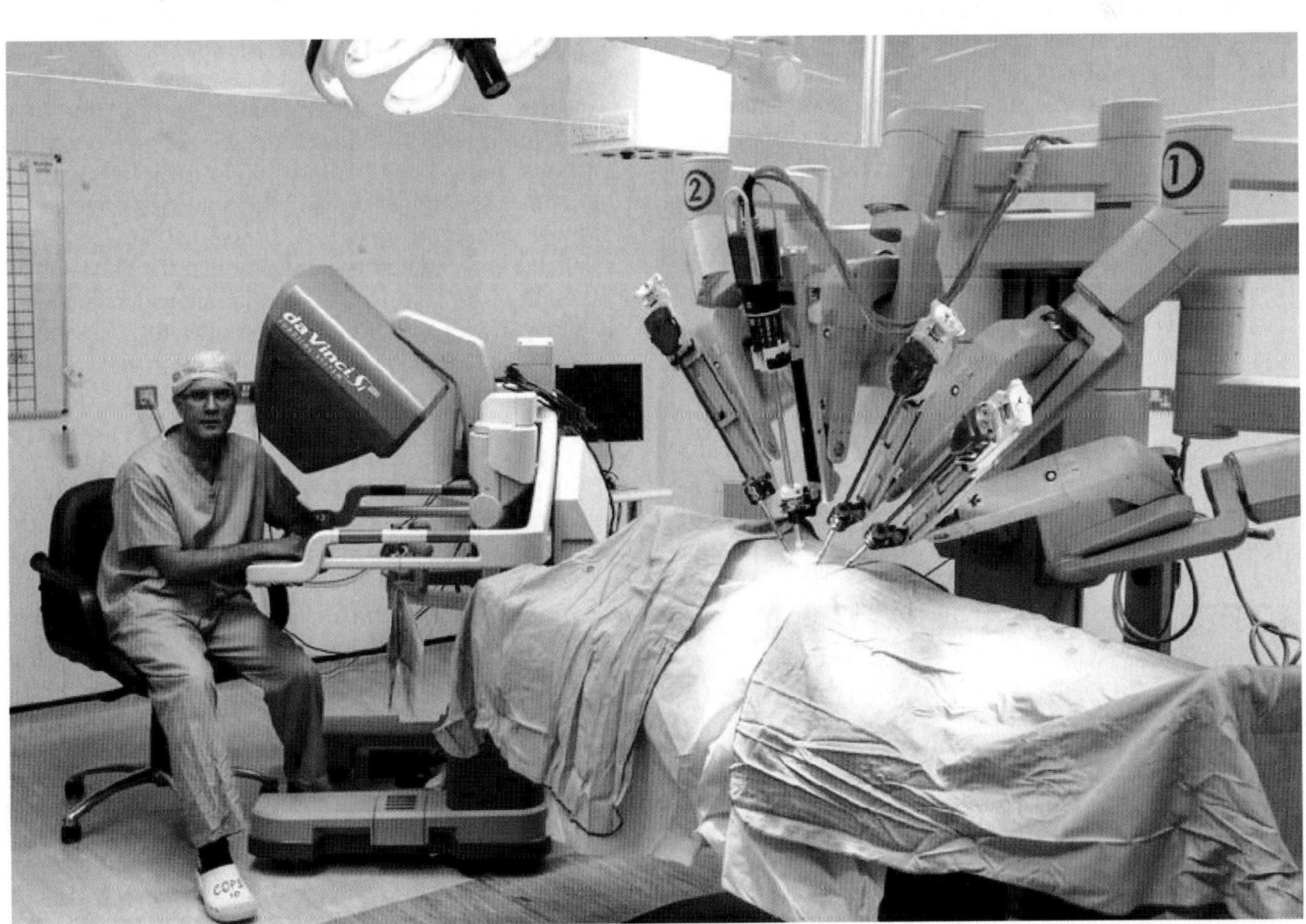

THE FALL OF MODERN MEDICINE

We've already covered a fair bit of medical history. The common theme among them is that medicines and their discoveries have always played a beneficial role. But can too much of good medicine ever become a bad thing? Let's take a look at the supposed 'fall' of modern medicine.

In 1949, as the NHS was newly formed, we had around 250 drugs. Today, we have over 18,000! This may sound great—with advances in the sciences and medical understanding, we have more drugs than ever to treat diseases and fight sickness. But what happens if doctors give too many pills to their patients? Well, they would suffer the side effects and could get sicker. In fact, it's estimated that now 10%–20% of hospital admissions are due to adverse drug reactions (that's when patients get sick from the drugs doctors prescribed to them). What's more is that 10% of drugs given by doctors in primary care are considered unnecessary. In other words, doctors are *overprescribing* medicines and causing preventable harm to patients.

But the harms from overprescribing go beyond the patient; it also affects health services. As more people get sick from unnecessarily prescribed medicines, more patients come into hospitals. Recent NHS figures show that in England alone, there is a shortage of 12,000 hospital doctors and 10% of hospital jobs are vacant. Furthermore, overprescribing reportedly costs £2 billion each year! So, at a time when our health services are overworked and underfunded, overprescribing is creating more patients and more ill-health and increasing spending on drugs we don't need.

Modern medicine has undoubtedly saved millions of lives and is, overall, a positive advancement. However, the paradox of modern medicine is that, at a time when we have more medicines, more therapies and more treatments, we are also creating more unnecessary illness. It's true what they say—too much of a good thing can become a bad thing.

Of course, when patients are ill, doctors must prescribe appropriate medicines. This is about those circumstances when patients don't require medicines for their recovery. What they need instead is a nonmedical intervention that addresses the root causes of their illness. For example, a patient could present anxiety and depression but these may be caused by stressful life events—like a death in the family, poor financial conditions or a divorce. In such cases, it is more important to improve the patient's wider determinants of health.

? What Is Health?

You might think that health means the absence of disease, or the normal functioning of the body. While this isn't a wrong understanding of health, it only considers the biomedical aspect. The truth is, health isn't just what's enclosed in our skin, the wider determinants of health exist outside the membrane of our biology. Health is made up of **bio-psycho-social** determinants. Think about how your mental health or social environment can affect your wellbeing. Every aspect of your life can shape your health. This also has implications on how doctors can treat patients. Instead of inappropriately medicalising health issues and overprescribing, doctors could use other nonmedical interventions. Keep on reading to learn about one of them (social prescribing).

Can you think of other issues or crises that modern medicine is currently dealing with? What could we face in the future and how could we prevent catastrophes from happening? Here's a list to get you thinking:

- Accident and emergency (A&E) waiting times: what is currently being done to reduce waiting times? Have you heard of the 'traffic-light' system?
- An ageing population leading to multimorbidity (people living longer with one or more chronic illnesses at the same time)
- Lifestyle factors leading to an obesity crisis and the rise of noncommunicable diseases (NCDs). What are the most important lifestyle factors to consider? How could you improve or change lifestyle choices for patients?
- Changes in public expectation
- Rising costs—what should be funded and what should take priority?

RISE OF COMMUNITY HEALTH AND PREVENTION

Now that we have covered the pitfalls of modern medicine, particularly overprescribing medicines when unnecessary, let's look at one of the most recent developments that's changing the way we think about medical interventions entirely. You may have heard of Sir William Osler; he is widely regarded as the Father of Modern Medicine. Over a 100 years ago, he said something that remains more relevant today in medicine than ever before. He said: '*A good physician treats the disease; a great physician treats the patient who has the disease*'.

What Osler meant by this statement was that it is more important to understand the illness from the patient's perspective than it is to simply focus on the pathology and treat symptoms of illness. Today, we call this 'patient-centred care'. It's about taking the time to ask patients 'what matters to you' rather than just 'what's the matter with you'. Doctors are finding that, often, when patients answer that question, their health issue is nonmedical related. In fact, around one in four general practice (GP) appointments are due to nonmedical reasons!

So how can we treat something that, at its roots, is not related to medicine at all but still affects the health of the patient? The answer lies in looking at health as a bio-psycho-social construct. In 2019, the NHS in the UK introduced 'social prescribing' to its service. Social prescribing describes the process of referring patients to a range of nonclinical services and activities that are designed to improve health and wellbeing (e.g. walking groups for the elderly experiencing isolation and loneliness). They are typically offered by the local voluntary and community sectors. Doctors can refer patients to a social prescribing link worker if they feel their concerns would be better addressed through nonmedical interventions. The link worker takes time to understand the patient's individual needs and codesigns an appropriate intervention. You may be questioning how useful this is, but evidence shows that social prescribing improves health outcomes and can save the NHS 4.5 million appointments a year!

This approach to medicine is based on the idea that '*health is made in our communities, not in hospitals*'. If we focus on improving people's lifestyle, we can improve their health and prevent further diseases from occurring. There is a growing interest in medicine on disease prevention. Currently, our healthcare is actually 'sick-care'. We wait for people to get sick before treating them. But it's far more efficient to help people prevent getting common diseases in the first place.

So, the future of medicine is beginning to look 'social'. It's about understanding health in a more holistic bio-psycho-social way, enabling and empowering people to take care of their health, and focusing on disease prevention. That doesn't sound as snazzy as AI-powered robots, but its repercussions may just be more powerful.

The future of medicine contains many other possibilities. The medical field has made several predictions regarding future discoveries that would change the way we study and practice medicine. Here are a few things to consider:

- Printing organs—solving the organ-donor problem (3D printer using living cells)
- Virtual reality dissection tables and surgery—innovating medical education
- Ultrasound surgery—less invasive surgery
- Online doctors—increases accessibility to healthcare without affecting continuity of care
- Designer babies—should people be able to choose certain qualities for their babies? How about their sex or eye colour?

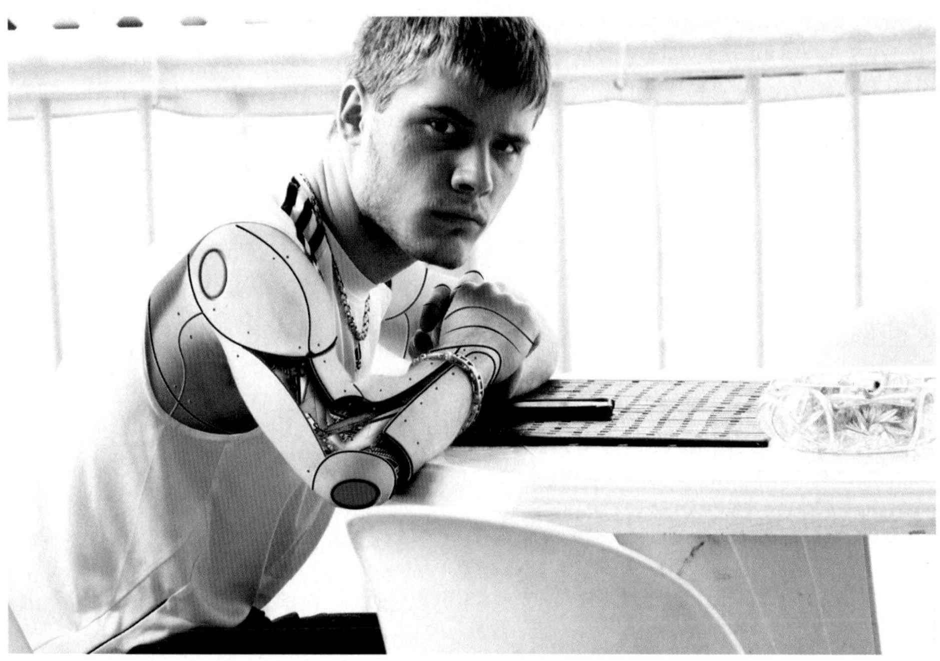

HOW CAN THIS HELP WITH YOUR MEDICAL SCHOOL APPLICATION?

- You can't fully understand something without following it back to its roots.
- If you want to be part of a profession, you must know what has been done before you.
- Previous discoveries lead to future innovations—you are not reinventing the wheel, but rather personalising and improving it.

> The value in learning about medicine's past history is to get a deeper appreciation of how we got to practice modern medicine today. Medical history is filled with incredible examples of discoveries and advancements, and those past achievements are important and relevant even today. It is important for prospective doctors to consider the history of medicine so that they can better understand present clinical practice and be a part of its future developments.
>
> **Hamaad Khan, First Year Medical Student**

PERSONAL STATEMENTS

Remember, knowledge is power as the saying often goes. If you decide to use any of it (although not necessary) in your personal statement, it may portray that you have a good understanding of the importance of previous discoveries and have done a bit of background reading.

INTERVIEWS

You could receive questions regarding the past, present and future of medicine, as you will soon find out in our interview section. Or you might want to use some historical examples when answering some questions. Make sure you take time to reflect on both the positives and negatives of each period.

> The history of medicine is full of incredible examples of discoveries, achievements and mistakes. Learning some key examples is a great way to improve your interview answers when practising. Top tip: pick your favourite examples from the past, present and future section and try to link them to a current health issue
>
> **Hamaad Khan, First Year Medical Student**

> Why, in your opinion, is medical history important? Which discovery is your favourite and why? Why does history matter, and why should you be familiar with the most famous discoveries?

SUMMARY, TEST YOURSELF AND REFLECTION

As we reach the end of our journey through the past, present and future of medicine, I want to leave you with a taste of YOUR future. Imagine being a medical student and a future doctor in a place where the biggest breakthroughs in history have been made. A place where the first accurate description of blood circulation was given by William Harvey. A place where Edward Jenner discovered the smallpox vaccine and potentially 'saved more lives than were lost in all the wars of mankind since the beginning of recorded history'. A place where John Snow located the source of cholera and successfully pioneered both anaesthetics and epidemiology. A place where Joseph Lister dramatically reduced postsurgical mortality by introducing antisepsis in surgery. A place where penicillin was discovered, where the CT scanner came from and where *Gray's Anatomy* (the first ever complete human anatomy textbook) was published.

But I also want to leave you with a taste of curiosity and uncertainty. When you join this army of heroes practicing medicine, how and in what way would you like to contribute to the ever-growing field of medicine? How will YOU use previous knowledge to shape the present and future of medicine?

A box for reflection and ideas has been provided here so you can jot down any thoughts you may have.

Test Yourself

- When was the NHS launched?
- Who discovered DNA? Don't rush; it may be more than one or two people.
- Who was Maria Sklodowska and what did she do for the world of medicine?
- What do we mean by 'medical stagnation in Middle Ages' and why did this occur?
- Who was Galen and what were some of his mistakes?
- What is the 'Channel Theory' and what civilisation contributed to its development?
- What is overprescribing and why is it bad?

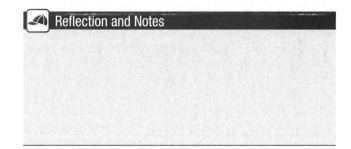

RESOURCES

Bynum, W., 2008. The History of Medicine: A Very Short Introduction. Oxford University Press, Oxford, UK.

Gawande, A., 2010. The Checklist Manifesto: How to Get Things Right. Profile Books, London, UK.

Ignotofsky, R., 2016. Women in Science: 50 Fearless Pioneers Who Changed the World. Ten Speed Press, Berkeley, CA.

Marmot, M., 2015. The Health Gap: The Challenge of an Unequal World. Bloomsbury Publishing, London, UK.

Marsh, H., 2014. Do No Harm: Stories of Life, Death and Brain Surgery. Hachette UK, Paris, France.

Porter, R., 2004. Blood and Guts: A Short History of Medicine. WW Norton & Company, New York, NY.

UK Medical Practice and Career Progression

3

Navin Mukundu Nagesh and Rachel Howard

Chapter Outline

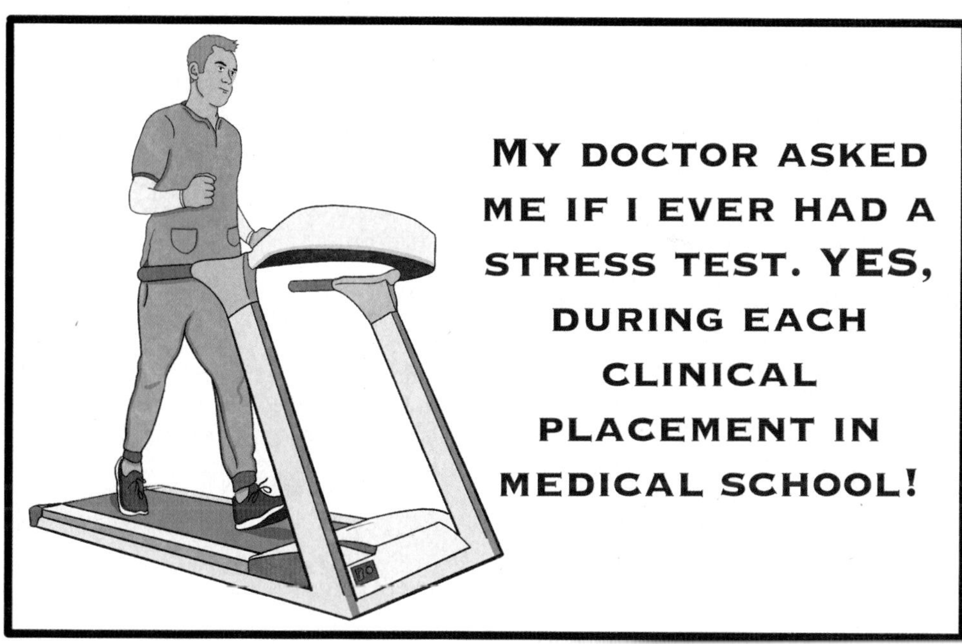

HEALTHCARE IN THE UNITED KINGDOM

Welcome to medicine in the United Kingdom! This chapter introduces you to medical practice in the United Kingdom. We will have a look at the history and development of the National Health Service (NHS) and the provision of services. The structure and functions of the NHS will be described in a simple and easy manner, and the key strategies for optimal patient care will be highlighted.

Once you understand the process of healthcare delivery, we will introduce you to the undergraduate medical curriculum in the UK. There is a vast variety in the medical school course structures and styles of learning. We hope to guide you through each style with reflections from current medical students. The aim is to provide you with a realistic understanding of the day-to-day life of a medical student in different medical schools. You will be able to summarise the pros and cons of each type of curriculum and decide which teaching method suits you the most.

The focus will then go towards your transition from a medical student to a doctor in various fields. The career progression will be outlined, and the vast range of specialities and career paths will be discussed. Testimonials from current students, medical, surgical and general practice (GP) trainees will provide you a glimpse into the specialties. This will allow you to appreciate the diversity, responsibilities and competencies that doctors require to become fully qualified.

Along your journey in medicine, several key medical organisations will play an important part in shaping your success, these will be introduced to you. You may be wondering, how will this help me now? Many of these organisations have a section dedicated to students and provide articles that can update your knowledge in medical practice and research. This will be a fundamental aspect of your preparation for medical school interviews and beyond.

'Once you're in medical school you're set for life'—I'm sure you've heard that before. The reality is that most doctors must continue professional development throughout their careers to ensure their knowledge and skills are up to date. We will introduce you to some examples of professional development and hopefully inspire you to start this process early by getting involved in similar activities at your stage. Don't worry, there will be reflections from current medical school applicants who will share their own experiences of professional development.

By completing this chapter, you will have a clearer understanding of how healthcare is structured in the UK and how you as doctors can play a role in working together to deliver high-quality patient care. You will be able to reflect in detail by imagining your own career path and seeing where you will be in the next 5 to 10 years. We hope you enjoy this informative chapter and make use of all opportunities provided.

THE NATIONAL HEALTH SERVICE

The UK has one of the most successful healthcare systems in the world. It is renowned for its quality, safety and clinical excellence. Understanding the roots and core principles by which the NHS operates is crucial for any medical school applicant. Whether you are a domestic or international applicant, understanding how the NHS delivers care to the nation will undoubtedly make you proud to be involved with such an incredible service. The following information has been carefully refined to allow students at your level to clearly understand the key points that will be raised within your interview. It is therefore crucial that you supplement this chapter by reading the healthcare news and updates from credible sources to further understand the current social, political and financial trends in the NHS. The NHS is changing every year, every month and even every day; therefore, it's vital to keep an eye on the news! We will now summarise how the NHS was started and some of the key changes over time.

> As aspiring doctors, we need to take responsibility and ensure that our knowledge is up to date and that we are constantly striving for the safest and best NHS that our patients deserve.

The NHS was launched in 1948. The NHS was not developed overnight. It was the product of over 50 years of debate, discussion and scrutiny. Some of the issues that delayed the introduction of the NHS were unstable finances, logistics and two world wars. Healthcare before the NHS was essentially unregulated and had a mixture of public, private and charitable sectors that delivered the appropriate services. Essentially, the quality of healthcare was directly related to patient location and accessibility to healthcare professionals.

5 JULY 1948

> Try your best to remember this date, as it's the NHS's birthday!

Mr Aneurin Bevan, the health secretary during this period, formally launched the NHS in Manchester at Park Hospital. This is now Manchester Trafford General Hospital, one of the premier hospitals in the UK. The idea was that good healthcare should be available to all, regardless of wealth. Remember this, as it's one of the NHS's core principles, which we will cover later. This was the first time ever that hospitals, clinics, doctors, nurses, opticians, pharmacists and dentists worked together under the same organisation. Sounds like a dream, right? This was the overarching vision that would develop over many years of innovation. For the purposes of your medical school application process, we would like you to have an awareness of the following timeline of developments within the NHS and England overall (Table 3.1). Of course, there is no need to memorise it all, but it is always nice to go down memory lane and admire how far we have come.

> It's a daunting prospect to try and remember the full history of the NHS; the way I did it was to simply remember what I found most interesting. This way I was able to find this learning process more fun and less monotonous. I found the change in NHS structure in 2012 particularly interesting, as the Health & Social Care Act was a significant moment in the NHS's history. I was able to talk about this with passion and depth during my medical school interview.
>
> **Dr Navin Nagesh, Academic Doctor, Oxford University**

THE SIX CORE VALUES OF THE NHS

Now that we have covered the history of the NHS, our focus turns to why the NHS works. This can be attributed to the NHS's six core values. Being aware of these values is crucial for any medical school applicant, as it defines how one should act and behave as a NHS doctor. Let's go through them now.

Working Together for Patients

The idea of 'working together for patients' is the simplest and most meaningful idea the NHS believes in. We must put patients first, and everything conducted in the NHS must ensure that the best interests of everyone are met. This can involve admitting to mistakes, striving to become better, acting within your competence and continuing your professional development. The NHS also ensures that health service providers involve their staff, carers and local communities in improving the delivery of healthcare to ensure the needs of the local regions are met.

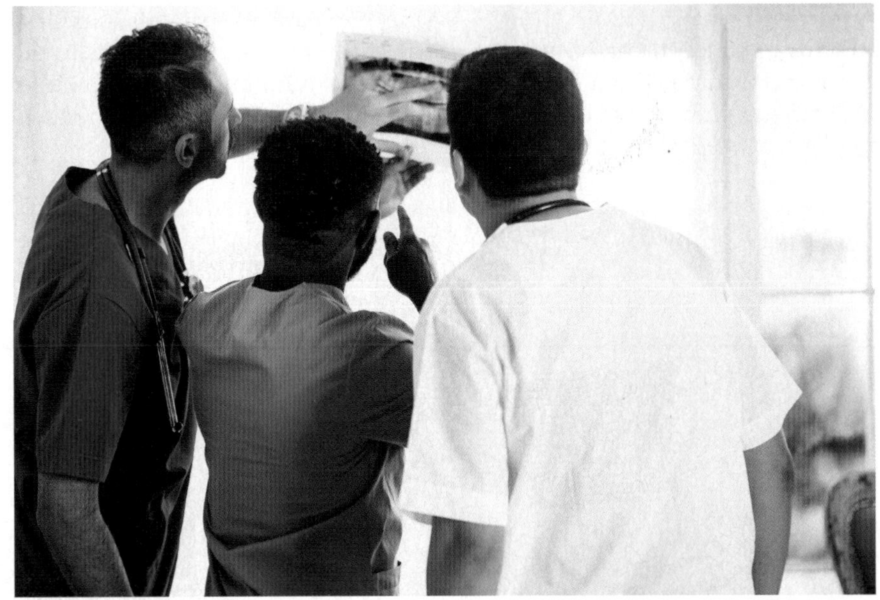

Table 3.1 **Timeline of the NHS**

YEAR	DEVELOPMENT
1948	NHS is created
1952	Fixed charge for drug prescriptions is introduced at 5p
1956	Clean Air Act is established by parliament to tackle air pollution in the UK's urban areas
1957	Willink's report proposes 12% reduction in number of training places for doctors
1958	Vaccination programmes for polio and diphtheria launched
1959	Mental Health Act replaces existing legislation on mental health service provision in England
1960	First successful kidney transplant
1961	Oral contraceptive pill made widely available
1962	First hip replacement
1967	The Abortion Act—Legal abortion up to 28 weeks' gestation
1968	Department of Health and Social Security is formed from the merge of Ministry of Health and Ministry of Social Security
1968	First British heart transplant
1972	Introduction of CT scans into medical imaging
1973	NHS Reorganisation Act
1978	World's first baby born via in vitro fertilisation
1979	First successful bone marrow transplant in a child
1980	The 'Black Report' demonstrates the gap in health inequalities is widening
1983	The Mental Health Act 1983 legislates those 'at risk' who have a mental illness can be detained with or without their consent
1985	Laparoscopic surgery developed
1988	NHS breast cancer screening launched
1990	New GP contract incentives health promotion
1994	NHS organ donor register set-up
1998	National Institute for Health and Clinical Excellence (NICE) is established
2000	NHS plan establishes a ten-year programme of investment and reform for the NHS
2002	First successful gene therapy
2004	NHS Foundation trusts created to allow financial independence for hospitals
2006	NHS bowel cancer screening programme launched
2007	Smoking ban in public places
2008	NHS HPV vaccination programme
2009	Care Quality Commission (CQC) launched
2012	Health and Social Care Act
2013	The 'new' NHS
2016	New contracts for junior doctors agreed
2020	UK leaves EU and COVID-19 emerges
2022	Health and Care Act 2022

Respect and Dignity

This may seem like an obvious concept, but this essential value emphasises the point that every individual who interacts with the NHS should be treated with the same level of respect and dignity, regardless of whether they are patients, patients' families, carers or members of staff. This value also seeks to promote an open and honest environment where a culture of humility and effective communication is present towards patients and colleagues.

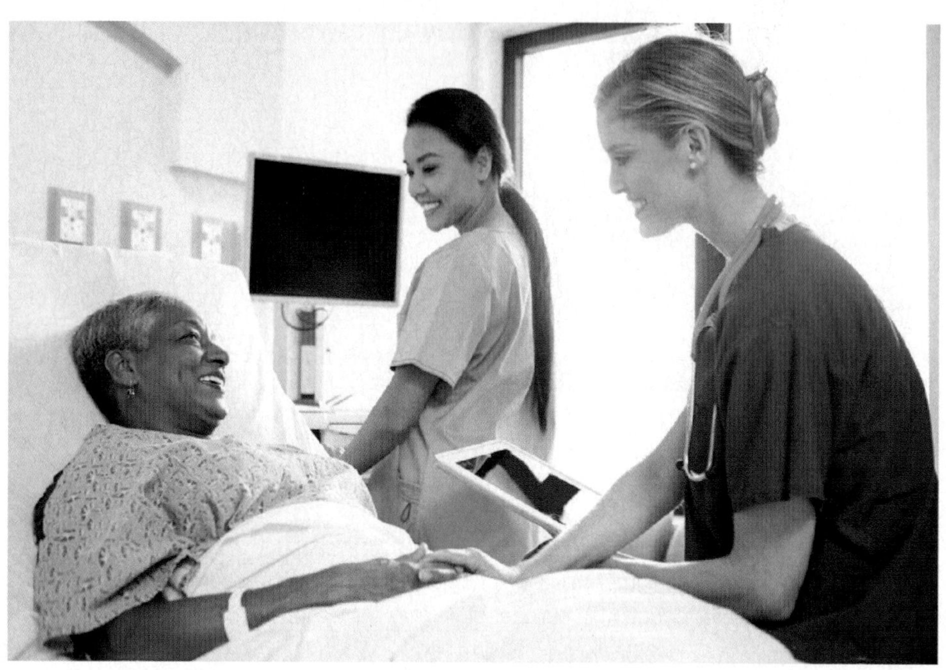

Commitment to Quality of Care

This value relates to the aspiration of the highest standard of professionalism, clinical excellence and provision of services that are safe and patient focused. With an ever-increasing population and burden on health services, the quality of care should not be compromised. Quality assurance should be based on feedback from patients and staff, and we should welcome this whether it is positive or negative. Organisations within the NHS should identify areas of improvement and drive changes towards ensuring that quality services are provided safely and consistently.

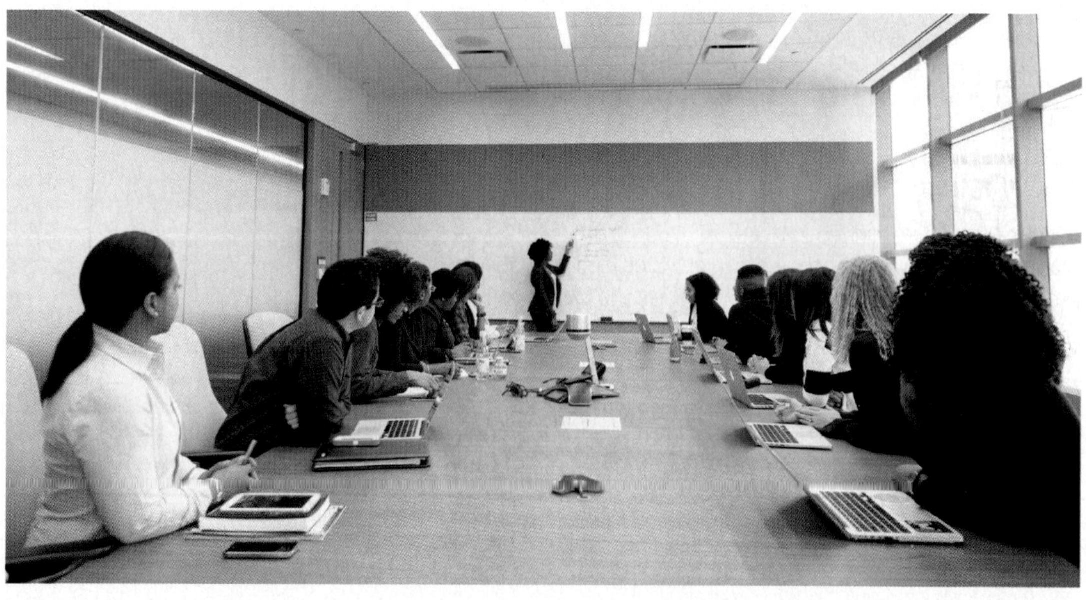

Compassion

Compassionate care ties closely with respect and dignity in that individual patients, carers and relatives must be treated with sensitivity and kindness. The business of the NHS extends beyond providing clinical care and includes alleviating pain and distress and ensuring that people feel valued and heard and that their concerns/autonomy is respected.

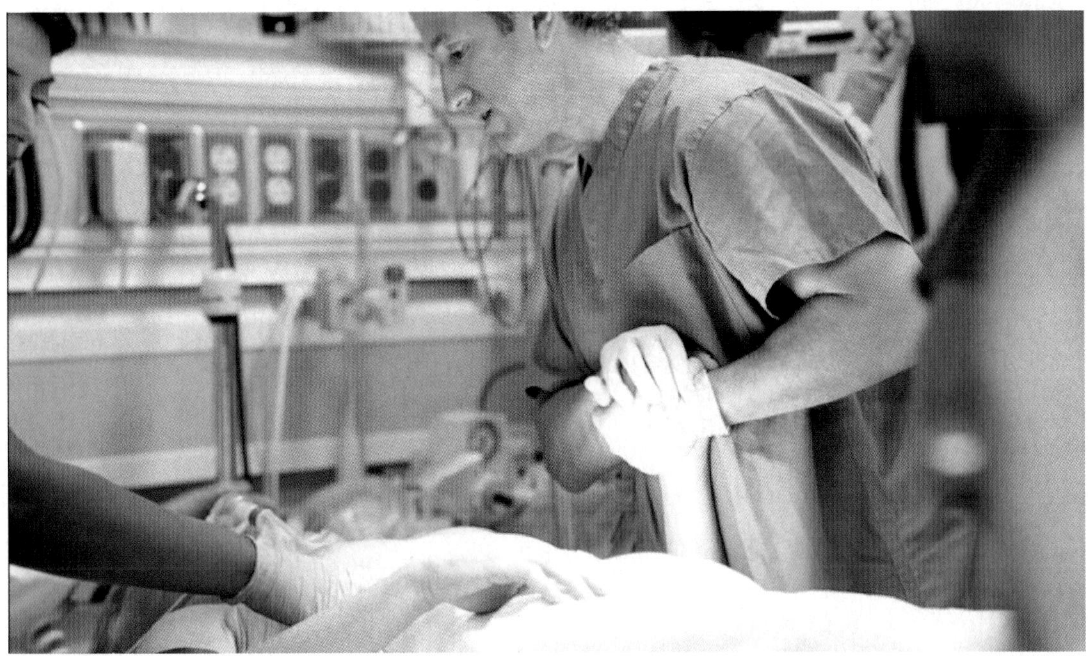

Improving Lives

This is perhaps the most important value of the NHS. Improving and adding value to people's quality of life is the core reason the NHS exists. This can be expanded to seeking improvements in wider public health and wellbeing of communities and populations. This can be achieved through its excellence in medical care, but also in understanding the need of preventative measures to ensure the health of the community and empowering patients to take ownership of their health and lifestyles.

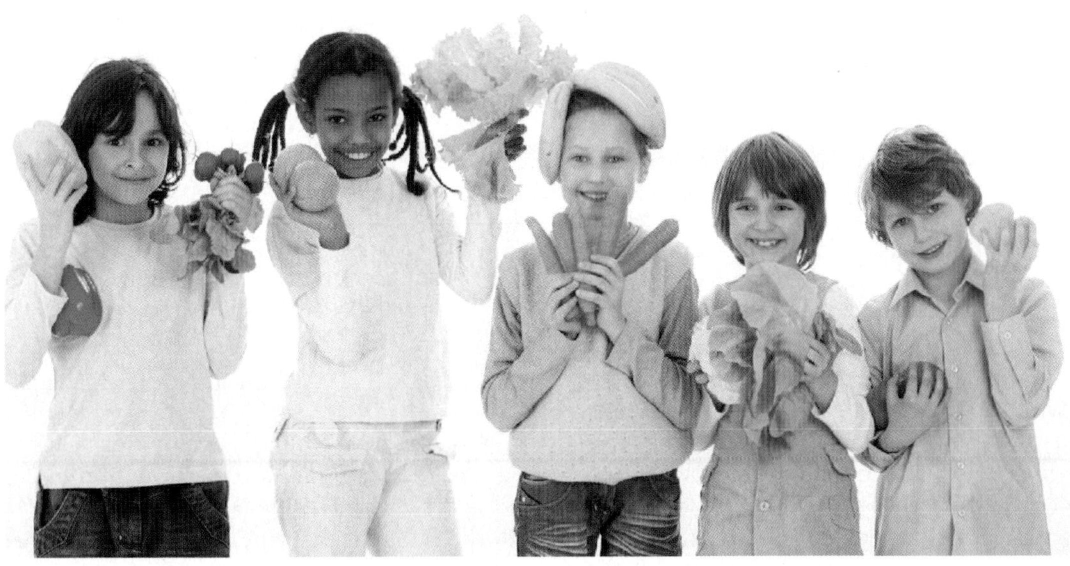

Everyone Counts

Of course, we must treat every patient with the same level of respect and dignity, but this value also relates to the distribution of NHS resources. This is to ensure that patients are not disadvantaged or discriminated against in any way due to their demographic or geographic background.

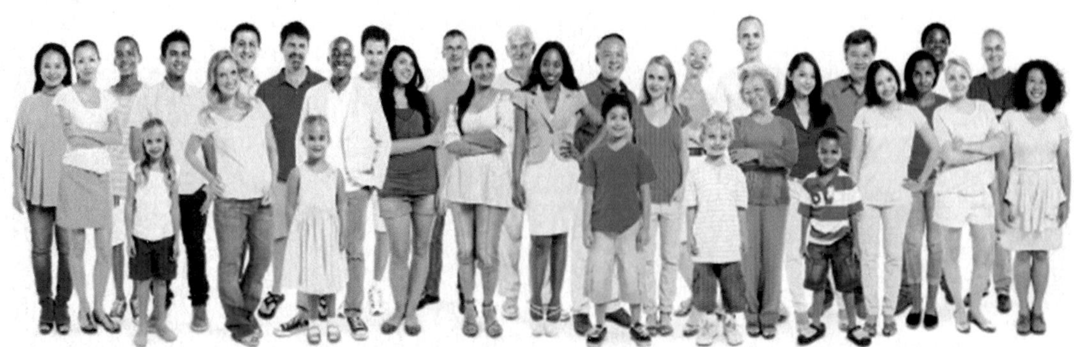

> If you sit back and reflect a moment, you can see that the NHS's core values correlate with the core values of a good doctor. If you learn these values and apply them to your thinking and behaviour, you will have the right frame of mind when you attend work experiences.

> I found it quite difficult to remember all six core values of the NHS initially, as I personally thought they were sometimes repetitive; for example, 'improving lives' and 'commitment to quality of care' seemed like the same thing to me. What I did in my interview was state that there are six core values of the NHS and that I will talk about three of them in relation to my work experiences. The values I chose were 'everyone counts', 'compassion' and 'working together for patients'. I was able to relate to what I had seen in clinical practice to these values and the interviewer seemed very impressed.
>
> **Andrel Yoong, Medical Student, Exeter Medical School**

NHS ORGANISATION

Let's look at the organisational structure of the NHS, how it is funded, and the various services within it.

Scale

The NHS interacts with over a million patients every 36 hours. Take a moment to think about that. That means in 1 week, the NHS would have interacted with more people than the population of the city of Manchester.

Patient care encompasses almost everything in healthcare from antenatal screening, management of long-term conditions, elective and emergency surgeries, all the way to end-of-life care. This sounds like a tremendous task, and you may be wondering, this surely cannot be sustainable or efficient. Well, the 2021 Commonwealth Fund stated that in comparison with the healthcare systems of 10 other countries, the NHS was rated fourth. This was in terms of efficiency, quality of care, safety, coordination of care and patient-centred approach. This means the NHS has a better healthcare system than:

- United States
- Canada
- France
- Germany
- Sweden
- Switzerland
- New Zealand

This truly remarkable feat has been achieved by a workforce of nearly 1.4 million people. This puts the NHS as one of the world's largest workforces.

> You may be surprised to find out that of the 1.4 million people employed by the NHS, around 130,000, are doctors and 300,000 are nurses. The remaining 1 million people are the outstanding support staff members, including allied healthcare professionals, ambulance staff, administrative staff, cleaners, maintenance staff and the managers.

The Organisational Structure of the NHS

Here comes the money. You'd be right to think that providing such a world-class service must be a very expensive business. The funding and structure of the NHS have always been rather complicated to fully understand, but for the purpose of your medical school application, we will cover the basics to ensure you can at least talk about it.

> In summary, the funding for the NHS comes directly from taxation set by the UK government. When the NHS was started in 1948, the annual budget was £437 million (£17 billion in today's value adjusting for inflation). The current NHS budget for 2022/23 is now £153 billion!

As you saw in the developments timeline from earlier, the NHS had a transformation in 2013 underpinned by The Health & Social Care Act. This essentially changed the way health services are funded (Fig. 3.1). The most recent reorganisation of the NHS was the 2022 Health and Care Act.

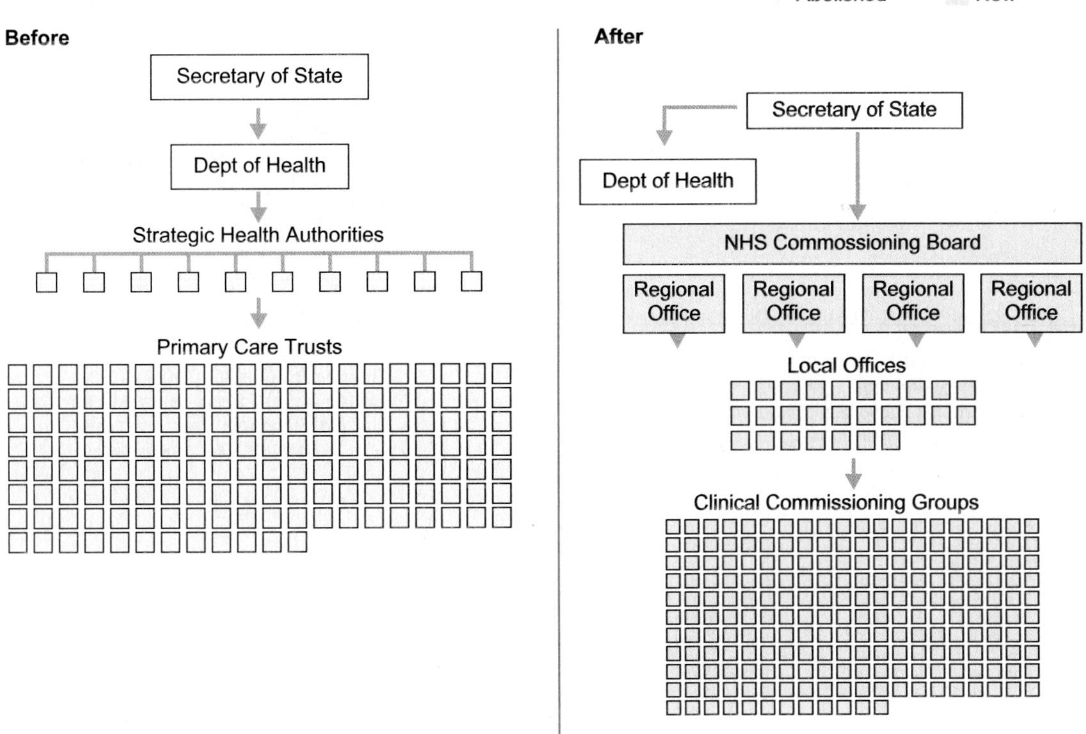

Fig. 3.1 Reorganisation of the National Health Service following the 2013 Health & Social Care Act.

The Health and Care Act (2022) has brought about the introduction of integrated care systems (ICSs). The new framework is designed to encourage the integration of services for patients through the collaboration of partnerships. On 1 July 2022, 42 ICSs were established across England. Each ICS is made up of integrated care partnerships (ICPs), integrated care boards (ICBs), local authorities, place-based partnerships and provider collaboratives. The introduction of ICBs resulted in the abolishment of clinical commissioning groups (CCGs).

Summary of Changes

- In April 2022, the Health and Care Act (2022) came into force, bringing with it many new structures and arrangements for the NHS in England (Fig. 3.2).
- The new integrated structure to the NHS promotes collaboration between organisations as opposed to previous competitions.
- The Health and Care Act aims to promote the abolishment of a one-size-fits-all approach allowing for flexibility at the population level.

Well done for getting through the administrative side of the NHS! As you see from the developments timeline, the NHS is an ever-evolving organisation. Therefore, it is crucial that you keep up to date with new developments and check the news regularly.

> We recommend the BBC News app, which can be accessed through your smartphone. If you read one or two articles per day, you will be very well informed for your medical school interviews.

HEALTHCARE SERVICES

So now that we understand the history and the basic structure of the NHS, we can finally talk about the healthcare services that it provides. It is crucial for you to understand the different pathways patients can go through to obtain medical attention, as it is a little more complex than simply primary care and secondary care. The following sections have the basic definitions and key information that you need to know about the NHS healthcare services. Fig. 3.3 gives an overview of access to unscheduled care.

Emergency Medicine

Emergency medicine is what most people relate to in medicine, with patients requiring urgent medical treatment to manage illness and trauma. The NHS employs a multistep process to allow patients with varying levels of illness to ensure they are seen by the appropriate healthcare professionals.

NHS 111 Service

- This is a telephone service for patients who can call to obtain medical advice and determine which health service to attend.
- This is generally for non-life-threatening illnesses and injuries.

NHS Walk-in Centre

- This service consists of doctors and nurses who primarily treat patients with non-life-threatening illnesses and injuries.

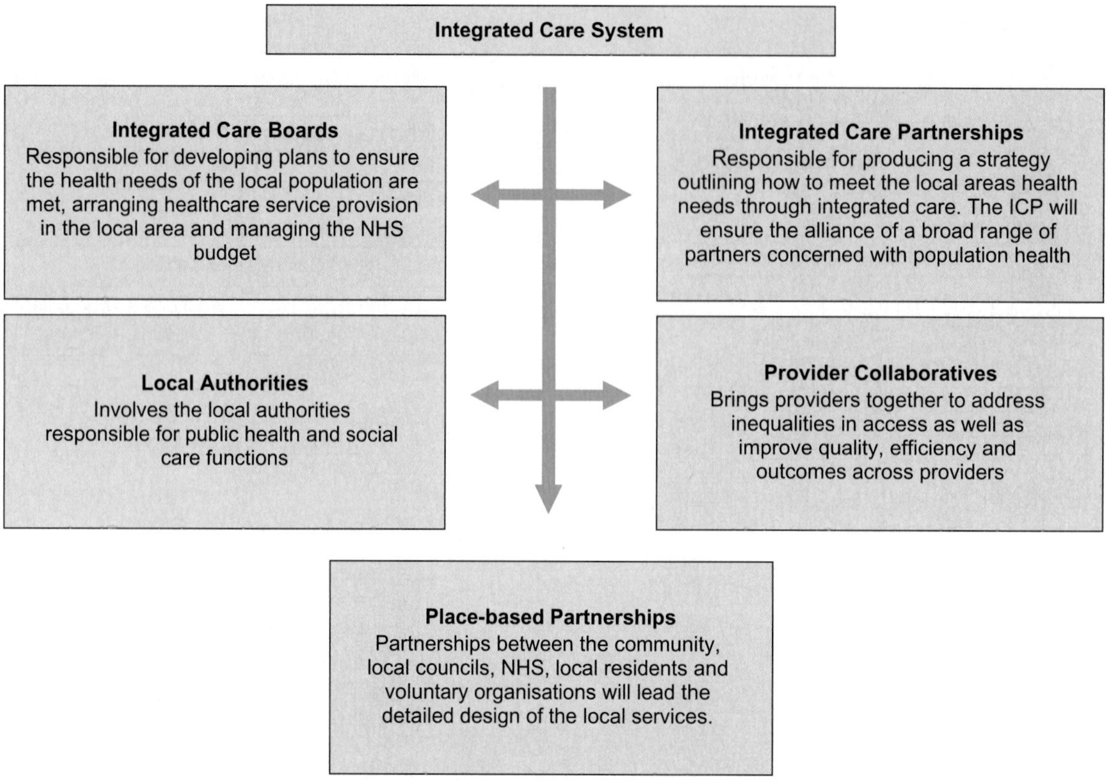

Integrated Care System

Integrated Care Boards
Responsible for developing plans to ensure the health needs of the local population are met, arranging healthcare service provision in the local area and managing the NHS budget

Integrated Care Partnerships
Responsible for producing a strategy outlining how to meet the local areas health needs through integrated care. The ICP will ensure the alliance of a broad range of partners concerned with population health

Local Authorities
Involves the local authorities responsible for public health and social care functions

Provider Collaboratives
Brings providers together to address inequalities in access as well as improve quality, efficiency and outcomes across providers

Place-based Partnerships
Partnerships between the community, local councils, NHS, local residents and voluntary organisations will lead the detailed design of the local services.

Fig. 3.2 Organisational structure of the National Health Service following the Health and Care Act 2022. *ICP*, Integrated care partnership.

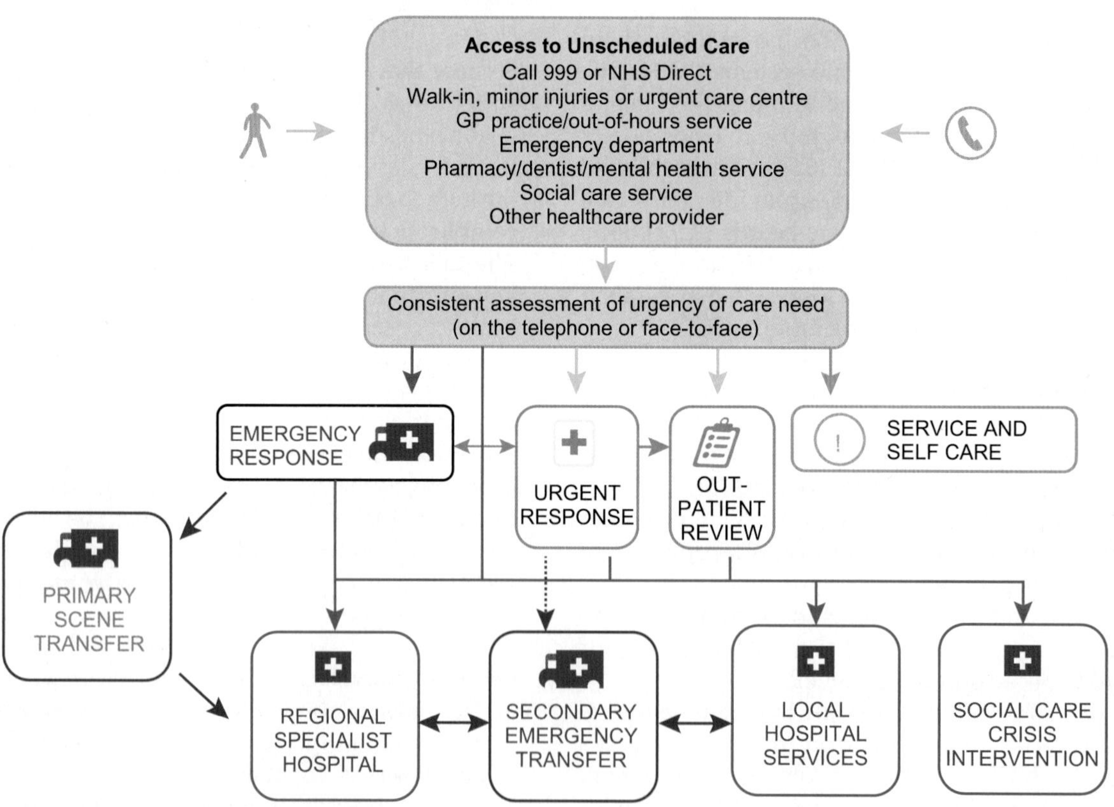

Fig. 3.3 Overview of access to services.

- Chronic diseases and infections are also generally managed within the walk-in centre.
- Genitourinary medicine services that specialise in sexual health and contraception services are also integrated into the NHS walk-in centre.

999 Emergency

- This is the main telephone service for patients who are seriously ill or injured and require immediate medical attention from ambulance and healthcare professionals.

- This is specifically for life-threatening illnesses and injuries.

Emergency Department

- The emergency department deals with patients who arrive via ambulance or voluntarily for serious illnesses and injuries.
- Once registered, patients are triaged (via a preassessment) by a doctor or nurse and a priority rating is given to ensure patients who require immediate attention are seen first.
- The current NHS emergency waiting time target is 4 hours.

> It was very overwhelming when I was reading about the types of healthcare services available in the NHS, especially the different levels of urgency of illness. For example, I found it sometimes confusing to differentiate when to call 111 or call 999. I can now understand how difficult it must be for patients who are going through an illness to decide when they are worried about their health but don't want to be a burden on the NHS.
>
> **Clarence Chen, Medical School Applicant**

General Practice

- GP has the largest number of doctors in its workforce in the NHS.
- GPs deal with a wide range of illness and diseases and offer medicine, counselling and advice for patients.
- Patient education is a big aspect of GP, and the notion of preventative medicine is key for long-term patient management.
- GPs can conduct tests, order imaging investigations, refer patients to hospital services and recommend nonmedical alternatives such as homeopathy.
- GPs work with a varied team of nurses, healthcare assistants, practice managers, secretaries and receptionists on the premises.
- They also work with allied healthcare professionals such as midwives, physiotherapists, health visitors, mental health workers and social care workers. This multidisciplinary approach allows for the holistic care of patients in the community.
- Patients who cannot be managed in the community are referred to hospital services for specialist medical attention.

NHS Pharmacy Service

- The pharmacists have a very crucial role in the NHS, as they are the experts in medicine and drug therapeutics. They combine their knowledge of pharmacology to ensure patients are well educated and take medications appropriately.
- Their everyday role is to dispense medication to patients in the community and hospital setting.
- As of 2022, the NHS prescription cost is £9.35. Please make sure you check the current cost if you are reading this well into the future.
- Pharmacists can also advise on common problems in the community such as management of colds, aches, pain, diet and smoking cessation.

NHS Dental Services

- Dentists work in a slightly different way than most other healthcare professionals in the NHS. Patients do not need to be in a geographical location to register at a dental practice, unlike the registration for GP.
- Dental practice in the UK is predominantly private practice, which means the capacity for patients may be reduced for NHS patients. This can cause health inequality and a phenomenon called the postcode lottery, where patients in different regions receive better healthcare than others.
- For dental emergencies, patients can attend the emergency department. Patients will be charged for this service at the band one rate of £23.80 (as of 2022). Patients who are entitled to free dental care may claim the cost back at a later date.

Mental Health Services

- Patients need to be specifically referred to mental health services by their GP.
- This service helps patients with underlying mental health disorders and drug and alcohol problems.
- There is a separate service for children with specialised healthcare professionals who are highly trained.
- Patients can undergo cognitive behavioural therapy as an alternative to taking medication.
- The following are the most common mental health services offered:
  - Anxiety services
  - Depression services
  - Eating disorder services
  - Alcohol and drug misuse services
  - Psychological therapy

Hospital Services

We're finally talking about the services within the hospital. The point of this section is for you understand that there is an extensive set of services in the community that care for the majority of patients within the UK. The hospital services are part of the secondary care pathway, which requires specific referral from the community services.

- As we mentioned previously, the services are regulated and commissioned by the CCGs. The hospitals are managed by their own NHS trusts, which ensure cost effectiveness and patient safety.
- There is a wide range of medical and surgical specialities in the NHS, some of which are illustrated in Fig. 3.4.

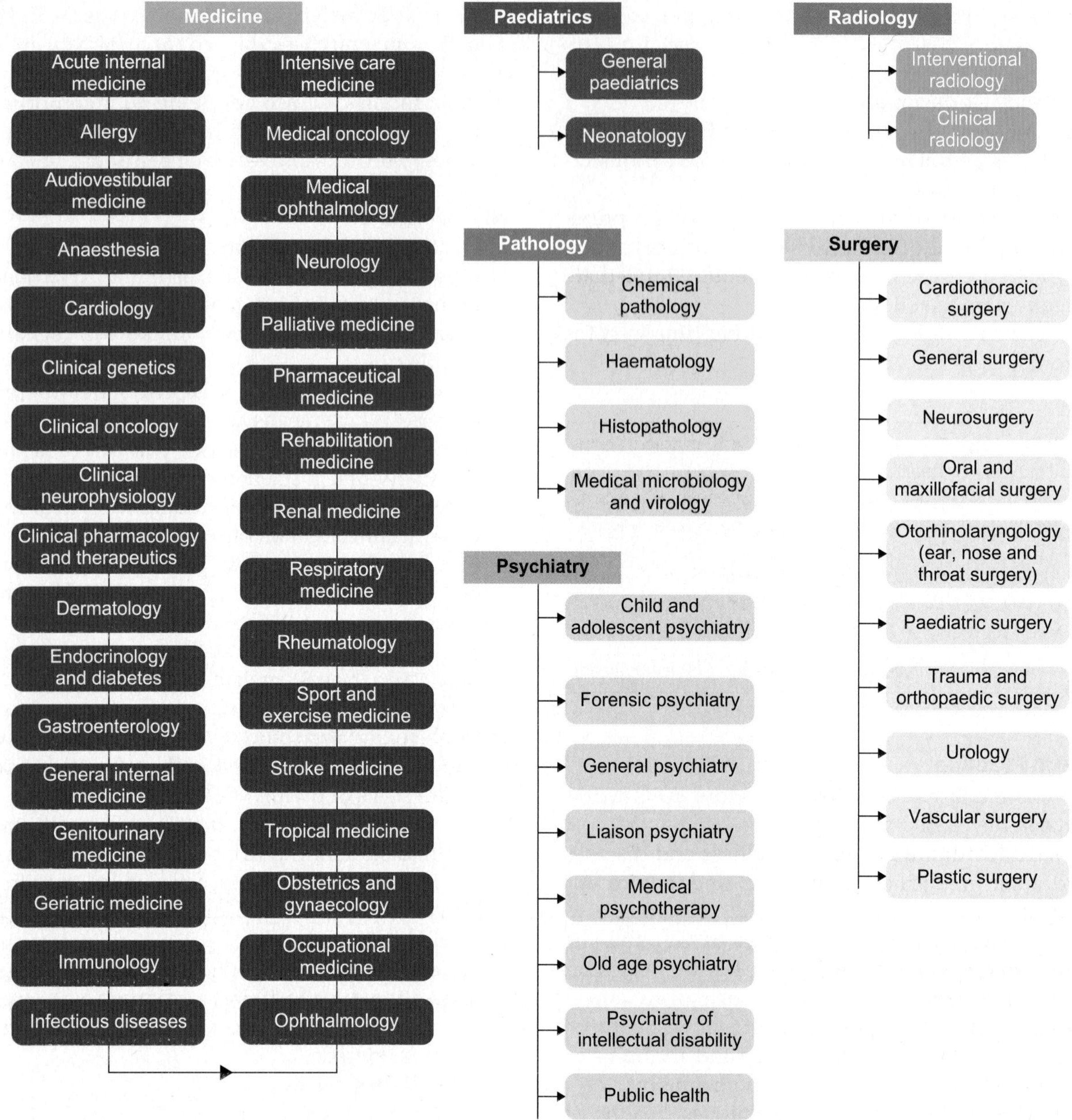

Fig. 3.4 Specialities in medicine.

> There are a vast number of specialities in medicine and surgery. Don't worry about learning all of them, as in reality during medical school training you are only exposed to the main branches of medicine and surgery. However, you should be aware of how specialities can vary in terms of their day-to-day jobs. For example, doctors in pathology and public health may decide to take on nonclinical jobs where they hardly ever see patients, and some surgeons will develop subspeciality interests where they only operate on a particular part of the body. The best way to articulate yourself is to find some profiles of doctors in GP, medicine, surgery and nonclinical medicine.
>
> **Dr Navin Nagesh, Academic Doctor, Oxford University**

UK MEDICAL SCHOOL CURRICULUM

Well, you're almost there! The purpose of this section is to provide you with a basic insight into the different types of medical curriculum currently available in the UK. What we don't want to do is provide information that is readily available online as you are all capable of finding that yourself. Here, we will go over the basics so that you have the confidence to go ahead and read for yourself later.

You should be aware of the following types of medical curriculum structures. We will go through each in turn:

- Traditional course
  - Preclinical and clinical years separated

- Integrated systems-based course
- Problem-based learning (PBL)
- Case-based learning (CBL)

The reason you should be aware of these types of course structures is for you to develop an understanding of which type of learning you are personally better suited for. Of course, most applicants will only attend the medical school that accepts them and may not have much choice. But during interviews, you will be expected to show an understanding of how your learning skills can be applied to the course curriculum. Now let's look at each course structure in a little more detail.

> You may think that you can find the following information online and on each medical school's website, and you'd be exactly right. This is why we have only provided a basic introduction to the learning styles so you get used to what each one refers to, and we urge you to check the medical schools' websites individually for any recent changes or innovations. Course curriculum can be updated very often, and you want to make sure you are aware of the latest changes that set one medical school apart from another.
>
> **Dr Navin Nagesh, Academic Doctor, Oxford University**

TRADITIONAL COURSE

This has been the structure of medical education for hundreds of years and has produced many Nobel Prize-winning physicians and surgeons. It follows the philosophy that one must understand medicine before practicing medicine. Students in this course structure will spend 2 years studying basic medical sciences with research techniques to develop a firm foundation of knowledge. This is delivered primarily by lectures, tutorials, laboratory sessions and dissections. This is followed by 3 years of clinical medicine with patient contact, supplemented by lectures and modules that you will study alongside. This type of course structure is slowly being phased out of medical schools as emphasis is being placed on patient-centred care; only Oxford and Cambridge medical schools still offer the classic course structure.

INTEGRATED SYSTEMS-BASED COURSE

The majority of UK medical schools use this course structure. This incorporates the integration of medical theory, clinical application and practice together so that students can apply their knowledge during their learning process. The GMC recommends this type of learning, as it combines many aspects of medicine such as anatomy, physiology and pathology into one focus, such as the cardiovascular system. This allows students to focus fully within this system and learn the clinically relevant aspects through lectures, small group sessions and clinical skills sessions.

PROBLEM-BASED LEARNING COURSE

This is the most patient-centred approach of any course structure, as students are exposed to patients from the very beginning of the course. Example medical cases are given to students to work on in a small group to identify the relevant key aspects, for example, the development of questions to study the anatomy, physiology, pathophysiology, pharmacology and social impacts of the case. Students generally have 1 to 2 weeks to conduct self-directed learning study on these topics and report back to the group for formal discussion. This is an almost entirely student-led approach supplemented by lectures and clinical skills sessions to ensure that all aspects are covered.

CASE-BASED LEARNING COURSE

This type of learning is very similar to problem-based learning; the key difference is that rather than a specific patient case study, there is a range of cases focusing on a particular problem. Students have 2 to 3 weeks to conduct self-directed learning for the cases; they will simultaneously attend seminars, lectures, dissection, clinical skills sessions and small group learning to facilitate their learning. The small group sessions are led by experts in the particular fields. There is a wrap-up session at the end of the case period where the key messages are discussed and reflections are made on how it may affect their future clinical practice.

Now you have been introduced to the main types of learning, let's see what types of learning medical schools employ (Table 3.2). Please note, these are subject to change each and every single year, so do make sure you check for updates on the official websites.

> During my medical school interview training, I asked myself, 'Why do I want to study at this particular medical school?' My answer mainly concerned the curriculum's learning style. I gave examples of how I worked in teams and enjoyed communicating my ideas in group projects, and therefore I would enjoy a PBL learning style through medical school. It's very important to give real-life examples to provide some context for your answers.
>
> **Claudia Young, Medical School Applicant**

CAREER PROGRESSION FOR UK DOCTORS

Congratulations, you're now a doctor!

We will now look at the career progression of doctors in the UK. You may be wondering, this is so far into the future, 'I'm just trying to get into medical school!' But it's very important that prospective medical students are aware of the career pathways and appreciate that medicine is a lifelong learning process. So let's imagine we have just finished medical school and are looking to get formal registration to practice as a doctor. Let's meet the General Medical Council (GMC).

WHAT DOES THE GMC DO?

- Maintains a register of qualified doctors
- Disciplines, suspends and rehabilitates doctors
- Regulates doctors' fitness to practice
- Monitors complaints against doctors by patients

Table 3.2 Medical Schools by Course Type

	TRADITIONAL	INTEGRATED	PBL	CBL
Aberdeen		✓		
Anglia Ruskin		✓		
Aston		✓		
Barts (Queen Mary, University of London)			✓	
Birmingham		✓		
Brighton and Sussex		✓		
Bristol		✓		
Brunel			✓	
Buckingham		✓		
Cambridge	✓			
Cardiff				✓
Dundee		✓		
Chester				✓
Edge Hill		✓		
Edinburgh		✓		
Exeter		✓		
Glasgow		✓		
Hull York			✓	
Imperial		✓		
Keele		✓		
Kent and Medway		✓		
King's College London		✓		
Lancaster			✓	
Leeds		✓		
Leicester		✓		
Liverpool		✓		
Manchester			✓	
Newcastle		✓		
Norwich (East Anglia)		✓		
Nottingham		✓		
Nottingham Lincoln			✓	
Oxford	✓			
Plymouth			✓	
Queen's Belfast	✓			
Sheffield		✓		
Southampton		✓		
St Andrews		✓		
St George's		✓		
Sunderland		✓		
Swansea		✓		
Ulster			✓	
University College London		✓		
University of Central Lancashire		✓		
Warwick			✓	

'To Protect, Promote and Maintain the Health and Safety of the Public'—Principles of the GMC

The GMC is the main regulatory body of doctors in the NHS. It ensures the highest level of quality and safety of medical practice in the UK. They are also heavily involved in the regulation of the UK medical school curriculum and have published a number of recommendations for both students and teachers. They also provide the key competencies and outcomes that graduates of medical school should be expected to accomplish throughout their training. The GMC have the following key publications that you should ideally read before your medical school interview. These can be found on the official GMC website, www.gmc-uk.org:

- Outcomes for graduates
- Promoting excellence: Standards for medical education and training

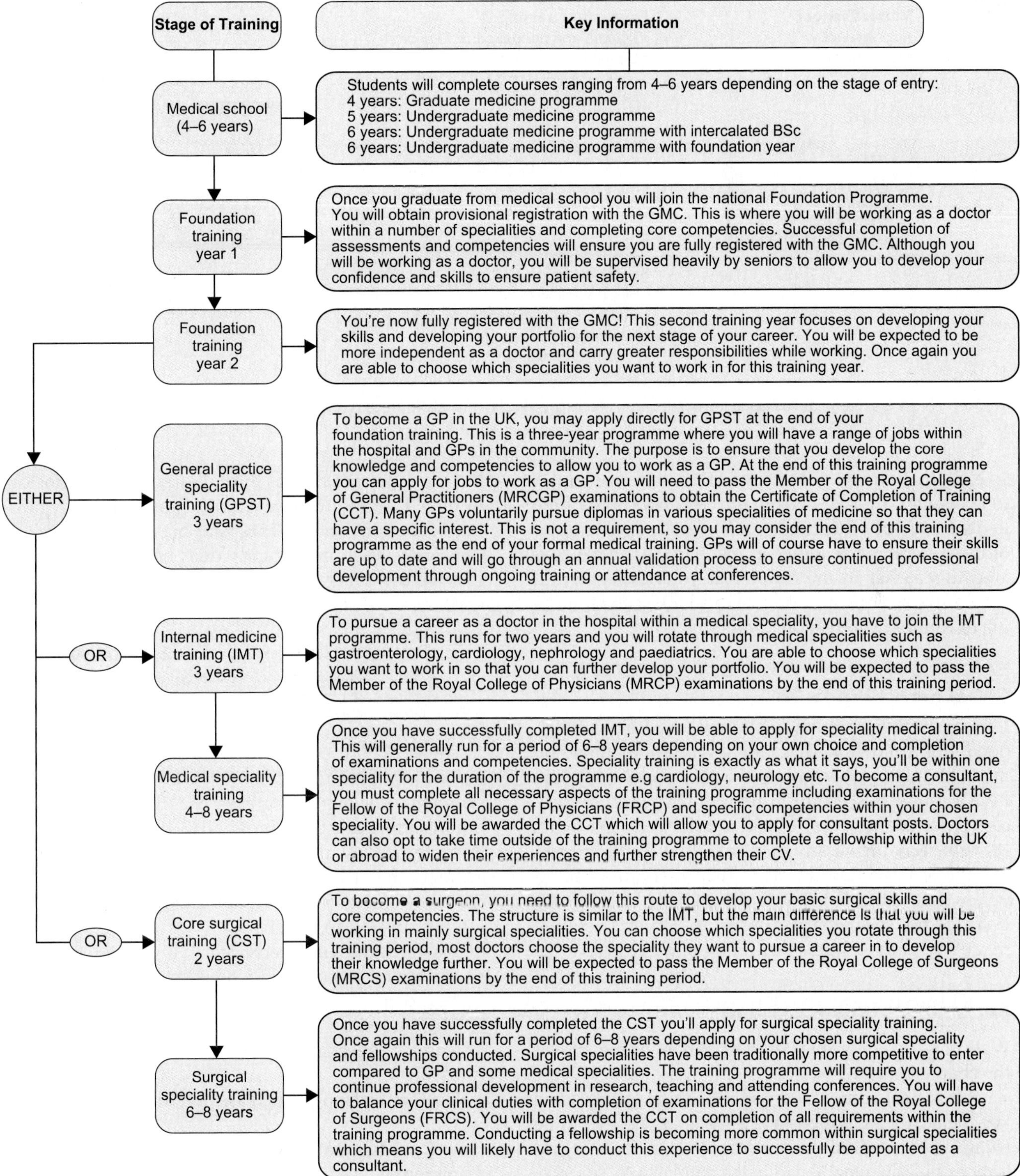

Fig. 3.5 Medical school and foundation years; core training in surgery, medicine and GP. *CCT*, Certificate of Completion of Training; *GMC*, General Medical Council; *GP*, general practice.

- Achieving good medical practice: Guidance for medical students
- Professional behaviour and fitness to practice: Guidance for medical schools and their students

Of course, there is no need to memorise all of the information in these publications, but it is important that you are aware of the basic standards required for UK medical school graduates and the professional behaviour expected.

Now, you may be wondering, how do I get registered with the GMC so I can start my career? This is a good question. We will now take you on a journey from medical school to becoming a GP, medical consultant, surgical consultant and alternative career paths doctors can take (Fig. 3.5).

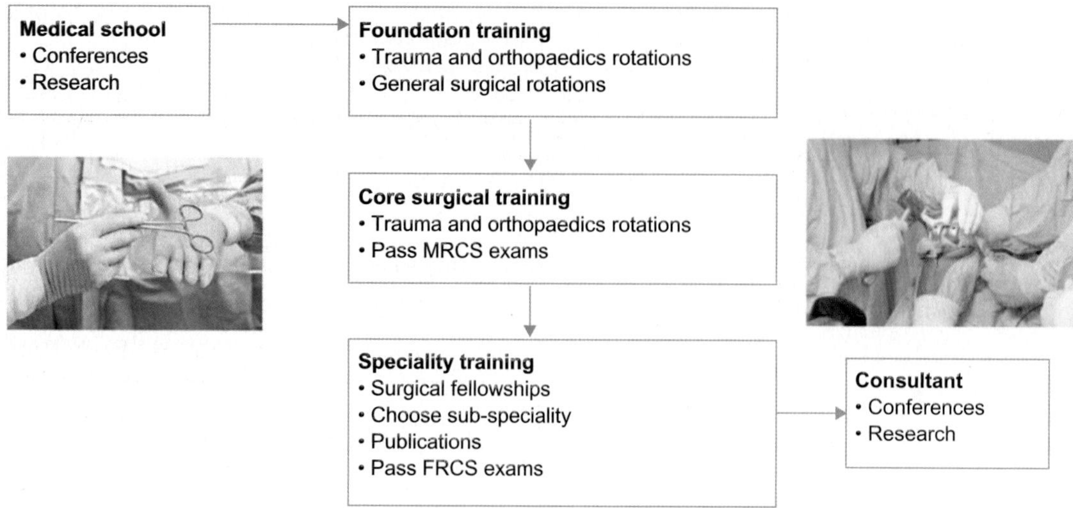

Fig. 3.6 Diagram illustrating the path to orthopaedic surgery. *FRCS*, Fellow of the Royal College of Surgeons; *MRCS*, Member of the Royal College of Surgeons.

Now that you've got an idea of the different routes to becoming a GP or consultant, let's take some time to dream of your future career! If you need a reminder of the different specialities in medicine, we have covered this earlier in the chapter. If you're unsure and would like some inspiration, take a look at the following examples from real doctors.

EXAMPLE OF AN ORTHOPAEDIC SURGEON'S CAREER PROGRESSION

I am a fourth-year medical student and I have developed this following diagram (Fig. 3.6) to illustrate my ambitions of becoming an orthopaedic surgeon. I have found this useful in reminding me of the process required and what I need to achieve to get there. I would recommend any medical school applicant create one of these flow charts to help them understand where they will be 5 or 10 years from now! Don't worry if you're not sure what you want to do yet, I actually made five of these at the beginning of medical school.

KEY MEDICAL ORGANISATIONS

Well done—keep going—you're almost at the end of the chapter!

In this final section, we will introduce you to some key medical organisations in the UK that you should be aware of as a medical student and a doctor. These organisations play an integral part in the regulation of practice, medical research and publication of medical literature and collectively are a forum for discussion in medicine. As a prospective applicant, you can gain an appreciation of these organisations and how they can help you as a future doctor, but they also allow you to learn more about current affairs in UK medical practice.

BRITISH MEDICAL ASSOCIATION

The British Medical Association (BMA) is a professional association and registered trade union for doctors in the UK. They are seen as the collective voice of doctors in the UK in discussions with the government regarding economics and politics that may affect the NHS. This association importantly does not regulate or certify doctors' practices; this responsibility belongs to the GMC as we discussed earlier.

> The British Medical Association does not regulate or certify doctors, a responsibility which lies with the General Medical Council.

As of 2022, there were 160,000 doctors and 20,000 medical student members of the BMA. The UK government officially recognises the BMA as the only organisation that represents NHS doctors. Therefore, they are heavily involved in discussions with the government regarding changes to working conditions, contracts and employee rights. The BMA offers the following support to members:

- Expert employment advice
- Advice for job planning, pay disputes and personal relations
- BMA provides assistance to doctors in the armed forces represented by the Armed Forces Committee (AFC)
- Doctors working in private practice

How Can You Get Involved as a Medical School Applicant?

- Visit https://www.bma.org.uk.
- Click under the 'Medical Student' tab, and you'll find current news and updates relevant to medical students.
- Click under the 'Patient and Public' tab, and you'll find current news and updates targeted at the lay audience.

THE BRITISH MEDICAL JOURNAL

The *British Medical Journal* (*BMJ*) is a peer-reviewed medical journal published on a weekly basis. It is considered one of the oldest and most prestigious journals. The journal's primary focus is to provide high-quality, evidence-based medical publications that can be accessed globally. It is available online and in print in the full *BMJ* journal and student *BMJ* versions. The *BMJ* also hosts events for healthcare professionals in the UK and internationally. The *BMJ* also provides other service, such as BMJ Careers and BMJ Learning to support members in employment and education.

Significant events in the *BMJ* timeline:

- 1840: *Provincial Medical and Surgical Journal* (later renamed the *British Medical Journal*) first published
- 1847: James Simpson uses the journal to publicise chloroform, which paved the way for modern anaesthetic techniques
- 1867: Joseph Lister publishes his introduction to the concept of antiseptic in wound healing
- 1950: Richard Doll publishes his discovery of the link between tobacco consumption and lung cancer
- 1958: Alice Stewart publishes her study of the risks of low-level radiation
- 1995: First website for the BMJ.com

How Can You Get Involved as a Medical School Applicant?

- Subscribe to the student *BMJ* to follow the latest discussions for medical students.
- Learn the common research trends in the UK.
- Find out about courses aimed at medical school applicants from the *BMJ* events tab.

As an applicant, the full *BMJ* was far too complicated and didn't seem relevant to me. But I was able to get hold of the *BMJ* student version and this was an excellent resource! Some editions have specific advice for medical school applicants such as writing a good personal statement, interview techniques and current issues in the NHS that we should be aware of. I would highly recommend anyone applying to medical school to subscribe.

Claudia Young, Medical School Applicant

THE NATIONAL INSTITUTE FOR HEALTH AND CARE EXCELLENCE

The National Institute for Health and Care Excellence (NICE) is a very important organisation in the UK that provides doctors with guidance and advice to improve the health and social care of patients. NICE acts as an external agency with the agenda of promoting clinical excellence by developing evidence-based guidance and recommendations for treatment and medical procedures for NHS England and Wales. If you are asked what the role of NICE is within the UK, you should ideally remember the following points:

- Development of evidence-based guidance for healthcare professionals in the management of disease.
- High-quality advice for health and social care professionals in long-term patient management.
- Development of quality standards and performance analysis of healthcare, public and social care services in the UK.
- Online information service platforms to allow individuals involved in patient care access to high-quality information and data including:
  - NICE Evidence Search for high-quality evidence-based medicine.
  - British National Formulary for providing up-to-date information on medications, dosages, interactions and complications.
- Medication and prescribing support.

How Can You Get Involved as a Medical School Applicant?

- Visit the NICE website: https://www.nice.org.uk.
- Click on the 'Clinical Knowledge Summaries' tab to find basic information regarding 330 common presentations of diseases in patients. Skimming through the presentation and management of a handful of these diseases will allow you to understand the importance of evidence-based medicine and the multidisciplinary nature of patient care.
- You could bring this up in your medical school interview, although please make sure you know the topic you mention inside out, otherwise they might pick on you!

When you're a clinical year medical student, NICE guidelines become your main source of information on how we should manage patients. They basically tell doctors what treatment or management plan patients should get based on the best available evidence. This is very useful, as there is usually a flowchart showing us different treatment options and when to use it. As an applicant, you should probably check out the management of asthma and diabetes, or any long-term condition for that matter! It will be a great talking point for the interview.

Andrel Yoong, Medical Student, Exeter Medical School

THE CARE QUALITY COMMISSION

The Care Quality Commission (CQC) is an independent regulator for health and social care in England. Imagine that they are the inspectors who go into hospitals, care homes, GP surgeries and dentist offices to ensure the care provided is high quality and effective. The CQC is a very important organisation that ensures patient safety in the NHS. They will provide detailed improvements and refinements for services if they are not the absolute best. The following ratings are used to provide services with a grade for their performance:

- Outstanding
- Good
- Requires Improvement
- Inadequate

To determine the appropriate rating for the healthcare service, they ask the following key questions:

- Is the service safe?
- Is the service effective?
- Is the service caring?
- Is the service responsive to people's needs?
- Is the service well led?

The ratings are published regularly on the CQC website, free for both healthcare professionals and the public to view.

Now, let's talk about what happens if a healthcare service is deemed 'Inadequate' and doesn't answer the five questions in a satisfactory manner. The CQC will label the service 'Special Measures', which requires action from the providers. The purpose of this state is to:

- Provide key recommendations for improvements.
- Give a clear time frame in which the healthcare providers need to show this improvement.
- Reassess the service to ensure that the recommendations have been satisfactorily implemented.

The CQC is an invaluable organisation that ensures both healthcare providers and staff are constantly working towards quality improvement and patient safety, to maintain the NHS's status as one of the best healthcare services in the world.

How Can You Get Involved as a Medical School Applicant?

- Visit the CQC website: http://www.cqc.org.uk.
- Click on the 'For Public' tab to find the latest news and learn more about how the CQC assesses healthcare services.
- Check the latest results of inspections to find out which healthcare services are deemed inadequate and see what measures have been put in place for improvement.

SUMMARY, TEST YOURSELF AND REFLECTION

Well done! You've successfully completed this chapter. The NHS is very complex, and you are not expected to know all information in-depth; a good overview as provided in this chapter can help you shine during the interview and may be the deciding factor in securing a place at medical school. It makes sense to be asked about the NHS: You'll be part of it one day. Furthermore, the NHS will be your employer.

It is important to remember that:

- The NHS structure and core values are key.
- There are three types of medical courses: integrated systems based, problem based and case based.
- The NHS and medical school training are complemented by several medical organisations, including the BMA, GMC, NICE, CQC, Royal Colleges and many more.

Reflecting on what you've learnt from this chapter is very important for your medical school application process. Having a basic understanding of how the NHS works, how doctors progress through their career, and organisations that are involved in medicine is essentially the most basic requirement when it comes to interviews. A box for reflection and ideas has been provided here so you can jot down any thoughts you may have. We've provided a few pointers to get you started.

Test Yourself

- How can the BMA help you as a medical student and a doctor? Think about your career progression and support during times of difficulty!
- Write or draw how the Health & Social Care Act reformed the structure of the NHS.
- In the history of the NHS, what do you remember as the most memorable developments/changes?

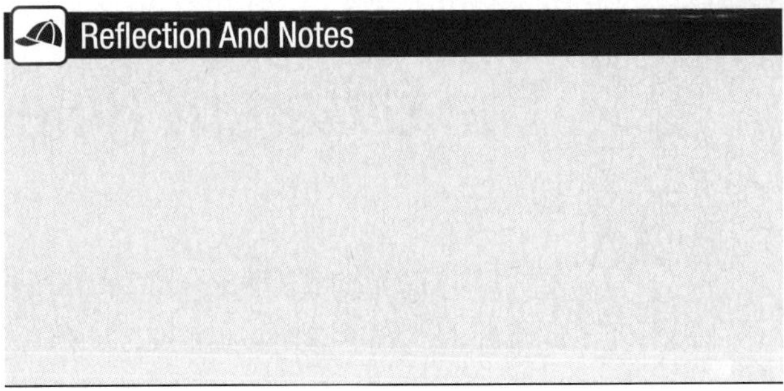

RESOURCES

BBC Health News. Available at http://www.bbc.co.uk/news/health.

British Medical Association. Available at https://www.bma.org.uk.

Care Quality Commission. Available at http://www.cqc.org.uk/.

General Medical Council. Available at www.gmc-uk.org.

NHS history. Available at https://www.nhs.uk/NHSEngland/thenhs/nhshistory/Pages/the-nhs%20history.aspx.

The BMJ. Student. Available at http://student.bmj.com/student/student-bmj.html.

The National Institute for Health and Care Excellence. Available at https://www.nice.org.uk.

NHS Choices. History of the NHS. Available at https://www.nhs.uk/NHSEngland/thenhs/nhshistory/Pages/the-nhs%20history.aspx.

4 The Different Roles of a Doctor

Bogdan Chiva Giurca, Ida Saidy and Alisha Sharif

Chapter Outline

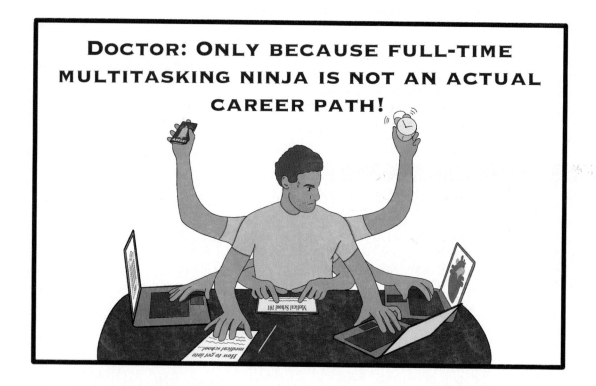

THE DIFFERENT ROLES OF A DOCTOR

Many times, when we say the word 'doctor', we imagine a person wearing a white coat with a stethoscope hanging around their neck, running around the hospital and jumping on peoples' chests to save their lives. This is, however, far from the truth—very far in fact, since white coats are not even used anymore in the UK, but that's not the point I wanted to make.

Depending on the setting, doctors wear different masks. Often, when asking students or the public about the duties of a doctor, we only (or mostly) hear things related to their clinical job. Doctors take histories, prescribe pills and carry out life-saving operations, yes, and we hear that doctors perform exotic tests and get to the bottom of rare medical cases (I think this latter group have watched the TV series 'House M.D.' a bit too much). It is not until students join medical school that they realise the other duties a doctor has.

The UK General Medical Council (GMC) has put together a document entitled *'Tomorrow's Doctors'*. This is essentially the holy bible of medical school, as it contains all the roles and responsibilities of student doctors in medical school and later on in the hospital as graduates. Here are some of the duties described by the GMC:

Doctors as Practitioners. No shock here, I hope. This is what everyone thinks doctors are meant to be doing. It is still, however, totally understandable given that doctors should place patients at the centre of their care.

Doctors as Scholars and Researchers. Hang on, did someone say research? But, but… I thought that's what biosciences or genetics students do? You would be surprised how often we hear that comment, not only from medical school applicants but also from medical students early on in their medical school training. Very often medical school students ask their colleagues interested in research whether they do it because they want to pursue a career as a scientist. Having an understanding of medical research from an early stage is key to getting into medical school. How about doctors as scholars? Well, this also shouldn't come as a surprise, given that the word 'doctor' comes from a verb in Latin which literally means 'to teach'. Doctors, therefore, have a duty to pass on knowledge and to teach.

Doctors as Teachers. As a doctor progresses through their training and gains more and more exposure to different patients with unique presentations, their 'bank' of what works best grows and grows. This allows them to be able to share their 'bank' with students and trainees, who do not have as much experience with patients, but rather have learnt the more theoretical sides of medicine first. Doctors can also teach other healthcare professionals, and vice versa. Inter- and multidisciplinary learning is crucial and so is realising that the doctor does not know it all but is rather supported by several colleagues within the healthcare setting. Doctors can also share their knowledge in an accessible way with the general public to equip them with the skills to either prevent illness from happening or manage their own illness and deal with emergency situations that may arise.

Doctors as Leaders and Managers. Leadership and management? Hang on, are we still talking about medicine or about business and management? This is another branch that shocks medical school applicants. What would happen if all healthcare decisions were made by politicians? Healthcare needs young, enthusiastic minds who are ready to challenge the system in order to benefit the patient. Having a basic understanding of how services are run, and getting involved in improving service quality, is key in medicine.

Doctors as Agents of Change. Doctors have much responsibility to stay on top of current medical advancements and implement these changes in their day-to-day practice. As well as being clinicians, researchers and teachers, doctors can influence and inform members of the public about different aspects of healthcare. Furthermore, doctors have to actively initiate change that is in the best interest of patient care and treatment. As agents of change, they should explore different perspectives and aim to develop healthcare by facilitating action among their colleagues and the public. This can be done by considering the different social, environmental, economic and environmental factors that impact patient health, not just their biological symptoms. Doctors have to remain observant of their patient populations to pick up on patterns and act on them accordingly, to ensure patients get the care and treatment that they deserve.

Doctors as Professionals. Although not commonly spoken about, the duty of being professional while undertaking your role as a medical student and doctor is assumed. We all carry the duty to respect our colleagues and patients, and to not act in ways that would make the public lose trust in us. To make things easier, we have summed up these roles and responsibilities, and we will take each of them one by one, outlining the key concepts that will prepare you to impress medical admission tutors. We won't dwell too much on the role of a doctor as a clinician, practitioner and professional, as these have been mainly outlined in the medical ethics chapter.

DOCTORS AS PRACTITIONERS

The duty of doctors as practitioners as summarised by the GMC is pretty much what good doctors have done and will always do. Fig. 4.1 provides a glimpse into the key responsibilities of clinicians.

Carry out consultations successfully and effectively
2
Diagnose and manage diseases
3
Communicate effectively with patients and colleagues

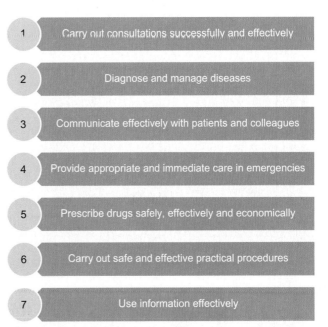

Provide appropriate and immediate care in emergencies
5
Prescribe drugs safely, effectively and economically
6
Carry out safe and effective practical procedures
7
Use information effectively

Fig. 4.1 Key responsibilities of doctors as practitioners, according to the UK General Medical Council.

DOCTORS AS SCHOLARS AND RESEARCHERS

The discovery of DNA, insulin, antibiotics or unmasking a new illness—each one of these revolutionary discoveries (some of which we covered in detail in Chapter 2) was only possible through research. Research has played a key role throughout history and has been with us since the dawn of humanity. From ancient Greece to the Middle Ages, up to the 21st century, physicians have experimented with new techniques and methods for improving human life expectancy and overall quality.

Fig. 4.2, adapted from the BBC archives, fully emphasises the dramatic shift and improvement in life expectancy throughout history.

There are several ways in which medical research can help patients and the healthcare system. In simple terms, medical research can facilitate the:

a) **Prevention** of a disease
b) **Diagnosis** of a disease
c) **Care** of a disease
d) **Cure** of a disease
e) **Cause** of a disease
f) **Link** between diseases
g) **Patterns** of disease

Okay, okay—you probably got it already, it's very important and all doctors should appreciate it, but how is this relevant to your medical school application? Or in other words … Why should you care?

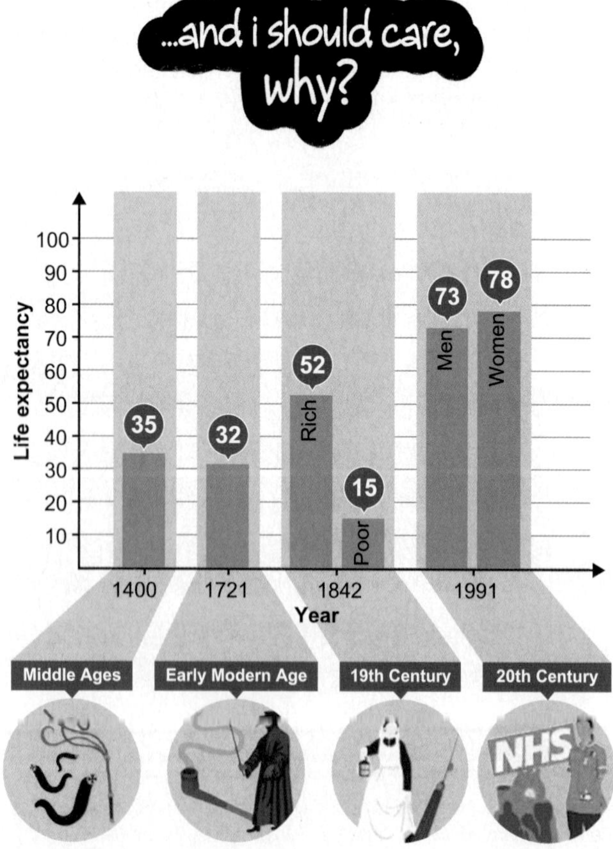

Fig. 4.2 Life expectancy through the ages.

Our experience has taught us that a good applicant is able to answer questions related to the importance of research in medicine, and to show awareness of a doctor's different responsibilities. This could be tested during the medical school interview or shown in your personal statement. Be careful though, too much emphasis on research and you may be asked, 'Why not get a degree in biomedical sciences if you're so passionate about research?' We'll save this question for later in our Interview chapter.

Research is a compulsory part of undergraduate medical programmes in the UK. This is mostly in the form of 'Student Selected Components' or 'Special Study Units'. These are a couple of weeks where you are assigned to a specific field and supervisor of your choice, and have to undertake a short research project—either by looking at existing literature and analysing it or by doing hands-on investigations in the clinic or lab.

> Perhaps more important than doing research is **understanding** it. This way you can follow the best treatment or best practice to date. Please don't feel overwhelmed by the various research terms. As long as you understand the basic principles, there's no need for a formal definition.

Several medical schools in the UK also offer the opportunity to do an extra year to complete a BSc degree in an area of your interest. Many medical schools have this year already integrated it into their curriculum. Examples include University College London, Oxford and Cambridge Medical Schools. Instead of 5 years, they offer a 6-year programme that integrates an extra year for research. Being aware of these opportunities is key to scoring Brownie points at the end of the interview when you may be asked if you have any questions regarding their medicine programme.

To further emphasise the importance of understanding the role of research in medical school, find further in the chapter the official guidelines from the UK GMC.

Medical students are tomorrow's doctors; they are expected to be able to apply biomedical scientific principles, methods and knowledge to medical practice. Graduates are expected to:

1. Critically appraise (i.e. analyse something with a critical mind) the results of relevant medical research papers present in the scientific literature (i.e. stay curious and question everything).
2. Formulate simple, relevant research questions in the fields of:
   - biomedical science;
   - psychosocial science; and
   - population science

   … and successfully design experiments to address their questions.
3. Apply findings from scientific literature to answer questions raised by clinical problems (i.e. don't just Google symptoms like the rest of the population!).

4. Understand the ethical issues involved in medical research (e.g. patients must consent to taking part in research, don't just assume they are happy to do so) (GMC, 2009).

Hang on, did they just say GRADUATES? But graduation seems like a very long time away, right? So why bother now? Because admission tutors want to make sure that you have researched online and know clearly where you are heading. They don't want you to join the medical school to later find out that you hate research or worse, that you don't understand its purpose in medicine.

You would be surprised at how many of our students and colleagues are reluctant to accept the positive benefits of research to medicine. There is a common misconception among medical students that doctors only see patients, and that if they wanted to do research, they should have joined a science course. The truth is all doctors do research at some point in their careers.

By understanding the purpose of research at this point, you can easily prove during the interview or personal statement that you have clearly explored your career path and see yourself in the future, not only as a doctor, but also as a researcher, teacher, leader and innovator.

> I did my A-level Extended Project Qualification research project on depression and the impact of social media on teenagers. I wasn't sure how to bring this up in my medical school interview, but when I learned about the various roles of a doctor, I thought this might be a way to illustrate my understanding of the subject.
>
> During my interview at UCL I had the chance to talk about doctors as researchers and how I had already started working on this during my EPQ. The panel complimented my answer and seemed to enjoy that I saw doctors as more than just clinicians!
>
> **Marie, Medical School Applicant**

> Other benefits that come from doing research include the development of teamwork and leadership skills. You learn not only to work with a team, but also to work towards deadlines, deliver presentations and write scientifically. You also have the opportunity to think critically and find answers for yourself. The answer 'because that's what it says in the textbook' or 'that's how things are done' simply isn't good enough.
>
> **Dr Zeshan Qureshi, Paediatric Registrar**

Enough with what you should do, however. Let's focus now on some research terminology. As boring as this may be, I am afraid you must have a basic understanding of some of these concepts.

RESEARCH TERMINOLOGY

To get you started, the following table includes a description of each type of research design, their advantages and disadvantages and when that particular type of design should be used (Table. 4.1).

Although we don't think you should know any specifics regarding study design and research methodology yet, we have had students encounter questions about this in their interviews. Therefore, we thought we'd prepare you for the worst-case scenario!

> Research affects all doctors' practices, from a primary care physician in a rural practice to a professor in a large teaching hospital. Knowing how a clinical problem is translated into a research question is a challenge that both clinicians and researches need to be involved in.
>
> **Dr Zeshan Qureshi, Paediatric Registrar**

CLINICAL AUDITS

A clinical audit is defined as a quality improvement process that seeks to improve patient care and outcomes through a systematic review of care against explicit criteria, and the implementation of change. In other words, assess the current situation, create a study to examine your performance, compare your performance to the national standards, reflect and make some changes, then re-audit to examine your progress.

The following diagram should make things easier (Fig. 4.3).

CLINICAL TRIALS

These are studies to evaluate the safety and effectiveness of medical devices and medication. They are conducted by monitoring the effects of drugs or devices on large groups of people. Depending on their size and expected outcome, clinical trials are usually structured over three or more phases (Fig. 4.4). Before the start of the clinical trial, several studies must be undertaken to prove the safety of the drug/device in a controlled laboratory environment. If it receives approval, it moves into the first phase of the project. If, for example, the drug is considered safe during the first phase, it gets approval to reach the second phase, which includes a larger population, and so on until the end of the clinical trial.

Qualitative vs Quantitative Research

The differences between qualitative and quantitative research are summarised in Fig. 4.5.

Retrospective vs Prospective Studies

An easy way to remember and distinguish between these two is by looking at their names: 'Pro' + spective vs 'Retro' + spective.

Pro = pro-ceeding or pro-jecting forward. Prospective studies look for an outcome in the future. Prospective studies examine the development of disease over time and into the future. For example, you can design a study where you examine the impact of smoking on the development of lung cancer.

Table 4.1 **Different Types of Research**

TYPE OF RESEARCH	DESCRIPTION	ADVANTAGES	DISADVANTAGES	WHEN IT IS USED
Case report/case series	A report or series of reports on the disease presentation or treatment effect in an individual	Possibility of contacting individuals for further information is probably easier than in larger study designs Low cost Quick to complete	Unlikely to be representative of the entire population Inferences about prevalence or causality are difficult to establish	For rare diseases, rare presentations of diseases, new treatments or new reactions to known treatments for a disease
Ecological study	Comparison of different populations that have different exposures (e.g. high vs low air pollution)	Practical because participants do not have to be uprooted to be put into a different study group May be able to use existing data	No randomisation to each study group so populations may differ in characteristics other than the exposure	Useful for studying relationships involving the natural environment (e.g. relationship between lead in water supply and cancer) or in behaviour (e.g. salt intake in urban or rural populations)
Cross-sectional study	An outcome is studied in a representative sample of the population as a snapshot in time	Relatively cheap Results are generalisable to the source population	Will naturally exclude the most severe/fatal disease presentations Causality is difficult to establish in a snapshot	Good for measuring prevalence of disease and disease risk factors
Case control study	Comparison of people with the disease/outcome (e.g. Cushing's disease) with another population (e.g. those without Cushing's disease) in terms of their exposure to possible risk factors	Good for studying uncommon diseases, where you would need to follow up a very large population sample to observe even a few cases Relatively quick and cheap to perform	Identification of a suitable control group may be difficult Susceptible to bias (such as recall bias) Less strong causal evidence as more difficult to establish that exposure preceded outcome	Useful for establishing associations with a disease or risk factor
Cohort study	A population with a range of risk factors is followed up at multiple time points	Produces large amounts of data over a lifetime Information about exposures (risk factors) is collected before outcomes happen, so concerns about temporal relation of exposure to outcome is less of a problem	Expensive and time-consuming Difficult to prevent loss to follow up	Good for identifying premorbid markers of a disease, measuring prevalence of disease and determining disease risk factors

Economic evaluation	Comparison of the relative cost of one intervention over another, relative to the gains	Provides objective data to inform healthcare decision makers	Can be complex to calculate, and data may be difficult to obtain	Useful for healthcare planning since different interventions can be compared in terms of value for money
Qualitative research	Describing and understanding phenomena that are not easily summarised by numbers (e.g. exploring why people behave in a certain way)	Helpful to understand participant perspectives in relatively unexplored areas Studies can evolve based on initial results, allowing new data to be continually collected from different sources until the researcher is satisfied	Difficult to compare two qualitative studies because the methodology varies so much Difficult to validate the quality of data collection and analysis	Useful for exploring behaviour and understanding social phenomena
Randomised controlled trial	One group in the trial receives an intervention (e.g. medical treatment) and the other group receives a different intervention (e.g. placebo, alternative treatment). The allocation to groups is controlled by the investigator, and participants may be blinded	Allows blinding of participants, so that the results are not affected by participant knowledge of intervention Randomisation means that groups should be similar, allowing comparison of 'intervention' with 'no intervention' to be made meaningfully	Expensive May be difficult to recruit sufficient numbers May be difficult to ensure adequate blinding and complete follow-up	Excellent for looking at the effects of a new treatment for a known disease, or looking at primary preventative measures
Systematic review/ meta-analysis	Combines information from multiple independent studies to estimate the true effect size. Systematic reviews do this in a descriptive manner, whereas meta-analysis combines the data from multiple studies to get an overall effect	Ability to quantify and analyse the inconsistencies occurring across a series of similar studies Results can be generalised to a large population, but also contain subgroup analysis to cover atypical groups of the population Relatively cheap Regarded as the highest level of evidence	Meta-analysis of several small studies does not always predict the results of a single large study File-drawer problem: publication bias occurs due to the lack of published negative/insignificant results (though there are methods to assess this) It is possible to manipulate the results of a meta-analysis by cherry-picking favourable studies while excluding others	Best used to determine the true effect size in fields where some studies reject the null hypothesis and others do not

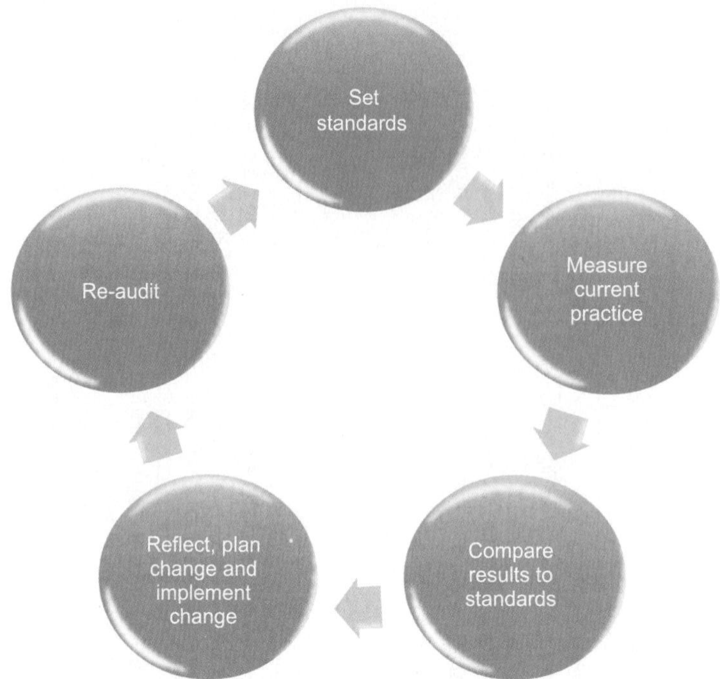

Fig. 4.3 Audit process.

Pre-clinical

Preclinical trial is designed for asssessment of safety, toxicity, pharmacodynamic and pharmacokinetic information

Phase 1

Drug or treatment is given to a small group of people (20–100) to evaluate its safety and identify side effects and safe dosage range

Phase 2

Drug or treatment is given to a medium group of people (100–500) for further evaluation

Phase 3

Drug or treatment is given to a larger group of people (300–3000) to evaluate its safety

Phase 4

Postmarketing studies delineate additional information including the drug risk, benefits and optimal use

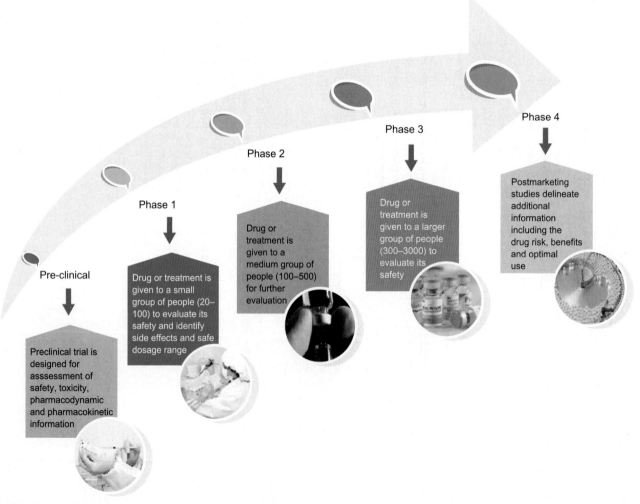

Fig. 4.4 Phases of research.

Qualitative	Quantitative
• Focusing on quality • Measuring feelings, opinions	• Focusing on quantity • Measuring numbers
In other words, you care more about *what* people think!	In other words, you care more about *how many* people think!
e.g. 1. What is it like to live with a condition/ disease?	e.g. 1. How many people in the UK want to give up smoking?
e.g. 2. How do you feel about this treatment?	
Methods • Interviews • Discussion groups • Focus groups	Methods • Objective measurements • Statistical/mathematical • Surveys, questionaire and polls

Fig. 4.5 Qualitative vs quantitative research.

Retro = backwards. Retrospective studies examine things that have already happened. For example, you may have access to a database of patients who died due to lung cancer. Hence, you can design a study to assess the risk factors that might have led to lung cancer in the first place.

In simple terms, you either examine things over time or look at things that have already happened.

EVIDENCE-BASED MEDICINE

The words 'evidence-based' have been used extensively over the present century. You will often hear great leaders talking about interventions or treatments that are 'evidence-based'. Quite often, these words are not only used for medicine but go beyond the domain of healthcare altogether. Variations of these words include (but are not limited to) evidence-based procedures, evidence-based practice, evidence-based social care, evidence-based teaching or evidence-based policy.

As the words suggest, each of the previous terms is based on the same core principles. These principles refer to making informed decisions based on accurate evidence. For example, in medicine, you would prescribe aspirin to someone who has had a heart attack because there is enough evidence (i.e. several studies and research) suggesting that aspirin reduces the clumping effect (i.e. stickiness) of platelets, therefore decreasing the risk of a future heart attack.

In medicine, each decision taken on behalf of, or together with, patients should be backed up by relevant evidence. One simple definition is:

Evidence-based medicine is the conscientious, explicit and judicious use of current best evidence in making decisions about the care of individual patients.

Let's take a minute to examine this definition so we can better understand the meaning of evidence-based medicine. Should the evidence be perfect and supporting? Of course not, as the definition suggests, we need to access the 'current, *best* evidence'—meaning the best evidence available at this point in time.

The definition also mentions making decisions about the care of **INDIVIDUAL** patients. This is key. As humans, we are all different from one another, not only in terms of genes, but also in terms of personal values. What may work for someone may not work for somebody else, and therefore, we should always make decisions based on individual cases and not a series of cases.

Most importantly, when possible, doctors should make decisions together with their patients—a concept known as 'shared decision-making'. By taking into consideration the values and wishes of the patient, you provide the best care available to them, as an individual.

DOCTORS AS TEACHERS

Did you know that the word 'doctore' in Latin basically translates as 'teacher'? The doctor's role as a teacher for students, trainees and the public is crucial. This role allows for the endless cycle of teaching that creates and perfects the good practice of doctors after training—one senior doctor trains a junior, who advances as a senior to train another junior and so on. This allows junior doctors to adjust from learning concepts theoretically in medical school to applying it to real-life, unique patients who sometimes have different presentations from what has been learnt. Needless to say, teaching starts as early as medical school (and for many of you even secondary school) through peer teaching and student-led conferences.

Furthermore, the role that a doctor has as a teacher not only applies to teaching other students or doctors. This also applies to teaching other healthcare professionals around them. This can manifest by sharing knowledge during a multidisciplinary team (MDT) meeting, or it can take place by teaching in a conference. This allows for the sharing of good practice across fields and characterises the teamwork that healthcare is known for!

Finally, doctors have a duty to teach and inform the general public. Public health campaigns throughout the years have proved to be extremely beneficial for teaching the public how to save their lives, or the lives of others, in emergency situations. One example of this is the COVID-19 broadcasts that would keep the public updated on the pandemic, and also remind them of the symptoms of the disease and what can be done to stop the spread. Another example of this is the 'FAST' campaign, which teaches the main signs of a stroke so that the general public can contact emergency services immediately if they suspect one. Due to the life-threatening nature of a stroke, this can be extremely beneficial to increase survival rates. And this is just one example besides many, not to mention valuable teaching delivered by doctors regarding self-management of chronic conditions such as diabetes, mental health and cardiovascular disease, where patient involvement is crucial.

DOCTORS AS LEADERS AND MANAGERS

A common notion is that being a good doctor is just about being a good clinician. This is far from the truth. Being a good doctor also entails working effectively in teams, providing leadership to colleagues, and sharing a vision with the organisations and hospitals in which they work. You may be wondering—why do we all need to learn about leadership if only some of us will eventually become formal leaders accountable for the performance of our team, department or organisation? Well, the simple answer to this is that we are all leaders, and we all share the responsibility of leadership.

Let's clarify the previous statement further. Imagine yourself as a medical student during one of your surgical placements. While shadowing a surgeon, you get the opportunity to watch a leg amputation. If you're a geek, I bet you have already started shouting, 'Wow, how awesome!' Before the surgery, because you are a keen student, you go and have a chat with the patient to find out what happened and ask for permission to watch the surgery. You enjoy having a half-hour conversation with Mr Smith, and even help him prepare for the operation. Before the operation starts, you notice that the wrong leg has been marked for the procedure. The theatre assistants, anaesthetists, auxiliary nurses and other members of the team are ready to begin. No questions asked, no concerns raised. Your eyes and mouth open wide when you see the surgeon is ready to operate on the wrong leg. Convinced by your conversation with Mr Smith that the ***left*** leg was the problematic one, you raise your hand politely and raise your concerns.

'Erm … Excuse me Mr/Ms Surgeon, but from my conversation with Mr Smith, I know that the left leg should be amputated. I wanted to raise my concerns before you chop his leg off!' You may be wondering whether the surgeon will kick you out of the operating room, but instead, you will be happy to know that something like this could lead to you being known as a hero for the rest of your medical school training programme.

You see, this example simply illustrates how it doesn't matter who you are or what position you hold, as long as you are ready to SHARE the responsibility of LEADERSHIP. This concept is known as '**Shared Leadership**', and it simply means that the responsibility for identifying problems, solving them and implementing the appropriate action should be shared by the team as a whole.

> Shared leadership is crucial in healthcare. No matter what your role is (e.g. nurse, medical student, doctor, occupational therapist, etc.), you carry the responsibility to identify problems, solve them and implement the appropriate action. The safety of the patient ALWAYS comes first.

The GMC is pretty clear about the need for students and young doctors to learn about concepts such as medical leadership and management. They have even written a document for it entitled *'Leadership and Management for All Doctors'* (2012). The GMC states, 'Doctors are expected to offer leadership, and to work with others to change systems when it is necessary for the benefit of patients'. Other responsibilities include:

- Raising and acting on concerns locally and nationally
- Helping develop and improve services in local and national environments
- Effective planning, usage and management of resources within local and national organisations

Another model to be aware of is the *NHS Leadership Framework*, designed for medical students and doctors. According to the NHS Leadership Framework, individuals working in the NHS should be capable of (Fig. 4.6):

- Demonstrating personal qualities (i.e. you are responsible for your own development and progress)
- Working with others (i.e. you are responsible for being a good team member and leader)
- Managing services (i.e. you are responsible for contributing to ideas, planning and strengthening existing services)
- Improving services (i.e. you are responsible for encouraging transformation, innovation and improvement)

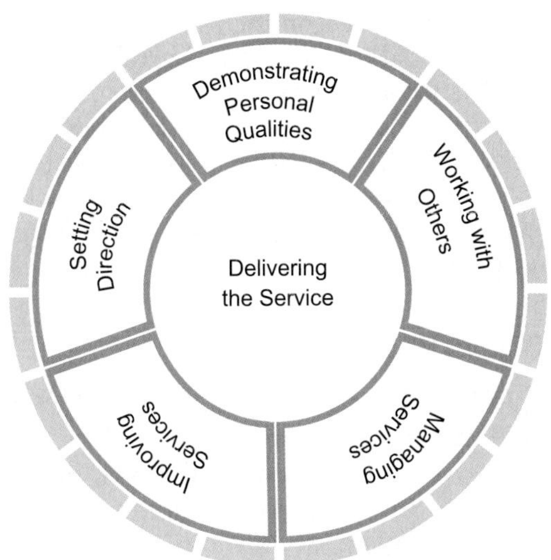

Fig. 4.6 Key components of delivering a service.

- Setting direction (i.e. you are responsible for making decisions, and applying evidence and knowledge to set future direction of services)

In the following, you will find a couple of examples of leadership at various stages of the medical career.

EXAMPLES OF LEADERSHIP IN MEDICINE

Undergraduate Stage

Third-year medical student Mandy was passionate about evidence-based medicine and wanted to improve the current way this concept was being taught at her medical school. Mandy decided to do a bit of research, took part in an audit to assess the quality of evidence-based medicine and then developed a whole teaching session based on her findings. Mandy shared the teaching session with senior academics from her medical school, who were happy for her to organise an extra teaching session for Year One and Year Two medical students.

Mandy successfully delivered her session and received positive feedback from her colleagues, who were eager to attend further sessions and get involved in promoting the concept of evidence-based medicine in the future. You can clearly see how Mandy helped develop and improve current educational materials at her medical school, therefore being a good leader and manager at her own institution.

Postgraduate Stage

Dr Cindy is a trainee in elderly care. In her hospital, there are numerous patients who are medically fit for discharge but, due to their home circumstances, remain in a hospital bed.

Her team on the ward, including physiotherapists, nutritionists and nurses, are always keen to help move such patients to other social services available, but the staff working in the community have done an initial assessment and think it may take several weeks or months before they can take care of each patient. Both parties meet up, but as you can imagine, the discussion is tense and leads to conflict between the two groups involved. Those working in the hospital blame community services and vice-versa.

Dr Cindy decides to take on an informal chairing role of future meetings between the community and hospital services in order to solve this problem. Dr Cindy successfully helps the team look at a range of ways to meet the individual needs of patients while also taking into consideration the limitations of each party. Dr Cindy bridges the gap between hospital and community services by acknowledging everyone's feelings, good intentions and concerns, and by helping them agree on a common point. Dr Cindy and her new team set goals that lead to the improvement of elderly care in her organisation.

Consultant Stage

Our final case is about Dr Apsey, who works as part of the Accident and Emergency (A&E) team in his hospital. One day, one of the patient's relatives complains to the hospital board about her sister, who was treated unfairly and ignored just because she was 'old and confused'. The relative apparently overheard a couple of upsetting comments from nurses and junior doctors, which indicated that her sister's condition was not taken seriously.

Dr Apsey was not appointed as the formal leader of the department, but he decided to assume responsibility and visited the family who made the complaint. Dr Apsey asked for feedback and apologised on behalf of the team. On his return, Dr Apsey involved his whole team in reviewing the attitudes of staff members towards confused patients. The team started a collaboration with the elder care department of the hospital. Together, both teams set up a series of workshops and feedback sessions on practices and policies designed to significantly improve the experience of the frail and elderly who are attending the A&E department.

Bonus Stage: School and College

We've added an extra example—the stage below undergraduate study, a stage through which YOU are going right now. Kiyara is a successful medical student at Bristol Medical School and also one of the authors of this book. She's originally from Sri Lanka and a few years ago she established a medical society at her previous school through which she delivered presentations and hosted debates and discussions for her peers who were hoping to get into medical school.

As you can see, you don't have to be a doctor to demonstrate leadership skills. When I was a student, nobody in my school even thought about having a medical society, although there were hundreds of students interested in studying medicine. Everybody lacked the vision, the motivation and the resources to do it. The resources are no longer a problem—we can help with that. I wish I did this when I was a medical school applicant.

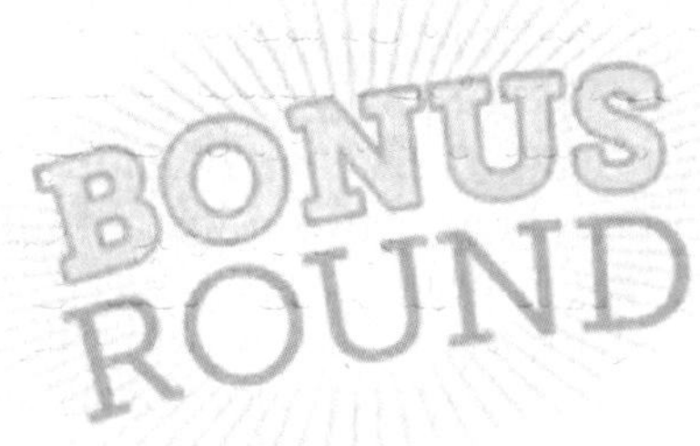

How can you become a better leader? Through our organisation, we have already helped students from all over the world establish a medical society in their school of origin. This is run by students, sometimes under the supervision of a willing teacher. Full resources and starter packs are freely provided—all you have to do is be enthusiastic, take on a leadership role and find students who share a similar passion for medicine like you do. You can imagine how much this could enhance your 'Getting into medical school portfolio'. If you would like to hear more about this, drop us an email!

DOCTORS AS AGENTS OF CHANGE

A very important aspect of leadership is setting an example for others to follow, by being a good role model. This can manifest in many different ways, but usually, what these different ways have in common is change. To be a good leader, you must be observant enough to identify what could be improved and how and then actively implement these things yourself.

What is an example of this? Well, let's say that diabetes is a common issue in your local area, and many patients are unaware of how to manage their chronic disease best. As an agent of change, do you observe that and brush it off? Absolutely not. An agent of change is equipped with the skill set to recognise this pattern and then implement something to improve it. So, you could make a clinic to support those with diabetes and help them to manage their chronic illness. You could also advocate and campaign for certain rights and give a voice to those vulnerable who need your help the most.

Another example of this can be in the workplace. Being a doctor is characterised by consistent teamwork with both your patients and your fellow colleagues. Imagine a colleague is making inappropriate jokes, ones which are making both your other colleagues and your patients within earshot uncomfortable. As an agent of change, you would say something about it to ensure that the space remains safe and comfortable for everyone around you.

Alongside their roles as physicians, researchers, teachers and professionals, doctors can advocate for the wider public by becoming agents of change. This is a vital role as it takes various factors into account and attempts to make a positive difference to healthcare. As part of this role, doctors can promote action to improve patient care, they can inform the public of ways to prevent disease and they can empower their colleagues to also act as agents of change to facilitate improvement in healthcare.

DOCTORS AS PROFESSIONALS

As medical students and doctors, we all carry the responsibility of acting professionally. This includes the times when we are serving patients, but it isn't only limited to this. Take for example a medical student who loves having fun. Say John goes out to a club, starts partying and drinking with his friends. Nothing wrong with this so far, right? There's nothing wrong with having fun—we're human after all, and need ways to relax after a full week of tasks and assignments. This becomes a problem, however, when our medical student takes photos and records videos 'portraying unprofessional behaviour' (e.g. John takes off his T-shirt) and later posts them on Facebook, where everyone can see them. This may not seem like a big thing, but would you like your doctor to post drunk topless pictures online? The topic of social media and professionalism is very hot at the moment and specific guidelines have been created for this area.

Apart from this example, there are several other responsibilities of medical students and doctors under the umbrella term of 'professionalism'. Here are some of them, as outlined by the GMC in their ideal outcomes for graduates.

Medical school graduates should be able to:

- Respect and follow the GMC's ethical guidance and legal principles (we talk about these in detail in Chapter 5)
- Reflect, learn and teach others
- Work effectively and professionally in a team
- Protect patients and improve care

During COVID-19, the role of doctors as professionals was emphasised greatly and challenged. Doctors were not only responsible for providing care to others around the clock, they also had to ensure the safety of everyone around them (including their own safety too!). This was highlighted with the importance of vaccination. Doctors had the responsibility of advocating for patients and the public to take the vaccine, while offering information for those who were unsure about it, to ensure the safety of the public. Doctors were also trusted by the public, especially patients who were vulnerable and without family members due to the pandemic, so their role as professionals was highlighted to all at a time of national fear and instability.

SUMMARY, TEST YOURSELF AND REFLECTION

Next time you hear someone say that doctors are just clinicians, give them the evil eye and explain how many other amazing things doctors are responsible for. Doctors are much more than clinicians. Apart from practicing, doctors also get involved in research and the advancement of science.

Doctors are at the forefront of driving change in their organisations and in their nations. Doctors teach and pass on everything they've learnt. Doctors lead and provide vision for the future. Doctors innovate and improve current services.

Finally, doctors act professionally to build trust, maintain relationships with their patients and provide the best care available to each individual patient.

How has this chapter influenced your perception of doctors? Is there anything you are thinking of doing in the future that is related to these four duties? Have you been involved in any type of research so far?

A box for reflection and ideas has been provided here so you can jot down any thoughts you may have. Use these as reminders for when you start planning your interview preparation—these are common topics that almost always come up.

Doctors Are …

A. Practitioners
B. Scholars and Researchers
C. Teachers
D. Leaders and Managers
E. Agents of Change
F. Professionals

Test Yourself

- What do we mean by 'shared leadership'?
- Why is research important? How does it help patients and the healthcare system?
- What is a clinical audit?
- What is the difference between qualitative and quantitative research studies?
- What is professionalism and why is it important?

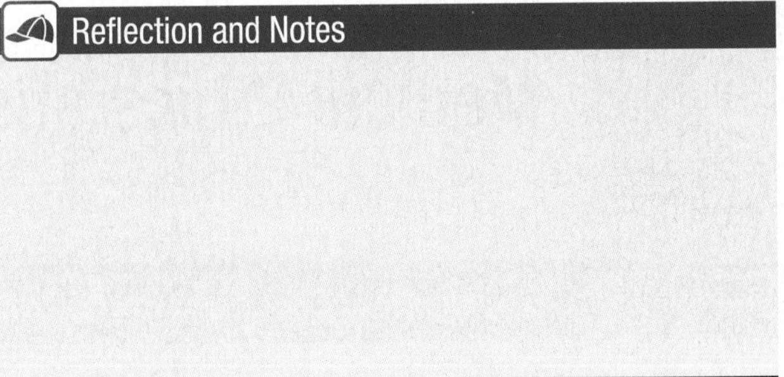

Reflection and Notes

RESOURCES

Evidence-Based Medicine. Available at http://www.students4bestevidence.net/start-here/what-is-evidence-based-medicine/.

General Medical Council (GMC) Guidelines. Tomorrow's Doctors (2024). Available at http://www.gmc-uk.org/Tomorrow_s_Doctors_1214.pdf_48905759.pdf.

General Medical Council (GMC) Guidelines. Leadership and Management for all Doctors (2012). Available at http://www.gmc-uk.org/guidance/ethical_guidance/management_for_doctors.asp.

Medicine Through Time. Available at http://www.bbc.co.uk/education/guides/zb6bkqt/revision/2. Accessed 2019.

NHS Institute for Innovation and Improvement and Academy of Medical Royal Colleges (2010). Medical Leadership Competency Framework, 3rd Edn, Coventry: NHS Institute for Innovation and Improvement. Available at https://www.leadershipacademy.nhs.uk/wp-content/uploads/2014/11/Leadership-Framework.pdf. Accessed 1 September 2023.

Sackett, D. L., Rosenberg, W. M., Gray, J. M., Haynes, R. B., Richardson, W. S. (1996). *Evidence based medicine: what it is and what it isn't*. BMJ. Jan 13;312(7023): 71–72.

Tang, T., Fischbacher, C., Qureshi, Z., 2015. *The unofficial guide to medical research, audit, and teaching*. London: Zeshan Qureshi Ltd.

5 Medical Ethics and Law

Bogdan Chiva Giurca and Charlotte Stoll

Chapter Outline

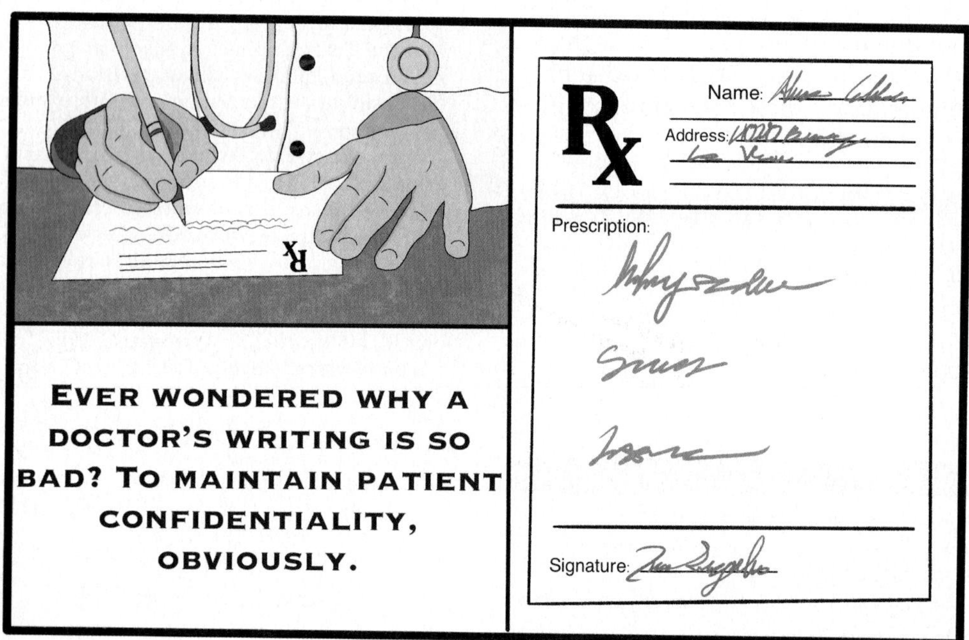

EVER WONDERED WHY A DOCTOR'S WRITING IS SO BAD? TO MAINTAIN PATIENT CONFIDENTIALITY, OBVIOUSLY.
Rx
Name:
Address:
Prescription:
Signature:

INTRODUCTION AND DEFINITION

Right, let's get the boring stuff out of the way first so we can have fun using real-life scenarios.

DEFINITION

One definition states: 'Medical ethics represent a system of moral principles that apply values to the practice of clinical medicine and in scientific research. Medical ethics allow for people, regardless of race, gender or religion to be guaranteed quality and principled care'.

Now that we've just thrown some fancy words at you, let me explain further. In plain English, medical ethics are concepts, values and standards that each doctor should respect when dealing with people. As simple as that.

IMPORTANCE OF MEDICAL ETHICS

What's the difference between someone working as a mechanic and an orthopaedic surgeon? Both fix things up, both lift things up, both use screwdrivers, hammers and other tools to make things work, but both can also mess things up. An orthopaedic surgeon may have the same abilities as a mechanic, but you see, blood vessels, skin, muscles and bones are made of 'stuff' that's much more important than aluminium. The chassis of a car holds its engine. The chassis of the human body (muscles, skin and bones) is home to the heart and the soul. Ruin the human body chassis and you could also ruin the soul.

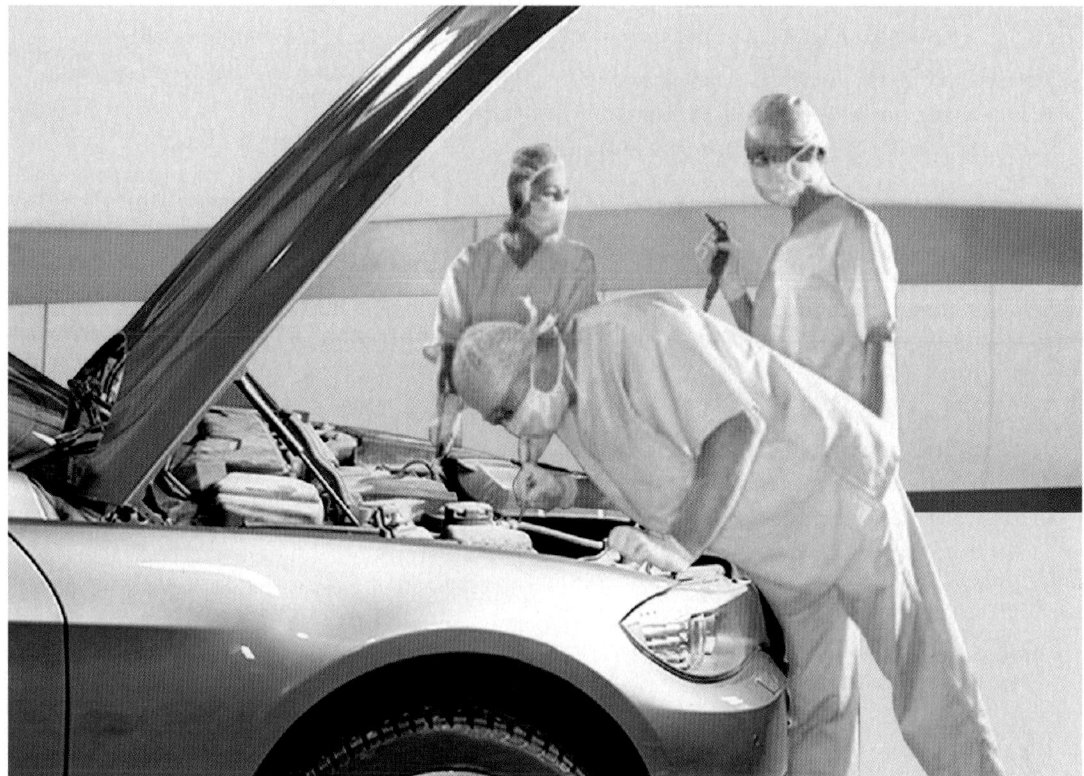

It is an extraordinary privilege and honour to operate on people's 'chassis' and even get paid for it. It does, however, entail an enormous responsibility. A common analogy is to think of doctors and surgeons as priests. Priests are devoted and pious to their faith. Priests pray in churches and answer to the gods they pray to. Similarly, doctors work in 'churches' too. They are called 'hospitals'. Doctors, however, answer to their patients, the 'chassis' owners or those looking after them. In order to minimise power imbalance and suboptimal patient care, medical ethics and moral codes have been around since the dawn of time.

Do you remember the ceremony we interrupted during our visit to ancient Greece in Chapter 2? You see, Hippocrates was a big fan of medical ethics. He even decided to lay down a moral code of conduct for physicians on which all modern ethical principles and laws have been based. Some of the main points of the old Hippocratic Oath are summarised here:

'A solemn promise:

- Of solidarity with teachers and other physicians.
- Of beneficence (to do good or avoid evil) and non-maleficence (from the Latin 'primum non nocere', or 'do no harm') towards patients.
- Not to assist suicide or abortion.
- To leave surgery to surgeons.
- Not to harm, especially not to seduce patients.
- To maintain confidentiality and never to gossip.'

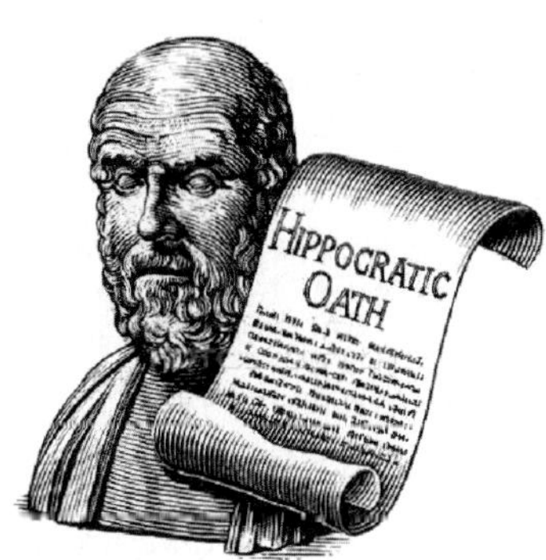

The Oath has been adapted over time, with the newest version in 2017.

Is the Hippocratic Oath still part of the graduation process? Some countries still do it, while others use different versions that have similar core values. For example, some medical schools use the 'Declaration of Geneva' physician's oath.

You may be wondering what's happening in the United Kingdom since this is where you want to practice. Well, sadly, there are no white-coated doctors making any solemn promises, but we do have some values and principles laid out by the General Medical Council (GMC). These are called 'Good Medical Practice', and they represent the gold standard of how medical students and doctors are expected to behave when doing their duty. These duties are organised into four different domains and categories. All four domains are summarised in Fig. 5.1.

Domain 1. **Knowledge, skills and performance**	Domain 2. **Safety and quality**

› Make the care of your patients your first concern.
› Provide a good standard of practice and care:
  › Develop and maintain your professional performance.
  › Apply knowledge and experience to practice.
  › Recognise and work within the limits of your competence.
  › Record your work clearly, accurately and legibly.
	› Contribute to and comply with systems to protect patients.
	› Respond to risks to safety.
	› Protect patients and colleagues from any risk posed by your health.

Domain 3. **Communication, partnership and teamwork**	Domain 4. **Maintaining trust**

› Communicate effectively.
› Work collaboratively with colleagues to maintain or improve patient care.
› Teaching, training, supporting and assessing.
› Continuity and coordination of care.
› Establish and maintain partnerships with patients:
  › Listen and respond to their concerns and preferences.
  › Give patients the information they want or need in a way they can understand.
  › Respect patients' right to reach decisions with you about their treatment and care.
  › Support patients in caring for themselves to improve and maintain their health.
	› Show respect for patients.
	  › Treat patients as individuals and respect their dignity.
	  › Treat patients politely and considerately.
	  › Respect patients' right to confidentiality.
	› Treat patients and colleagues fairly and without discrimination.
	› Act with honesty and integrity.
	› Never abuse your patients' trust in you or the public's trust in the profession.

Fig. 5.1 Duties of a doctor.

Consider all four domains and take notes regarding the key features in each area, since you're most likely to encounter these during your medical school interview. By quoting and explaining key features as emphasised by these domains in your answers, you will come across as knowledgeable and considerate (which basically means extra points!).

DIFFERENCE BETWEEN ETHICS AND LAWS

A common mistake is to think that laws and ethics are the same. Although similar, the two are very different. Let's consider them individually (Table 5.1).

Laws are rules and regulations set by the government. Laws are fairly strict and rigid, meaning that they clearly state what one must or must not do. Laws are set after taking ethics and moral values into consideration.

Ethics, on the other hand, represent a guide for the population, portraying what's good or bad. Ethics are not as rigid as laws, and there is a lot of variation. Ethics attempt to illustrate an ideal human character, and they inform people to make better choices. In other words, ethics are a code of conduct set by people or professional bodies (such as the GMC in medicine in our case).

The relationship between ethics and law has often been described as a 'tense marriage'. The two often overlap, making this topic very confusing. Don't worry too much about it at this point—you will understand more as we go through the chapter. One thing we can assure you is that admission tutors don't expect you to know the exact details of a law—after all, you are trying to become a doctor, not a barrister.

THE FOUR ETHICAL PRINCIPLES

You may want to take out a pen and scribble these down, as these four principles are among the most important pieces of knowledge you require in order to tackle hard problems in a clinical and nonclinical setting. Let's take them one by one, describing what each stands for.

AUTONOMY

Autonomy refers to the need to take into consideration and respect the decisions/desires of independent individuals.

Easy way to remember: Autonomy refers to the word 'autonomous', which means 'having the freedom to act independently'. Autonomy therefore means that patients have the freedom to choose their fate, and that you, as the doctor, should respect that.

BENEFICENCE

Balancing the benefits of care against the risks. The clinician should always be on the patient's side, always attempting to do good.

Easy way to remember: Beneficence. Some of you may know that 'Bene' in Latin means 'good'. Therefore, DO GOOD!

Table 5.1 **Laws vs Ethics**

COMPARISON	LAWS	ETHICS
Definition	Set of rules governing actions of the whole society	Set of guidelines suggesting how to behave in certain situations
Nature	Rigid, strict	Flexible, debatable
Regulated by	Government (leading body)	Professional bodies/people
Easy way to remember	What doctors should do, OR ELSE!	What doctors should do…

NONMALEFICENCE

Healthcare professionals should avoid causing harm to their patients. It can be argued that all treatments involve harm to some extent (for example, the sharp needle scratch when taking blood), but the harm should not outweigh the benefits of treatment.

Easy way to remember: Nonmaleficence is fairly easy to remember. Just think about the recent Disney film 'Maleficent'. Maleficent is based on Latin and means evil. Nonmaleficent would mean nonevil; therefore, DO NOT HARM your patients.

JUSTICE

Always treat everyone fairly and equally. Fair distribution of benefits, risk and costs.

Easy way to remember: Does anyone like superheroes? What about Justice League? Justice is easy to remember when thinking about superheroes who always fight for equality and restoring the balance between good and evil. As a doctor (and medical student/aspiring medic), you should respect every individual's rights.

Now that you know the four pillars of medical ethics, let us consider a very important letter in the alphabet … C, before jumping into ethical dilemmas and how to use this valuable information to solve them.

THE 4 C'S (AND IT ISN'T COFFEE, CROISSANTS, CAKE AND CHOCOLATE)

Before we move on, I recommend grabbing one or more of the above and, using this list, have a guess at which are the 4 C's:

- Confidence
- Confidentiality
- Courage
- Communication
- Consent
- Competence
- Compassion
- Creativity
- Capacity

Read on to C (do you C what I did there) if you've got them correct!

CONFIDENTIALITY

Although there is no legal requirement for this, and it is not considered one of the four core ethical principles, confidentiality plays a key role in the doctor–patient relationship and should always be taken into consideration. Over the years, the GMC has developed guidance regarding confidentiality. You see, this concept is not part of the core ethical principles because it overlaps with the first ethical principle: Autonomy. According to autonomy, patients have the right to control their own life, which includes the right to choose whether someone should have access to their personal information and if so, who.

Earlier on, we talked about the history of medicine and the famous Hippocratic Oath. Confidentiality has been considered one of the Hippocratic pillars (not the same as the four ethical pillars) holding together the trust between doctors and patients since the beginning of medicine as we know it.

> *All that may come to my knowledge in the exercise of my profession or in daily commerce with men, which ought not to be spread abroad, I will keep secret and will never reveal.*
>
> Hippocrates, 5th Century BC

In other words, anything I'm told that the person doesn't wish for others to hear, won't be told.

Food for thought: Take 5 minutes to consider the following questions before reading further.

> ? Why is confidentiality so important and what would happen if doctors did not maintain confidentiality? What is the purpose of this duty that we all carry and have to respect?
>
> Try to answer this question in your own words before reading further.

In short, without assurance about confidentiality, fewer patients would be willing to seek medical attention or provide personal information required by doctors to properly understand and manage their current situation.

By ensuring privacy, you encourage patients to visit healthcare professionals when in need, and to be sincere with their doctors. This benefits not only patients individually but also society as a whole. Take for example communicable diseases. If people were scared and concerned about who might find out from their doctor, several communicable diseases (such as malaria, smallpox, yellow fever, etc.) would go unchecked and untreated. This was exemplified during the COVID-19 pandemic (before laws were put in place in some countries that encourage people to manage their symptoms at home if possible).

Maintaining patient confidentiality encourages patients to be honest, therefore allowing doctors to make an assessment based on all information available.

Although a recurring theme in medical ethics, the complexity of confidentiality continues to challenge applicants like yourself, medical students, doctors and healthcare professionals. Have a look at this example of where confidentiality can get a little confusing:

John has tested positive for HIV and was made aware of his diagnosis 6 months ago. He is continuing to have unprotected sex with his wife despite the diagnosis and is refusing to tell her the truth. As John's general practitioner (GP), do you still respect his patient confidentiality or do you tell his wife?

Even Hippocrates was stunned by certain cases, as emphasised through his question, 'What ought not to be spoke abroad?!'

And, no, this does not mean that Hippocrates was debating sending patient notes to America. In more simple terms, he was asking what the exceptions to the general duty of confidentiality are.

Thankfully, the GMC has some guidelines in place to help you make difficult decisions so that you don't have to struggle like Hippocrates did. The following image shows four scenarios that make confidentiality 'not absolute'.

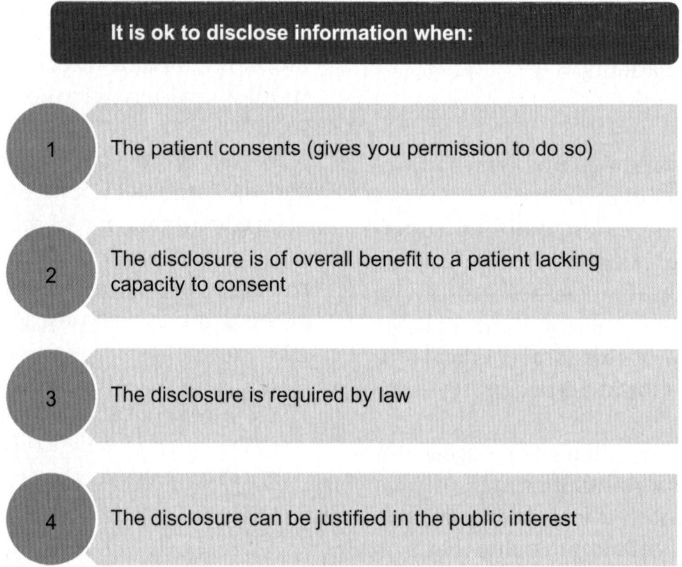

It is ok to disclose information when:
1 The patient consents (gives you permission to do so)
2 The disclosure is of overall benefit to a patient lacking capacity to consent
3 The disclosure is required by law
4 The disclosure can be justified in the public interest

In the case of John and his wife, as she is at risk of contracting HIV, it would be in her best interest for the GP to tell her if they cannot get John to. This would come under exception 2 as the wife doesn't have the capacity to consent to unprotected sex with John and she is not fully informed (this will make more sense when we get onto consent … luckily for you, that's next!).

Confidentiality and its clash with some of the other ethical principles can freeze your brain during the medical school interview. To ensure you get it right, we'll illustrate confidentiality and its interaction with other principles through ethical dilemmas later in this chapter. Let us now explain a few other useful concepts (or should I say let's C some more C's) that play a pivotal role in clinical decision-making.

Consent, competence and capacity are some of the other key concepts in medical ethics. Let us tackle them one by one. You must be warned, however, that these concepts are heavily intertwined with one another so it can be easy to mix them up. Try to come up with your own ways to remember the differences! Here's one way to remember them:

1. Consent has the word 'sent' in it and it's something that, as a doctor and medical student, you will need to receive from patients (sent and received are opposites).

2. Competency is a longer word and competence can be seen as a more all round assessment of a person's right to make decisions.
3. Capacity is a shorter word than competence and is less all round—it is a functional assessment.

Come back to these reminders once you've read about them!

CONSENT

In simple terms, consent represents the concept that a person must give permission before undergoing any test, treatment or medical procedure. Consent must be sought for things as simple as a discussion on the ward (i.e. 'Hello, my name is John Smith, I am a medical student, is it okay to have a chat with you sir?'), all the way to life-saving procedures such as organ donation and surgery.

To be legally valid (we call this valid consent—creative, I know), consent must be:

- **Voluntary**—the decision must be made by the patient and not influenced by medical professionals, relatives or acquaintances.
- **Informed**—full information regarding the procedure/test/examination must be given to the patient prior to seeking consent (e.g. benefits, risks, side-effects, alternatives and so on).
- Given by a **Capable** individual—meaning that the patient must be able to understand the information presented and reach an informed decision.

An adult (this is super important—we'll talk more about young people and children later) who understands the information presented and has **Capacity** (don't panic, we'll expand on this concept soon) has the right to decide what happens next, even if this means refusing a treatment that may result in their death.

There are three ways of giving consent:

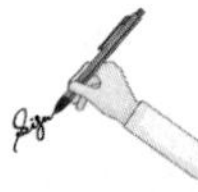

Written (i.e. consenting by signing a surgical procedure)

Verbal (i.e. consenting by saying 'Yes' to an examination)

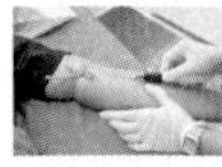

Nonverbal or assumed (i.e. consenting by pulling your sleeve up and placing out your arm for a vaccine)

Should your patient change their mind, they are entitled to withdraw their consent.

Cases when consent isn't necessary:

- Emergency treatment to save their life—when the patient is unconscious, therefore unable to make a decision
- Emergency need for an additional procedure during surgery, e.g. if a tumour is being removed and another is found during the surgery that also needs to be removed
- Severe mental health conditions (such as bipolar, dementia, schizophrenia) impairing the patient's decision making—patients are allowed to be sectioned under the Mental Health Act
- Patients who are a risk to society and public health (communicable diseases such as rabies, cholera or tuberculosis (TB))

COMPETENCE AND CAPACITY

The coffee and cake of the 4 C's because let's be honest ... they are just not as good without each other.

Although competence and capacity are often used interchangeably, there is a slight difference. This isn't something you are expected to memorise nor do you need to worry about which one you use as they are extremely similar. However, to clear up any confusion, competence refers to a person's ability to perform actions needed to put decisions into effect. In other words, it is being mature enough to follow through with a decision, e.g. a 16-year-old girl deciding to go on the oral contraceptive pill is deemed competent, unless proven otherwise, to take the pills. On the other hand, capacity is a less all round assessment of a person, limited to a functional test. In other words, it is the ability to make a decision. It took me a while to get my head around these two concepts so let's have a look at how competence is assessed in order for us to understand both terms much better.

Assessing competence is a two-stage process: Stage 1 is referred to as objective evidence and stage 2 is a functional test.

Stage 1 (objective evidence)—this is a diagnosis of a physical or mental condition that can impair a person's mind.

Examples of how a person's mind may be impaired include but are not limited to:

- Mental health conditions—such as schizophrenia or bipolar disorder
- Dementia
- Severe learning disabilities
- Brain damage—for example, from a stroke or other brain injury
- Physical or mental conditions that cause confusion, drowsiness or a loss of consciousness
- Intoxication caused by drug or alcohol misuse
- Temporary things:
  - Shock
  - Panic
  - Fatigue
  - Medication

Stage 2 (functional test)—patients are considered competent if the answer is 'yes' to all the questions in the following image.

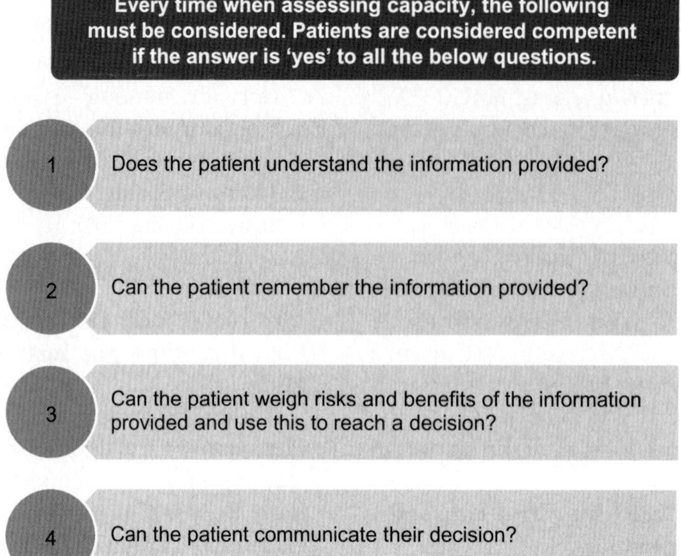

Every time when assessing capacity, the following must be considered. Patients are considered competent if the answer is 'yes' to all the below questions.
1
Does the patient understand the information provided?
2
Can the patient remember the information provided?
3
Can the patient weigh risks and benefits of the information provided and use this to reach a decision?
4
Can the patient communicate their decision?

A patient can be deemed incompetent in stage 1 and still be deemed to have capacity to make a certain decision if they pass stage 2. This is very important to remember! It is also crucial to bear in mind that capacity often changes over time due to physical or mental conditions (this is called fluctuating capacity). For this reason, **capacity is assessed at the time when consent is required**. If a person has been deemed incompetent in the past, that does not mean they are incompetent now.

The four questions on this page for assessing capacity seem pretty simple, right? Things get complicated when you also consider personal beliefs. It doesn't necessarily mean that someone lacks capacity if they make a decision that seems irrational to most people. The best example to clarify the previous statement is a person holding certain religious beliefs preventing them from having a blood transfusion. They understand the consequences of their actions, and you must respect their personal beliefs. Stick around for more examples like this one!

Conversely, let's consider the case of a severely malnourished, anorexic 18-year-old who is refusing help because (from their point of view) there's nothing wrong. In this case, the patient cannot make sense of the reality of their situation. They cannot understand the consequences of their disease and therefore cannot be deemed competent.

In short, as long as someone understands the reality of their situation, they are entitled to make their own decisions.

TREATING PATIENTS WHO LACK CAPACITY

If patients aren't competent to make their own decisions, a 'best interest' decision will need to be made on behalf of the patient.

If no one can reach a decision regarding medical treatment of a patient lacking capacity, an independent mental capacity advocate (IMCA) should be consulted. In difficult situations where best interests cannot be determined, cases can be referred to court for a ruling.

Sometimes, it is possible to predict whether someone's capacity will be affected in the future. In such cases, patients can make an 'advanced decision' regarding treatments and procedures that they refuse to undergo in the future. Similarly, they can arrange for a family member to have lasting power of attorney. This can be a close family member or relative who can make important decisions for the patient.

For example, if John's GP diagnoses him with dementia, a consultation can be booked with John and his family to discuss who can have lasting power of attorney to make decisions for John in the future. In certain cases, for patients approaching end of life, there are certain forms that can be used called 'DNAR' (do not attempt resuscitation). These forms, as shown here, notify the medical team regarding the wishes of a patient not to be resuscitated if they go into cardiac arrest.

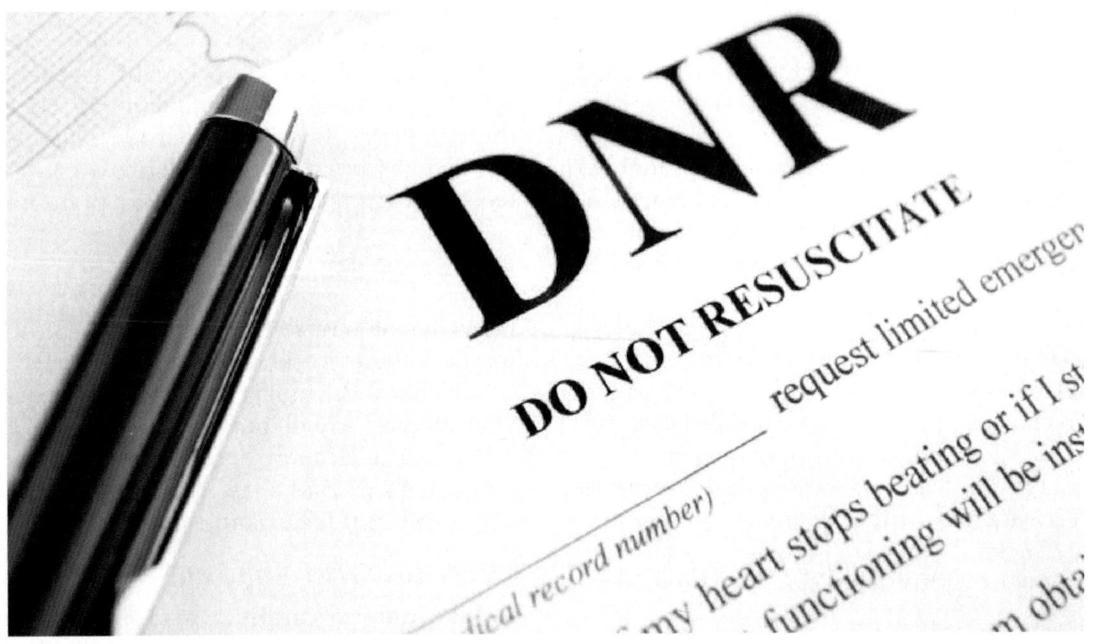

Another concept worth mentioning here is the so-called 'Principle of Double Effect' or 'Doctrine of Double Effect'. This refers to when something is done or given to a patient with good intention that ends up having a harmful side effect. This may sound confusing at first, but take for example patients who are in severe pain due to cancer. It is considered morally appropriate to give morphine to such patients, even though this makes them drowsy, because the overall benefit improves quality of life through making them comfortable.

CONSENT IN YOUNG ADULTS AND CHILDREN

In the UK, all adults are presumed to have the capacity to make decisions relating to their healthcare, unless they are proven incompetent using objective evidence. Conversely, children are presumed incompetent unless proven otherwise. This is where it can all get a little bit confusing. But, using the 4C's, we can make sense of this.

Age	Competence
18+	Legally able to consent and refuse treatment
16–17	Legally able to consent and refuse treatment. Can be overridden by parents/the law if in their best interest
Under 16	Can consent to own treatment if believed to have enough intelligence, competence and understanding to appreciate what's involved in their treatment
Parents of under 16	If the parents are competent, they can consent. If they refuse treatment for their child, the court can overrule in the best interest of the child. If they disagree about what is in the best interest of their child, the courts can make a decision.

Remember: In **emergency situations**, if waiting for parental consent could place the child at risk, healthcare professionals can proceed without consent.

Victoria Gillick and Fraser Guidelines

Do you want the good news first or the bad news? Bad news it is … time to make things a little more complicated. But, the good news is, after reading this, you'll hopefully have a really good understanding of consent in young adults and children! And if that wasn't already the best news you've heard all day, we're going to tell you a story…

Victoria Gillick was a British activist campaigning against prescribing contraception to under-16-year-old girls. Victoria was a mother of five daughters who believed that contraception should only be prescribed if parental consent is given. In the 1980s, the government published guidance for practitioners for offering contraception and family planning to those under 16. Frustrated by the new guidelines, Victoria sued those proposing these laws, including a GP who prescribed oral contraception to an under-16-year-old girl.

This case became famous and you will soon find out why. Victoria's argument was that 'parents should have duties to their kids, and rights over them, as long as they are in the developing years of their life'. This meant that parents should be involved in the family planning of their children.

Doctors were often faced with under-16s requesting oral contraception. In such cases, doctors would be afraid to prescribe contraception as they could get into serious trouble from a legal point of view. One brave GP, however, said the following:

'The girl I have spoken to was indeed under 16. Did I prescribe oral contraception? Yes, I did, and here's why …

- I tried persuading her to tell her parents, but she said she cannot do so under any circumstances
- I tried explaining and advising against unprotected sexual intercourse, but the girl said she will continue doing this anyway
- I assessed whether the girl is mature enough to make this decision and whether she is competent enough to understand the realities of this situation
- If the girl continued to have unprotected sex, without receiving oral contraception, she could become pregnant, leading to worse physical and psychological outcomes than if I didn't prescribe the pill'

Lord Fraser was the judge assessing the issues raised in court. His conclusions made Victoria Gillick famous:

'The following criteria MUST apply when medical practitioners are offering contraceptive services to under-sixteen-year-olds without parental consent and knowledge:

1. The young person must understand the professional's advice
2. The young person cannot be persuaded to inform their parents under any circumstances
3. The young person is likely to begin, or to continue having, sexual intercourse with or without contraceptive treatment
4. Unless the young person receives contraceptive treatment, their physical or mental health, or both, are likely to suffer
5. The young person's best interests require them to receive contraceptive advice or treatment with or without parental consent'

Assessing a young person's competence to receive contraceptive advice or treatment is referred to as 'Gillick Competence', while 'Fraser guidelines' is the term used to describe any other assessment of a young person's maturity and subsequent ability to make decisions about their own health. This includes decisions relating to abortion.

Please note that Gillick and Fraser guidelines are terms sometimes used interchangeably.

You may ask—well, what do we do if an 11-year-old girl comes and tells you about a sexual relationship with a 21-year-old male? As you'd expect, there is a limit when we should immediately involve social services, and this is when the girl is younger than 13 years old or in a relationship that raises concerns over age difference, assault, abuse (emotional, physical, sexual), etc.

MENTAL HEALTH ACT

The Mental Health Act (2005) is something that you should also be aware of, as many of the concepts outlined earlier are part of it. Essentially, the act lays out the legal framework for making decisions in patients who lack mental capacity to make decisions regarding their healthcare, personal wellbeing and financial situation. The Mental Capacity Act is only valid for those aged over 16 years.

Five big principles are leading legislation in this act. These have been illustrated in Fig. 5.2. As you go through them, you'll see how it all relates back to what we were discussing earlier in terms of consent, competence and acting in the best interest of the patient.

ETHICAL DILEMMAS

Now that you're equipped with the most powerful weapon there is (knowledge, obviously!), you can tackle ethical dilemmas like a pro and ensure you ace your medical school interview.

Having a weapon does not make you ready for battle. Let's discuss a few tactics before moving on to battle with real-life examples.

TACKLING AN ETHICAL DILEMMA FRAMEWORK

1. **Take time to carefully read and understand the scenario.**
   Instead of blurting out what first comes to mind after initially reading an ethical dilemma, try to abstain from this temptation and take time to get to the core of the issue proposed.
2. **Peel off each layer of the scenario by observing how the fundamental ethical pillars and other concepts are involved.**
   What are the core principles clashing in the scenario? Are there any other concepts such as Gillick competence or consent that should be considered? How about the confidentiality of the patient, is this respected or does it clash with anything else?
3. **Do not make assumptions based on your previous experience—only act with the information that you are provided with.**
   It is very easy to assume what the answer might be, based on some of your previous experiences. Instead, try to tackle the dilemma from different angles, taking into consideration different viewpoints and possibilities.
4. **Justify using arguments (based on the theory learnt) what the ideal solution to the scenario would be.**
   Mention what you would do if you were the one to decide and provide appropriate reasons regarding why this is the ideal solution, working in the best interest of the patient.
5. **Reach a conclusion by summing up your answer.**
   Ethical dilemmas rarely have a correct answer. As long as you can argue how and why you would do something, you should be fine. Remember, some scenarios put entire boards of doctors and lawyers at difficulty, so don't be disheartened if you struggle to come to a conclusion.

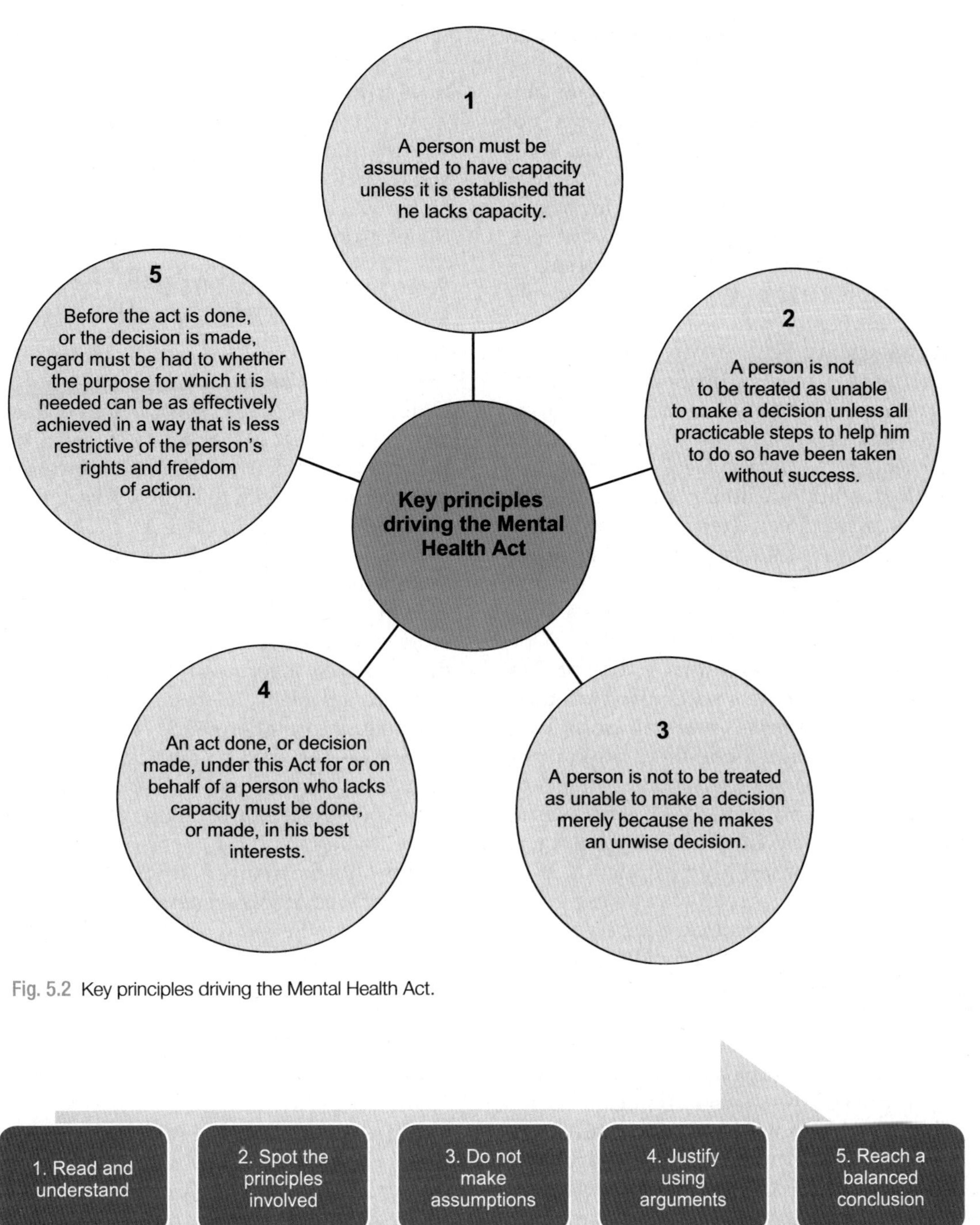

Fig. 5.2 Key principles driving the Mental Health Act.

1. Read and understand
2. Spot the principles involved
3. Do not make assumptions
4. Justify using arguments
5. Reach a balanced conclusion

> When answering ethical questions in interviews, don't be afraid to acknowledge your limitations, be honest and mention that this is a difficult ethical dilemma that requires discussion with the entire healthcare team. For this reason, one suggestion you should always make is that you would not attempt carrying this dilemma on your shoulders alone. You should always involve senior staff members such as consultants or members from other relevant services (e.g. social services).

Before testing your ethical knowledge, let's acknowledge some considerations that could have an influence on someone's decision making (such as a Jehovah's Witness potentially not wanting to go ahead with a blood transfusion). It is crucial that you are respectful and understanding of these beliefs, even if you do not agree with them. A person's decision influenced by these factors is still a decision that should be respected provided they have capacity.

Disclaimer: these are generalisations and do not apply to everyone from these groups.

- People from certain religions, such as Islam and Hinduism, as well as vegetarians/vegans may not want biological valves, skin grafts, medications, implants, etc., that contain animal products.
- Some women may not be comfortable seeing a male doctor (whether this be a religious reason or other).
- Some religious groups are against contraception.
- Some people do not agree with abortions for religious and/or moral reasons.
- The Amish are against heart transplants and reluctant to undergo most medical treatments.
- Seventh Day Adventists emphasise a mostly holistic approach to health.
- Christian Scientists discourage medical care.

Objections to medical treatment don't end with patients; doctors are also allowed to refuse providing certain treatments. This is called a conscientious objection. In order to protect patients from being discriminated against for their beliefs, values, lifestyle choices, etc., there are limits to what a doctor can object. The General Medical Council states that a doctor can choose to opt out of providing a particular procedure because of their personal beliefs and values, as long as it doesn't result in direct or indirect discrimination against, or harassment of, individual patients or groups of patients. In other words, the objection has to be something that goes against a belief you hold, e.g. believing that abortions or fertility treatment is morally wrong, and not against a group of people, e.g. not providing gender reassignment surgery. It is important that if a doctor has an objection to providing a procedure, they make the patient wanting or requiring the procedure aware. They must also refer the patient to a doctor who will be able to provide the procedure.

The topic of conscientious objections is a highly controversial one, with some people arguing that a doctor should be able to put all personal beliefs aside and others arguing that doctors are still human and entitled to their own opinions. It is worth considering that if a doctor was not allowed a conscientious objection, then they may still be biased against the procedure and so intentionally or unintentionally discourage the patient from having it. Conscientious objections allow these views to be valued and the patients to be referred to someone who can support them. It can still be argued, however, that despite having a conscientious objection, the doctor may still attempt to discourage the patient as some doctors believe that referring is just as bad as doing the procedure themselves.

As you can see, this is a very contentious area and not something that anyone can truly say is right or wrong. There is no need to have a definitive opinion on this topic, but being aware of both sides of the argument puts you in a good position to discuss it if it comes up in an interview question!

Now that we've got all the nitty gritty details covered, let us put into practice what we've learnt. We have chosen some topical scenarios/'hot topics' to highlight the relevance of medical ethics and help you to understand the importance of having a good understanding of the foundations that underpin ethical decision making. Following this are a series of case studies to help you test your newly acquired knowledge.

WHY ARE SOME CASES HOT TOPICS AND OTHERS ARE NOT?

Not every difficult decision is a news story, an X (formerly Twitter) debate or a hashtag—but why is this? Often, ethical hot topics are the ones that are controversial due to the age of the patient involved, the number of patients involved or a series of disagreements, e.g. parents disagreeing with the doctor's best interest decision, the court's best interest decision, etc. It is worth being up to date on medical news to show off your interest in current medical affairs (download a news app and change your preferences to health news). However, it is even more crucial that you are aware of ethical hot topics as these are likely to form some of your interview questions.

There are plenty of resources out there that have amazing information and facts on current ethical scenarios—just search 'medical ethics hot topics for interviews' on your preferred browser or YouTube and once you've done your reading, think about some of the following:

- What are the main ethical principles that need to be considered in this scenario?
- What are the sides to the argument and what is either side's justification?
- Who is/are making the decisions in this situation? Do their decisions or opinions clash?
- Who is/are the 'victim/s' in this scenario? Are there children involved, and if so, does this change anything?
- What was dealt with well in the situation? What could have been dealt with better? How could the way it was dealt with been improved?
- If you were to have an input in the progression of the situation, what would you do differently?

EXAMPLES OF ETHICAL HOT TOPICS

Here are a few in-the-news ethical dilemmas to delve a little deeper into—think about these questions and the ones above in relation to the following:

- COVID-19 isolation—Does mandatory isolation go against human rights? Is it for the greater good to prevent people from seeing their families in hospitals/care homes? What are the advantages and disadvantages to this kind of infection control?
- COVID-19 vaccinations—Is it morally right to enforce resignation for not being vaccinated? Should vaccinations be a legal requirement? What are the two sides to the argument? Did COVID-19

transparency for vaccination efficacy comply with regulations?

- Archie Batterspee—Was it in his best interest to be taken off life support? Did Archie have autonomy and/or capacity? Why were doctors and the court entitled to make a decision and not Archie's parents? What are other considerations that need to be taken in this case, e.g. psychological implications on Archie's parents?
- Abortion law changes in the UK to allow home abortions—Is this in the best interest of the person seeking the abortion and why/why not? If someone was under 16 seeking an at-home abortion, would the outcome be different?
- DNA from three parents to create an embryo—What are the advantages and disadvantages to this? Is it moral to carry out research on an embryo? Who consents for the embryo to be involved in medical research? Is it enough to suggest that something 'does not seem to affect development' of the foetus for the sake of medical progression?

Now that we've considered some of the tricky questions (and potentially no answers) that stakeholders in medical ethics are subject to, it's your turn to escape the maze of ethical dilemmas! As tempting as it may be to jump straight to the answers, racking your brains and reflecting on how you would handle the situation will help you become a master of medical ethics.

Ethical dilemmas rarely have a clear yes or no answer. It's not about the conclusion that you reach, it's about balancing the arguments and reminding yourself to always place the patient at the centre of your thoughts. Remember, it's not about your final answer; it's about how you got there by using the theory you've learnt.

Case 5.1 A Patient With a Learning Disability Who's Refusing Treatment

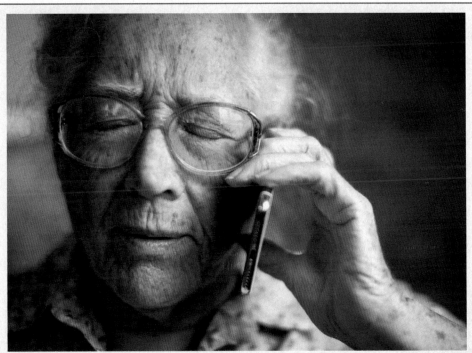

Mrs Ying is 56 years old and has a learning disability. She is admitted to hospital with a benign tumour blocking her ureter. Left untreated, this will result in kidney failure. Mrs Ying would need an operation to remove the tumour. Mrs Ying has indicated quite clearly that she does not want a needle inserted for the anaesthetic for the operation to remove the tumour. This is because she is uncomfortable in a hospital setting and is frightened of needles.

The doctor is concerned that if the tumour is not removed, Mrs Ying will develop kidney failure and require dialysis, which would involve the regular use of needles and be very difficult to carry out given her fear of needles and discomfort with hospitals. The anaesthetist is concerned that if Mrs Ying does not comply with the procedure, then she would need to be physically restrained. Mrs Ying's niece visits her in the care home every other month. The niece is adamant that her aunt should receive treatment.

Should the surgeon perform the operation despite Mrs Ying's objections?

Reflect on the answer. What would you do? Remember, this is not a yes or no answer.

How did that feel—not so straightforward, right? Did you spot any of the four pillars clashing with each other? What other key concepts were involved?

Case 5.2 Jane, a 15-Year-Old Who Just Had a Miscarriage

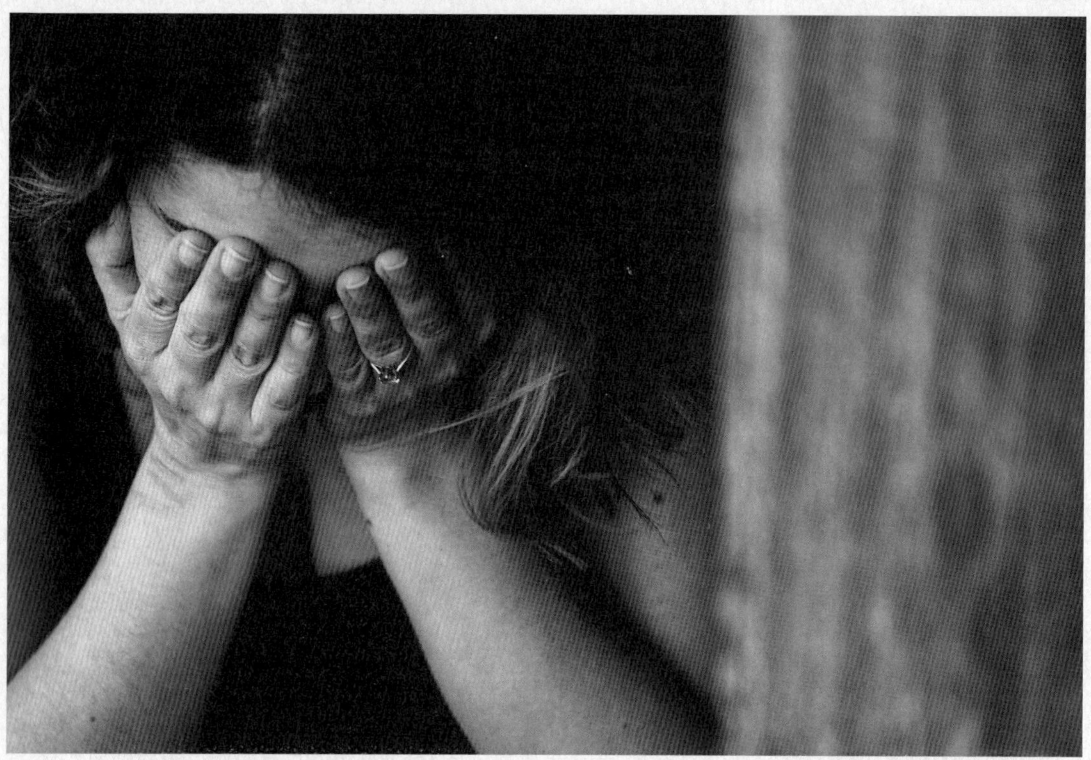

You are a junior doctor and Jane, a 15-year-old girl, had a miscarriage. She asks you not to tell her parents because they did not know she was pregnant. Her father finds out from a neighbour that his daughter is in the hospital, but he does not know why. Jane's father turns up on your ward requesting to see Jane immediately. What do you do?

? Write your answer here. Remember, this is not a yes or no answer.

Case 5.3 An HIV Patient Refusing to Disclose His Disease Status (Part 1 of 2)

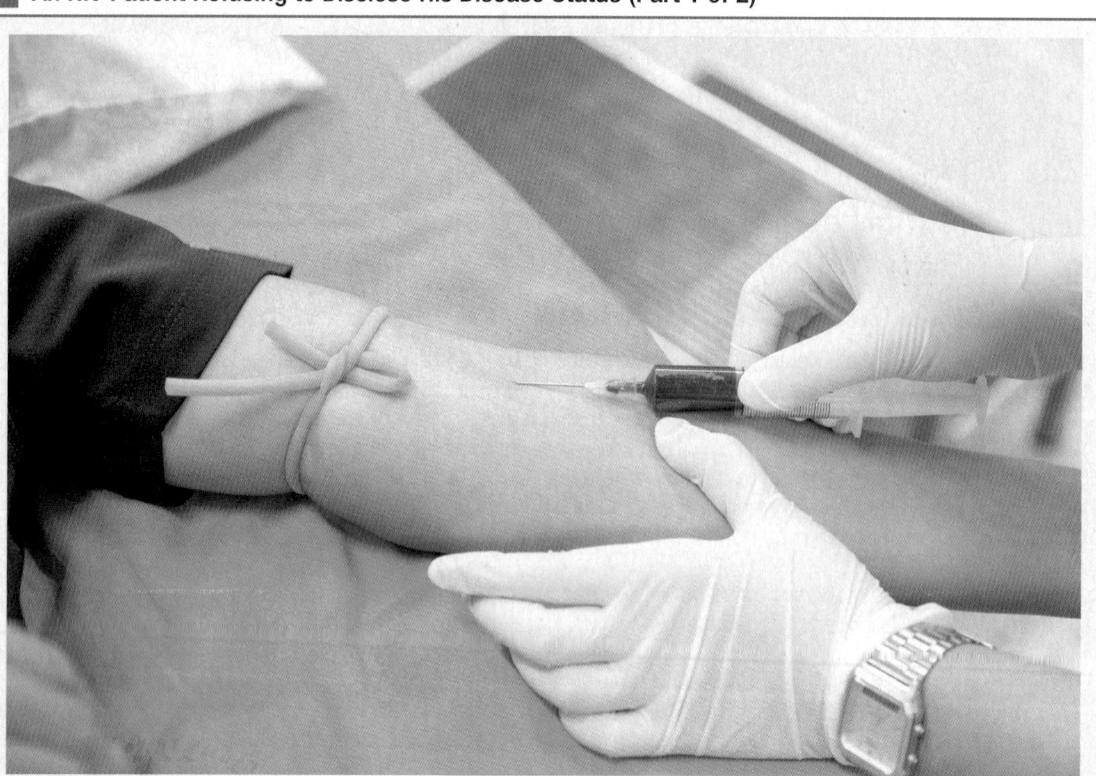

Martin visits a genitourinary medicine (GUM) clinic with what he suspects are genital warts. He is examined, provided with treatment for his warts and offered advice on how the medication should be applied and what to do in the event of complications. The clinic's policy is to offer chlamydia, gonorrhoea, syphilis and HIV tests to all new patients, in line with national guidance, and Martin is offered these along with information about the benefits of testing and how the result will be given. He consents, and the HIV test comes back positive.

Martin comes back to you to discuss the results. You order a confirmatory test and tell Martin about the likely stage of disease and how it is treated. You reassure Martin that HIV is a treatable medical condition and the majority of those living with the virus remain well on treatment. You ask Martin if he has any other immediate concerns and provide him with written information about HIV and about the services available to patients in the area. Martin arranges a follow-up appointment for the following week to discuss the results of the confirmatory testing, future treatment, partner notification, the risks of onward transmission of HIV, and the medico-legal issues associated with this.

Martin immediately expresses anxiety about his privacy, having witnessed a friend suffer discrimination following accidental disclosure of his HIV status. He is open to partner notification, although he has not been sexually active for a few months, but he says that he does not want his GP informed of his diagnosis. He has not got on well with his GP in the past and he fears discrimination in the practice as well as further, inappropriate disclosure of his status.

Do you…

a) Accept Martin's decision not to inform his GP in order to respect Martin's view and protect his confidentiality?
b) Explain the legal and ethical duties of nondiscrimination and confidentiality in an effort to reassure Martin about his GP, as well as the GP's need for information to provide safe, effective care, but ultimately respect Martin's decision?
c) Tell Martin that he's duty-bound to inform the GP, both because his GP wouldn't be able to provide safe or effective care without this knowledge and for the safety of the GP and his clinical colleagues?

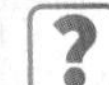 Choose and argue your choice.

Case 5.3 An HIV Patient Refusing to Disclose His Disease Status (Part 2 of 2)

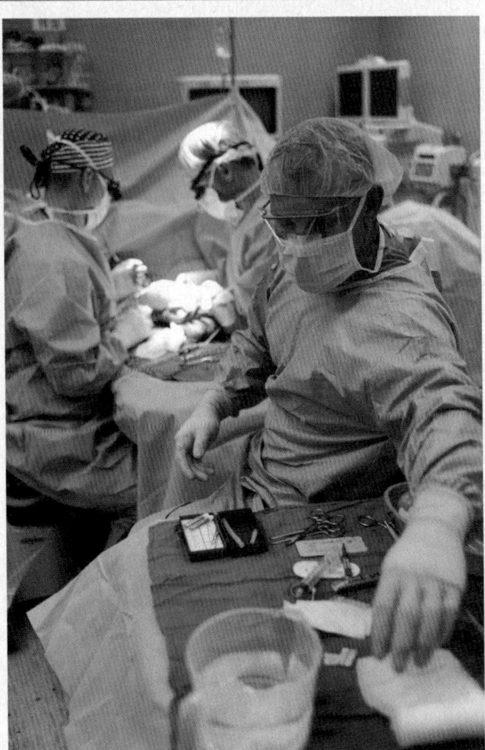

Two years later, Martin visits you for a routine appointment. Except for a knee injury, he is well. Martin mentions that his GP has referred him for orthopaedic surgery at a local private hospital. He has still not shared his HIV status with his GP, who he rarely sees, and he lets you know that he has not disclosed his status to the orthopaedic surgeon either. In addition to his concerns about discrimination and privacy, Martin is particularly concerned that information about his status might get back to his employer and that he could lose his job. His surgery is being paid for through a private health insurance scheme provided by his employer.

You tell Martin that surgeons sometimes take additional precautions with 'high-risk' patients, e.g. double-gloving and possibly a space suit for the surgeon, and gloves, aprons and face visors for the theatre staff. Furthermore, you tell him that HIV+ patients are sometimes put at the end of surgical lists to minimise the risk of infecting other patients. You urge Martin to tell the orthopaedic surgeon about his HIV status so that the surgeon and her team can take additional measures to protect themselves from the risk of infection. You also seek to reassure Martin of the surgeon's duty of confidentiality and that systems are in place to prevent inappropriate disclosures.

Martin refuses. He says he has been researching the issues on the internet and that the surgical team should be taking 'universal precautions' based on the assumption that all patients are potentially infected with blood-borne viruses. He becomes quite upset and says he will sue you if you break his confidentiality by informing the surgeon or anyone else about his HIV status. Martin adds that, in the event of a needlestick or similar injury to a healthcare worker, he would disclose his status.

Do you…

a) Accept Martin's refusal to allow his status to be disclosed?
b) Explain that you must inform the surgeon and that you will do so without Martin's consent if necessary?
c) Contact the orthopaedic surgeon and tell him that a patient with a blood-borne virus is booked in for surgery on the day for which it is planned, without disclosing Martin's identity?

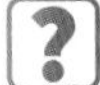 Reflect on the answer. What would you do?

Case 5.4 Informing Family Members at Risk—Ethics and Genetics

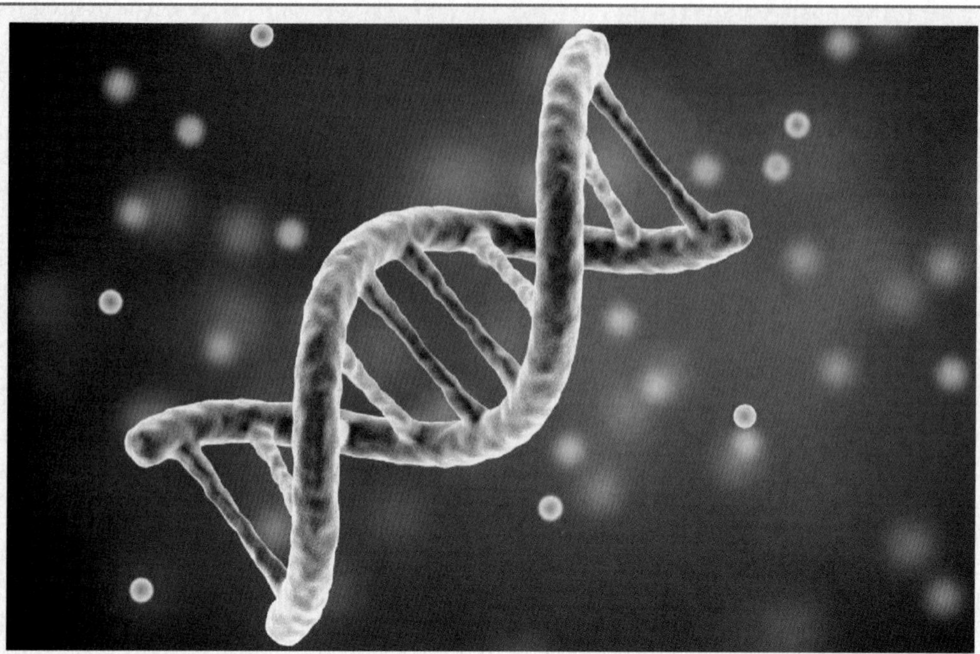

Adam is a 32-year-old man who has been referred to a cardiologist. His family medical history shows that a few of his family members died in their thirties due to a 'heart attack'. Because of the family history, Adam underwent a list of tests and the results proved that Adam has an inherited heart condition.

During a follow-up consultation of these tests, Adam is asked about other family members who may be at risk (given that this is an inherited condition). He mentions that he only has one sister, Rachel. Rachel is 27 and a firefighter. Adam asks the cardiologist not to contact Rachel, as he is scared that she would lose her job. He knows that things like this could jeopardise her whole career. Should the cardiologist inform Rachel?

Reflect on the answer. What would you do? Remember, this is not a yes or no answer.

Case 5.5 To Resuscitate or Not to Resuscitate?

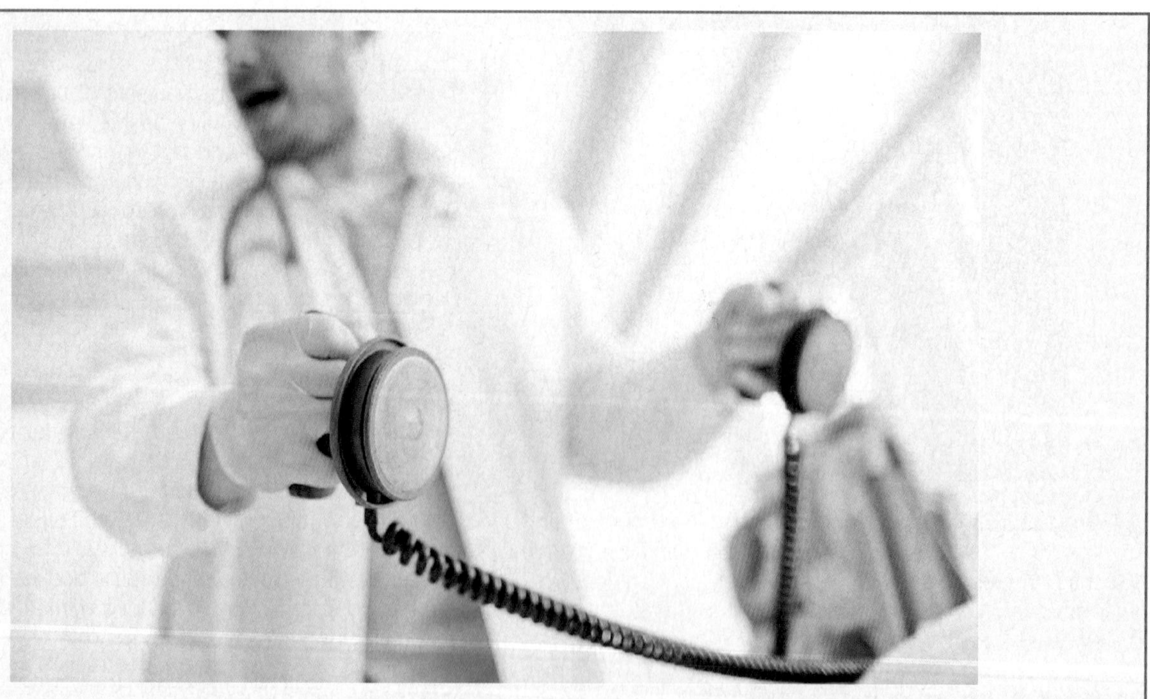

Lavender has multiple brain metastases. After several discussions with her family and doctors, she agrees to sign a Do Not Attempt CardioPulmonary Resuscitation form (DNACPR). She decided to spend her last days going on holiday with her family. As you walk away from the bed to prepare her discharge paperwork, the patient is choking on what you suspect to be a gummy bear. Back slaps and chest thrusts fail to dislodge the gummy bear. She suffers an arrest soon after.

Do you…

a) Perform CPR and call for help?
b) Call all her relatives to come and say goodbye?
c) Wait until there is no spontaneous response and declare the time of death?
d) Sue the gummy bear brand?

? Reflect on the answer. What would you do?

Case 5.6 Parents Refuse to Consent for Their Child

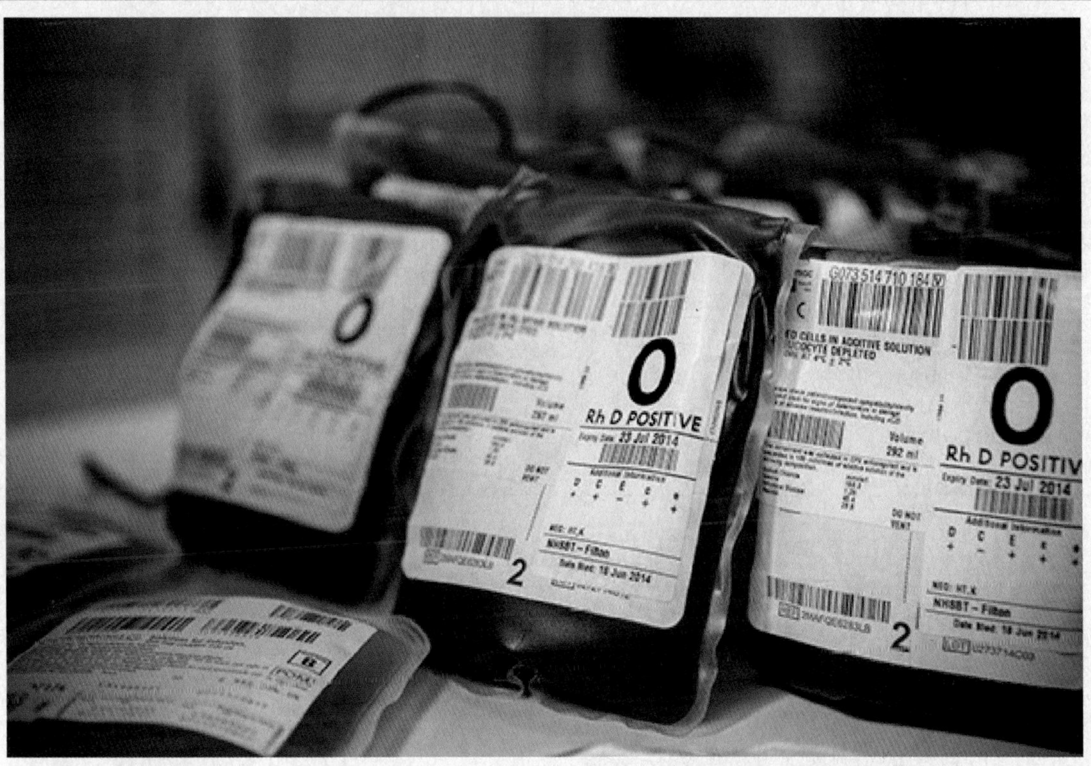

A 15-year-old child who has a life-threatening illness requires a blood transfusion. His parents refuse the transfusion because of religious reasons.

Do you…

a) Assess the child's ability and ask what he would like to do if he's competent enough?
b) Do the transfusion anyway as it is a life-saving procedure?
c) Get the court involved?
d) Follow the parents' wishes and put the child in palliative care?

 Reflect on the answer. What would you do?

Case 5.7 A 14-Year-Old Girl Who Does Not Want Her Mother to Know That She Is Pregnant

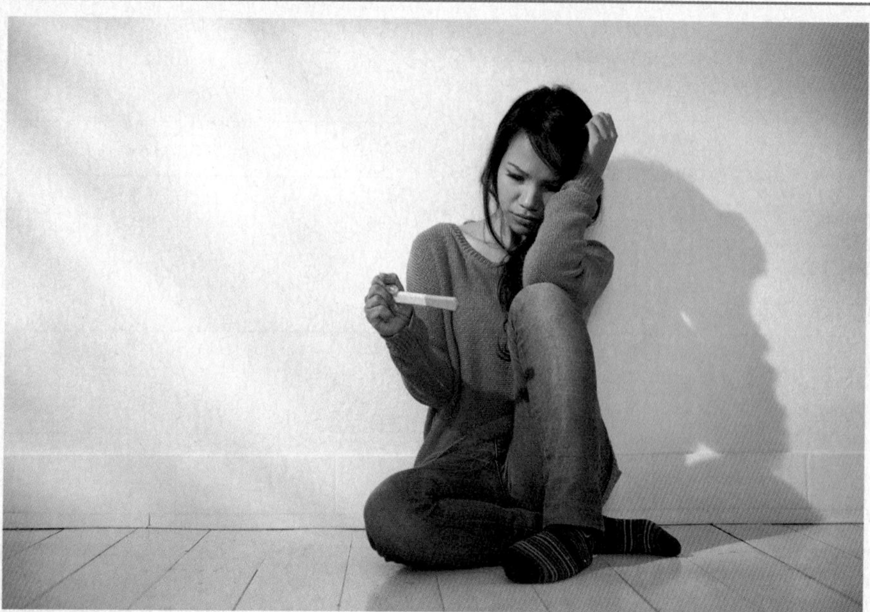

Geraldine is a 14-year-old girl who comes to you complaining of abdominal pain. You believe that she requires an abdominal X-ray for the sake of seeking the best treatment plan. However, she reveals to you that she is pregnant and that her mother (who is in the waiting room) does not know about it. She explicitly states that she does not want her mother to find out.

Do you…

a) Tell the mum as Geraldine is underage, but do not perform the X-ray and seek an alternative scan?
b) Tell the mum and perform the X-ray as the potential benefits may outweigh the risk?
c) Protect Geraldine's confidentiality, don't tell her mum and use an alternative scan to protect her baby from harmful radiation?
d) Protect Geraldine's confidentiality, don't tell her mum and perform the X-ray as the risk of harming the baby by radiation is minimal?

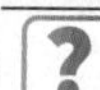 Reflect on the answer. What would you do?

Case 5.8 Safeguarding

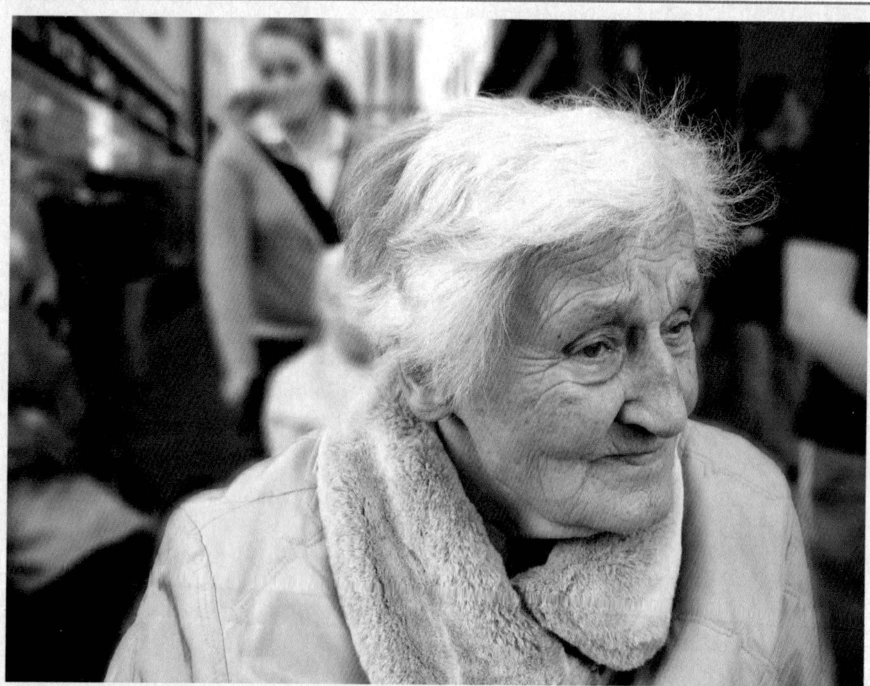

You discovered some bruises on an elderly woman's arm during a consultation. Mrs Smith insisted that it was an accident and asked you not to tell her daughter (who is her only carer) about this. Before the consultation, you also witnessed that her daughter was rude to her in the waiting area.

Do you…

a) Continue asking further questions and ascertain whether Mrs Smith should contact social services?
b) Report the incident to the police?
c) Bring the daughter in and have a consultation with Mrs Smith and her daughter at the same time?
d) Treat her and let her go, without documenting anything about this consultation?

? Reflect on the answer. What would you do?

Case 5.9 Reporting a Knife Wound

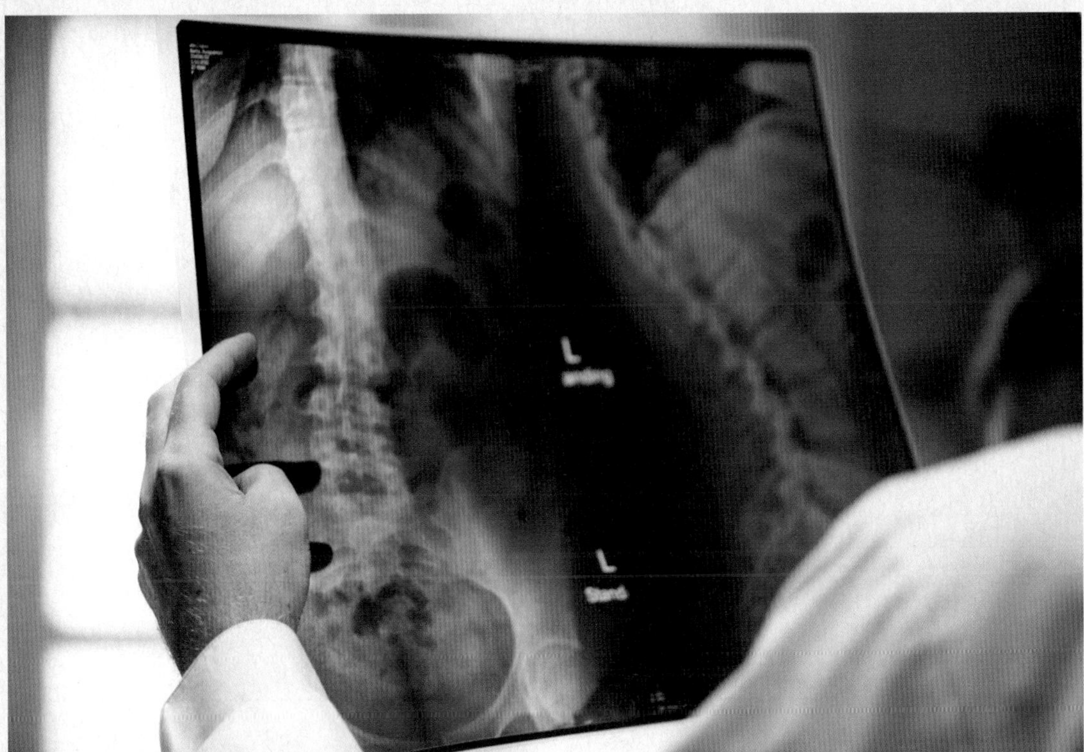

A teenager arrives in an ambulance on a Friday night. He reports being stabbed in the hand. His condition is not life-threatening. He explicitly expresses that he doesn't want the incident reported or the police involved, as it was 'just an accident'. The boy mentions that one of his friends was playing with a knife and it 'just happened' during a heated argument.

Do you…

a) Assess the patient's competence and decide whether to report the incident?
b) Phone the hospital's legal department for advice?
c) Report the incident to the police ASAP?
d) Respect the patient's wishes?

 Reflect on the answer. What would you do?

Case 5.10 **Relationship With Patients Outside Clinical Practice**

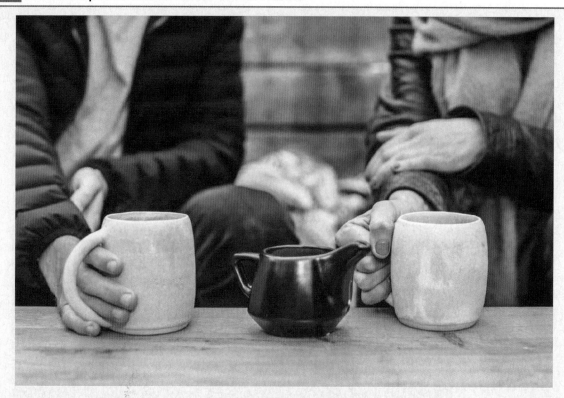

You are on placement in a surgical ward. Patrick, one of the patients, asks you if you would like to meet for a coffee once he feels better. He makes his romantic affections clear and you cannot help but show your happy feelings. Patrick is quite a nice guy too.

Do you…

a) Tell Patrick he'll have to wait until the end of your rotation?
b) Explain to Patrick that you can't meet outside the hospital in a nonprofessional capacity?
c) Ask Patrick if he'd be willing to switch doctors, if so then agree to go?
d) Go anyway as you are only working there temporarily as part of your training, i.e. #YOLO?

 Reflect on the answer. What would you do?

ANSWERS

ANSWER TO CASE 5.1

Let us work through the four ethical principles:

Respect for Autonomy

The principle of respect for autonomy means taking into account and giving consideration to the patient's views on her treatment. Autonomy is not an all-or-nothing concept. Mrs Ying may not be fully autonomous (and not legally competent to refuse treatment), but this does not mean that, ethically, her views should not be considered and respected as much as possible. She has expressed her wishes clearly. She does not want a needle inserted for the anaesthetic. An autonomous decision does not have to be the 'correct' decision from an objective viewpoint, otherwise individual needs and values would not be respected. However, an autonomous decision is one that is informed—has Mrs Ying been given enough information, in a manner that she can comprehend? There's a bit of information missing here—she may have a learning disability, but does she meet the criteria to be deemed competent to make decisions?

Beneficence

The healthcare professional should act to benefit his/her patient. This principle may clash with autonomy. This happens when the patient's decision is not what the healthcare professional considers to be in the best interest of the patient. Here we should consider both the long-term and short-term effects of overriding Mrs Ying's views.

In the short-term, Mrs Ying will be frightened to have a needle inserted in her arm and to be in hospital—this may lead her to distrust healthcare professionals in the future and to be reluctant to seek medical help. In the long-term, there will be a benefit to Mrs Ying in having her autonomy overridden on this occasion. Without treatment, she will suffer serious and long-term health problems that would require greater medical intervention (ongoing dialysis) than the treatment required now (operation). One bad (needle phobia) versus one good (benefit of the surgery)—does this sound familiar? Do you remember when we talked about the Principle of Double Effect?

The benefits of acting beneficently need to be weighed against the disadvantages of failing to respect Mrs Ying's autonomy. (From a legal point of view, the wishes of a competent patient cannot be overridden in their best interests.)

Nonmaleficence

Do no harm to the patient. Here, Mrs Ying would be harmed by forcibly restraining her in order to insert the needle for anaesthesia. On the other hand, if she is not treated now she will require ongoing dialysis a number of times per week. If she does not comply with dialysis, it would be impractical to administer it and may require restraint. Which course of action would result in the greatest harm? This assessment relies on assumptions such as: How successful is the operation likely to be? How likely is Mrs Ying to comply with dialysis?

Justice

Treating everyone fairly. Just because Mrs Ying has a learning difficulty doesn't mean she isn't competent to make decisions. The question also points out the fact that her niece is adamant about Mrs Ying being treated. If Mrs Ying cannot be deemed competent, you may enquire in this situation about power of attorney. Is the niece Mrs Ying's next of kin?

ANSWER TO CASE 5.2

As you may have spotted, autonomy is very important in this case, because your patient specifically asks you to keep the information confidential. Before moving forward, you would have to explain that you would check whether Jane is competent enough to make a decision. Can she understand and retain the information properly? If so, then you should respect her wishes.

The scenario becomes a problem when autonomy clashes with justice. Although you have to respect your patient's wishes, you need to treat everyone equally. Her father has the right to know what happened to his daughter. You may have noticed that beneficence and nonmaleficence also play a role in this scenario. You want to do good by respecting Jane's wish, but by doing so you will cause harm to her father.

As we said before, there are no right or wrong answers to these kinds of questions. You just need to take the interviewer through your thought process and explain why and how you have reached your decision. In this case, you could probably say that you would encourage Jane to tell her parents the truth because all parents love their children and they will eventually understand her situation. You could also try to calm her father down and apologise for not being able to provide an answer yet. A good thing to do is to tell the interviewers how you would feel at the time. Try and put yourself in the doctor's shoes and imagine you had to deal with this situation. I would certainly be frustrated because I cannot find a clear way to please both parties. Interviewers appreciate honesty and reflection!

Trigger warning (TW): Mention of sexual abuse

Can you think of any other important things to consider given that Jane is 15 years old? What about the father of the unborn child? How old is he and is he her boyfriend? Of course, if he's 30 years old, this could raise further questions as this may be sexual abuse. The law states that the age of consent to any form of sexual activity is 16. However, teenagers under the age of 16 will not be prosecuted if both mutually agree and are of similar age. The law clearly states that sexual acts involving children aged 12 and under are classified as sexual abuse.

ANSWER TO CASE 5.3, PART 1

Sharing information with other healthcare professionals is important for safe and effective patient care. That is why, when patients haven't been referred by a GP, specialists are advised to ask for patients' consent to inform their GPs before starting treatment. Specialists should also tell the patient's GP the results of investigations, treatments provided and any other information necessary for the continuing care of the patient, unless the patient objects.

That may be particularly important for a patient like Martin, who will be under medical care for the rest of his life and is likely to need antiretroviral (HIV) medication at some stage. Antiretroviral drugs have many potential serious interactions with other commonly prescribed medications, and it is important that his GP is aware of this if they are to provide safe and effective care. In addition, HIV-infected patients are at a higher risk of several chronic morbidities. GPs play a crucial role in the management of patients' long-term medical conditions in whose treatment knowledge of HIV status may be important.

In this case, Martin objects to you passing on the information to his GP. Confidentiality is important to all patients, but some patients who have or might have serious communicable diseases may have particular concerns. There is a clear public good in having a confidential medical service. The fact that people are encouraged to seek advice and treatment, including for communicable diseases, benefits society as a whole as well as the individual. Patients might avoid seeking medical assistance altogether if they do not believe the information they share with their doctors is secure. That could be dangerous both for the individual patient and the wider community.

In this case, you should strongly encourage Martin to consent, explaining the clear benefits of informing his GP of his status, and seek to reassure him about his GP's legal and ethical duty of confidentiality. All patients are entitled to good standards of care, regardless of what disease they might have or how they acquired it. If he cannot be reassured, you might suggest that Martin registers with a new GP practice.

Ultimately, Martin's decision must be respected unless there is an overriding public interest in disclosing the information without his consent. Doctors and nurses at his practice will not be at risk of infection if standard infection control procedures are followed. It is much less likely for exposure-prone procedures to be undertaken in primary care than in hospitals. It is important that all blood, body fluids and tissues are regarded as potentially infectious, and healthcare workers should follow precautions scrupulously in all circumstances to avoid contact with them.

ANSWER TO CASE 5.3, PART 2

You should certainly counsel Martin to disclose his HIV status, but ultimately you must respect his refusal unless you consider that failure to disclose will put the orthopaedic surgeon and her team at such a risk of infection that disclosure without consent could be justified.

You might also explain that:

- The risk to his surgeon and the other staff caring for him during his operation is negligible while he is on treatment so he should not stop taking his medicine.
- Postexposure prophylaxis is most effective if given as quickly as possible after exposure to the virus; if a needlestick or similar injury occurred in theatre, Martin would be unlikely to be made aware of it until some hours later, after he had recovered from his anaesthetic, if at all.

There may be circumstances in which appropriate infection control procedures are not followed, for a variety of reasons (not all of them justifiable). If you are seriously considering disclosing Martin's status without his consent, you could enquire about the usual infection control procedures at the hospital where Martin's surgery is to take place, without disclosing Martin's identity. You might be reassured by this, or revert to Martin if he still considers disclosure appropriate. Interference with Martin's privacy rights is, however, clearly less satisfactory than the implementation of appropriate infection control procedures by others. You should raise concerns if you encounter evidence of poor practice that leads you to breach your patient's trust.

In the event of a disclosure and a subsequent complaint, you might be able to justify your actions if you had good reason to believe that the surgical team were at risk, e.g. because they would not otherwise employ appropriate infection control procedures or if the nature of the procedure involved particular risks that are difficult to avoid (e.g. if Mr Jones's surgery involved the use of power tools to cut through bone).

Contacting the surgeon to say a patient with a bloodborne virus is booked in on the day Martin's operation is planned would not necessarily be a breach of confidence, but it would not be a sensible course of action. It might lead to disclosure of Martin's status (if he was the only person booked in for surgery on that day, for example), confusion if he changed the date of his operation or unhelpful speculation about who the patient is. It would also encourage and perpetuate poor practice: The use of universal precautions protects clinical staff from the risk of infection from all patients, including those who do not know their status.

ANSWER TO CASE 5.4

Issues to consider in this case:

- Perhaps a simple question to begin with: What is the pattern of this disease? Is it recessive, dominant, X-linked? This will give you an idea of the chance that Rachel might have inherited this condition too.
- Should Adam's right to make a choice about who is informed be respected? (Autonomy)
- Is Rachel at risk if the doctor doesn't inform her? Could this lead to a significant negative impact on her health and therefore does this justify breaching confidentiality? (Beneficence and nonmaleficence)
- Is Rachel's autonomy compromised if she isn't informed?
- Does Rachel have the right to know? (Justice)
- If confidentiality should be breached, who should be informed?
- What are the potential positive outcomes of disclosing the information?
- What are the negative consequences if the information is disclosed?
- Rachel is only 27; she might decide to have children in the near future. Doesn't she have the right to know in order to plan ahead of her pregnancy?

As always, start with the four core ethical principles and work your way through them.

Autonomy

It is your duty as a doctor to respect Adam's decision, as long as he is competent enough to make a decision. This does clash, however, with Rachel's right to know about her disease. At the same time, would she want to know? Employability, insurance policies and life planning are greatly determined by genetic conditions. Adam's thought is that not telling Rachel is in her best interest from a career perspective.

Justice

In this case, treating everyone fairly translates into 'Rachel has the right to know about her condition'.

This is important for many reasons, among others the most important being her long-term health implications and the possibility of passing on a faulty gene to her children.

Beneficence and Nonmaleficence

If you breach confidentiality and don't respect Adam's decision, he may lose trust in the healthcare profession and never seek help or support again. At the same time, although Adam's intention is to save Rachel's career, it may be the case that the health risks for Rachel are so high that she must be informed.

Now, what would you do? Well, in an ideal world, you'd be able to persuade Adam to share the information with his sister. Of course, this would be achieved by explaining that her safety and health are more important than her job. Be careful, however, people have different values and may consider their job or passion to be as important as their health—you need to show an understanding of this. In a less ideal world, if Adam could not be convinced, you would have to carry a few more investigations and find out whether the benefits of breaching confidentiality outweigh the negatives.

Here are a few of the many things to consider:

- The severity of the condition
- The sensitivity of the test
- Actions that can be undertaken by the family (including family-planning decisions)
- Potential harms caused because of the disclosure (don't forget about the damage to Adam and Rachel's relationship and the harm this could have on them psychologically)
- Potential benefits of the disclosure

If the potential benefits of the disclosure outweigh the harm, the cardiologist may consider telling the family, but according to the British Medical Association (BMA), this subject should be approached with sensitivity, taking enough time during the consultation to explain things properly.

It may simply be the case that Rachel doesn't even carry the gene. Either way, for family planning, it's important to establish the pattern of disease. This is relevant for all future generations.

> Our top tip once again is to not get tangled in the details. The main things to examine to get full marks are the four ethical principles, how they clash and what other concepts may be involved. Conclude your answer with 'In an ideal world…' and 'In a less ideal world…' examples and the interviewers will love it.

ANSWER TO CASE 5.5

DNACPRs are contextual to the anticipated cause of death, and as choking is not a common cause of death in terminal cancer, this is a 'not envisaged arrest'. Therefore, you should resuscitate according to the guidance. In simple terms, the gummy bear situation was just an unfortunate event unrelated to the true reason for which she agreed to sign the DNACPR.

In patients who may have several more months to live, an intervention like this is backed up by law.

ANSWER TO CASE 5.6

Once again, what do you do first? Yes, you are right, write down each of the four ethical pillars and look for other concepts that may come into play. Only after you've talked your way through the principles that clash will you be able to reach a conclusion.

Autonomy, Competence and Consent in Under-16-Year-Olds

First of all, what does the theory say about consent in under-16-year-olds? Children under the age of 16 can consent to their own treatment if they're believed to have enough intelligence, competence and understanding to fully appreciate what's involved in their treatment. Okay then, what else should we mention before thinking about the boy's right to decide for himself? What are the four key requirements for someone to be deemed competent (i.e. Gillick competent)?

In our case, the teenager is competent if they can:

1. Understand the information given.
2. Retain the information given.
3. Weigh the risks and benefits of having/not having this transfusion.
4. Communicate his final decision.

But what if the child refuses to have the treatment? When can consent be overruled? If a young person refuses treatment, which may lead to their death or a severe permanent injury, their decision can be overruled by the Court of Protection. The question is, do we have enough time?

Beneficence and Nonmaleficence

Respecting the parents' views and wishes while saving the teenager's life. It is in the patient's best interest to provide the transfusion. However, psychological harm may be caused to the parents and the child as a result of a damaged relationship with the parents due to the parents' concern about the religious implications to them and their child of the transfusion being carried out. Remember that you do not have to agree with someone's belief in order to respect and understand it.

Justice

Parents have the right to be involved in their child's health decision-making process. You could also argue that you should respect people's decisions regardless of their cultural and religious beliefs. There's various ways to think about it.

Other Aspects to Consider Before You Answer

Why are the parents refusing to consent? It may simply be because parents are scared or because they do not understand the significance of certain procedures. It's important to establish the reason behind the refusal. Once you explain the reasons in full, you may be able to persuade them to consent. Of course, this may not be possible due to certain religious beliefs.

Is This an Emergency or Not?

- In an emergency, where treatment is vital and waiting to obtain parental consent would place the child at risk, treatment can proceed without consent. You'll be able to defend yourself later in court.
- Not an emergency? We have enough time to go through the legal route to seek help. The decision should be made in court by respecting the religion the parents believe in while putting the child's best interest at the top of the list.

Again, conclude your answer by signposting and involving different members of the team, as well as mentioning what would happen in an ideal world and what you would have to do in a less ideal world. As you can see, there isn't really a clear answer as it is all situation dependent—which is why we asked you to give us your answer in a multiple-choice format. Applicants often rush to come up with a solution, when in fact the rationale behind the solution is more important.

ANSWER TO CASE 5.7

By now, you should be a master at this. What are the main ethical principles and relevant concepts involved?

Autonomy

You must respect Geraldine's decision, but only if she's deemed competent. What are the four requirements that she has to meet to be deemed competent?

Justice

Autonomy clashes with justice—the right of Geraldine's mother to know what's happening with her daughter.

Beneficence and Nonmaleficence

TW: mention of sexual assault

Tell the mum and you'll harm Geraldine, who may never seek support from you in the future. Don't tell the mum and if she finds out she'll be quite upset. What else is important here to make sure you do your job completely? One aspect you must enquire about is sexual abuse. Who is the partner and how old is he? (It would be suspicious if he was 28 years old!) Was this planned or unplanned? Is she still in a relationship? Is she going to keep the baby or not? What about contraception or future risk of sexually transmitted infections (STIs)? Lots of questions indeed.

Once you've considered these issues, the decision you will make is situation dependent. Is Geraldine competent? If yes, fine, don't tell her mother. If no, tell her mother. Is there evidence of sexual abuse? If yes, involve both her mother and social services.

The final thing to consider is the potential harm that could be induced by ionising radiation. There is a risk of causing cell mutation during the X-ray investigation. Reproductive cells as well as foetuses are more radiosensitive than other cells and body parts. Furthermore, young people (such as Geraldine) are still actively growing and immature cells are more radiosensitive than mature cells. In this case, an ultrasound scan to start with, and later an MRI, might be considered instead.

As usual, conclude by mentioning the ideal scenario of convincing Geraldine to tell her mother.

ANSWER TO CASE 5.8

If you chose answer a), well done. The dilemma does become more difficult if you imagine having to answer it without being prompted by multiple choices, as this answer is only half right. How would you approach this dilemma if the interviewers asked you to discuss it?

This is a tough one indeed, especially if you don't go through it in a structured manner. The best way to approach it is by going back to the four ethical pillars and other concepts that come into play. As usual, think out loud so the interviewers can understand your thought process.

Autonomy

You have to respect Mrs Smith's decision. Confidentiality also comes into play here. Is she competent enough to make her own decisions? What are the main requirements to deem Mrs Smith competent?

Beneficence and Nonmaleficence

Both principles are self-explanatory in this case. You want to do good and provide the best care available and social support for Mrs Smith, without upsetting her and involving her daughter. The challenge is that her daughter is in fact her only carer.

Justice

Justice is less involved in this scenario, although you can say that Mrs Smith has the right to receive support from social services given that her daughter is her only carer.

There are a few general things to consider too. Why does Mrs Smith not want her daughter to know? Is it because she's afraid that she would lose her only carer and doesn't know what help is available in that case from social services? Is it because she thinks her daughter will become violent if she finds out? Is it because she doesn't want her daughter to get into trouble? These and many other similar questions should be considered.

Either way, the interviewers will be interested in hearing how you would try to persuade Mrs Smith to accept your help and support. If that fails (i.e. in a less ideal world), at least mention doing your best to provide Mrs Smith with the information and support she needs to make a decision in her own interest, such as arranging contact with agencies that provide support for victims of domestic violence. Don't forget signposting to other relevant services, as well as documenting this encounter in your notes.

ANSWER TO CASE 5.9

What core principles can you spot here? The need to respect the patient's autonomy, the desire to do good and the desire to prevent any future harm from happening to the teenager—these are all valid points.

First of all, establish whether the boy is competent enough to make decisions. How do you assess if he's competent or not? Think back to the theory. You have probably realised that the clash here is between respecting the patient's autonomy and ensuring that this event could not repeat itself in the future and lead to serious harm to the boy or to any other parties involved.

If you went through all this and backed everything up with theory, you would have got top marks in your interview.

Here's what you need to think about when deciding whether to report such an event:

- Is there a risk of a further attack for the patient?
- Is there a risk of attack to the staff and visitors in the hospital?
- Is there a risk of attack to other members of the public?

All theses are worth considering when disclosing information; however, this scenario becomes trickier as it goes beyond the four ethical principles and uses specific guidance as emphasised by the GMC. The guidance states that any gunshot or knife (including any sharp object) wound should be disclosed to the police as soon as possible. Although this may seem out of scope, we've had several students encounter this scenario in the past. Remember, they are not assessing your knowledge of random GMC facts; they want to see HOW you think around the problem. The correct answer is therefore 'c) report the incident to the police ASAP', although you would not be penalised for choosing option a), as long as you take time to talk your way through the various ethical principles and theory concepts. Of course, you would impress them if you quote the GMC guidance with regards to knife/gunshot wounds. And, lucky for you—now you know it!

ANSWER TO CASE 5.10

According to the GMC, 'You must not use your professional position to pursue a sexual or improper emotional relationship with a patient or someone close to them'. Doctors need to act professionally to maintain trust within society. As a doctor, you should not pursue any improper emotional relationships with your current patients.

Of course, the answer would be different if you met Patrick outside the hospital and if he wasn't your patient—doctors can still have a life! There are still many other factors to take into consideration. One important question to ask yourself is: Are they vulnerable? It's important to realise that as a doctor you are in a position of high status, and it's unprofessional and unacceptable to take advantage of vulnerable people.

In this case, Patrick initiates the relationship and you should politely reestablish the professional boundary, or even consider ending the professional relationship with him if he is insistent. This is suggested by the GMC as part of their guidance on 'Ending your professional relationship with a patient'. However, they also state that ending a professional relationship with a patient solely to pursue a personal relationship is not acceptable.

Additional Ethical Dilemmas

Hungry for more? Here are some additional thought-provoking suggestions for you to cover as homework:

1. Euthanasia: A terminally ill patient asks you to give him an overdose of morphine as he's sick of suffering. What's the difference between euthanasia and doctor-assisted suicide? And how does the doctrine of double effect come into this?
2. Conflict of belief: A patient is enquiring about a fertility treatment that is against your own belief as a practitioner. What should you do?
3. Data handling: You receive a call from your patient's wife asking for her husband's appointment time and the details of his illness. Should you answer her question?
4. Screening for chromosomal conditions: Should screening for Down, Edward and Patau syndromes be an opt-out decision?
5. Necessary abortion to save the mother's life: Your patient has an ectopic pregnancy and requires an abortion in order to save her life. She refuses the abortion because to her that means 'murder'. What should you do?
6. Alternative medicine: Your patient suffers from lung cancer, and his wife comes to you and asks if alternative medicine would help alongside the chemotherapy and radiotherapy that her husband is undergoing. What do you tell her?
7. A decision made in advance: Tim had an official donor card and signed to donate his organs when the time comes. Upon his death, his family refuse to allow the healthcare professionals to harvest the organs. What should you do?
8. Justice: There is only one place available in a clinical drug trial. You have two patients with the same condition; they are the same gender and same age, but one of them has a low mental capacity. Who would you choose and why?

9. Confidentiality: A patient revealed their suicidal thoughts to you and asked you not to tell anyone. What should you do?
10. Racism: A patient is being aggressive to your fellow colleague who comes from an ethnic minority. He has asked you to change his doctor, as he does not want a non-British doctor to treat him. Your colleague is in great distress and asks you for help. What should you do?
11. Intimate examinations: You are a male doctor who is about to perform an intimate examination for a female patient, and she refused to have a chaperone or anyone else in the room during the exam. What should you do?
12. Receiving gifts: A patient gives you a cheque and a card as a gift. What should you do?
13. Malpractice: Your patient's relatives are not happy with your care and demand your name and GMC number. Should you give it to them?

HOW CAN YOU USE THIS INFORMATION?

I suppose there isn't much point to rambling on about how important the theories mentioned above are when tackling an ethical dilemma during your medical school interview. What you do need to know is that most interviews have at least one question involving ethical dilemmas. This is because they can easily reveal your suitability (or unsuitability) for becoming a doctor. This will further be emphasised in Chapter 9.

As well as equipping you with the right skills for your medical school interview, these concepts represent the basis of becoming a good clinician. You will encounter all these concepts as a medical student on the wards and during your future training as a doctor.

These intriguing notions dwelled and still dwell on my mind, but recently I realised I must come to terms with them; otherwise I may not be able to practice medicine. Once you get the main idea of each concept, you'll find them quite interesting, I promise.

My tip would be to keep an eye out for these principles during your placements. I tried integrating them during my work experience placement in the Emergency Department, where I would observe doctors from different specialities who must deal with what comes through the door. What I saw, besides the normal and extraordinary things they do that I look forward to doing myself in the future, was how doctors based difficult decisions on thorough reasoning. Guess what, the four pillars were the underlying principles to their decision-making, hence every medical applicant should be learning this piece of information no matter where they apply. It's not only relevant to your interview performance, but also to your future career.

Periklis, Medical School Applicant

If you have enjoyed working through this chapter and want to pursue medical ethics in the future, why not have a look into an intercalation in medical ethics!

SUMMARY, TEST YOURSELF AND REFLECTION

Ethics attempt to illustrate an ideal human character and inform people to make better decisions and better choices. There are four plus one core ethical principles:

- Autonomy
- Beneficence
- Nonmaleficence
- Justice
- Confidentiality

However, there's more to ethics than the core principles.

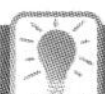

Other Useful Concepts to Remember

- Capacity
- Competence
- Consent
- Mental Health Act

When faced with an ethical dilemma, follow this algorithm, keep calm and carry on!

Steps to tackling an ethical dilemma:

1. Read and understand the text.
2. Spot the principles involved.
3. Do not make any assumptions.
4. Justify using arguments.
5. Reach a balanced conclusion.

A box for reflection and ideas has been provided here so you can jot down any thoughts you may have. Use these notes as guidance when preparing for the interview. Whether you like it or not, the interview will involve an ethical dilemma.

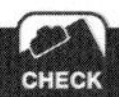

Test Yourself

- What is the difference between ethics and laws?
- What is the principle of double effect?
- What is consent? How many types of consent are there?
- What are the four requirements to deem someone competent?
- Can children accept treatment? What about refusing treatment?
- When can doctors breach confidentiality?

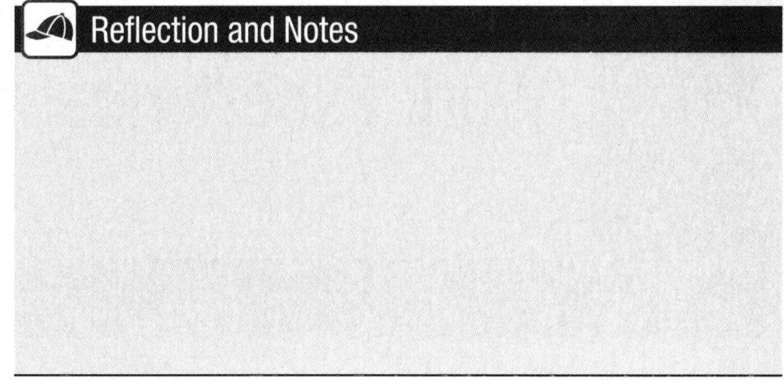

RESOURCES

General Medical Council, 2009. Tomorrow's doctors. Available at https://www.gmc-uk.org/Tomorrow_s_Doctors_1214.pdf_48905759.pdf.

General Medical Council, 2013a. Good medical practice. Available at https://www.gmc-uk.org/-/media/documents/good-medical-practice---english-20200128_pdf-51527435.pdf.

General Medical Council, 2013b. Maintaining a professional boundary between you and your patient. Available at https://www.gmc-uk.org/static/documents/content/Maintaining_a_professional_boundary_between_you_and_your_patient.pdf.

General Medical Council, 2018. 0–18 years: guidance for all doctors. Available at http://www.gmc-uk.org/guidance/ethical_guidance/children_guidance_27_28_lack_capacity.asp.

GP Notebook. Fraser Guidelines. Available at http://www.gmc-uk.org/guidance/ethical_guidance/children_guidance_27_28_lack_capacity.asp.

Hope, R.A., 2004. Medical Ethics: A Very Short Introduction. New York: Oxford University Press.

Hurwitz, B., Richardson, R., 1997. Swearing to care: the resurgence in medical oaths. Br Med J 315, 1671.

McManus, I.C., Gordon, D., Winder, B.C., 2000. Duties of a doctor: UK doctors and good medical practice. BMJ Qual Saf 9, 14–22.

NHS Choices. Consent to treatment. Available at https://www.nhs.uk/conditions/consent-to-treatment/.

Tyson, P., 2001. The Hippocratic oath today. NOVA. WGBH Educational Foundation. Available at http://www.pbs.org/wgbh/nova/body/hippocratic-oath-today.html.

UK Clinical Ethics Network. Ethical frameworks. Available at http://www.ukcen.net/ethical_issues/ethical_frameworks/the_four_principles_of_biomedical_ethics.

UK Clinical Ethics Network. Educational resources – Mental Capacity Act. Available at http://www.ukcen.net/education_resources/mental_capacity.

Special thanks to the GMC for kindly allowing us to use some of their useful learning materials and General Medical Practice in action tools.

6 Work Experience: Getting Involved

Bogdan Chiva Giurca, Ida Saidy and Kiyara Fernando

Chapter Outline

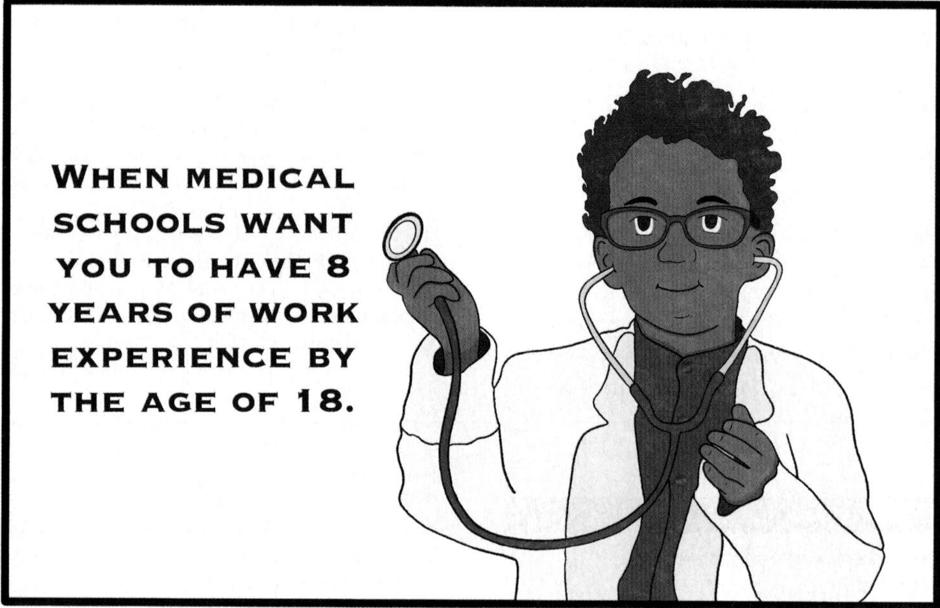
WHEN MEDICAL SCHOOLS WANT YOU TO HAVE 8 YEARS OF WORK EXPERIENCE BY THE AGE OF 18.

With thousands of applicants competing against one another, work experience is yet another important aspect of your application that can make a big difference and help you stand out from the crowd if done well. Work experience isn't JUST a tick box, however; it's not something that you should do just because medical schools say so. Work experience is something you should get involved in out of your own initiative, enthusiasm and pure interest. After all, you want to make sure that medicine is the perfect subject for you. In other words, you are not allowed to say, 'I love medicine' without experiencing it, being part of it and knowing what it entails.

This chapter covers some of the most frequently asked questions about work experience. We've also done our best to equip you with our top tips to make the most of your work experience placements. Upon completion of this chapter, print out a bunch of empty work experience templates (see 'How to get the most out of your medical work experience?') and stick them into your personal portfolio. When it comes to writing your personal statement and even preparing for your medical school interview, these templates will save hours and hours of work!

Let's jump right in!

THE WHY, WHEN AND HOW

WHY IS MEDICAL WORK EXPERIENCE IMPORTANT?

Work experience allows you to get first-hand experience in the medical field. Seeing if you enjoy the environment and the role of a doctor is critical to determining if you will enjoy a career in medicine.

Some find the experience eye-opening to the realities of the profession and it strengthens their desire to study medicine. Some students might realise that medicine is not for them, and it is better to learn this early on so that you can decide on a more suitable career path.

The more time spent in work experience, the better you will understand the realities of the profession. It will help you learn how hospitals, clinics and surgeries are run and what skills different medical personnel require. You will soon see that medicine is not what is portrayed on TV screens… it is more.

> Medical work experiences were essential in exposing me to the field of medicine in clinical settings and giving me insight into the collective work of healthcare professionals to successfully serve the community. It was these experiences that confirmed for me that my future lies in medicine. To obtain these experiences, I personally visited and wrote to the clinics/hospitals I believe reflected my interest and motivation. It wasn't easy and many of them turned me down, but I kept trying until a few replied.
>
> Shadowing healthcare professionals from different departments was also beneficial, as they presented me both the rewarding and the heart-breaking realities of medicine. (In my case, observing a gynaecologist provide the prognosis and options for abortion to a couple due to a foetal anomaly.) The hardest part for me was facing a language barrier while volunteering at a free clinic and dealing with several impatient patients; hence it was amazing to see the professional way the nurses dealt with the situation calmly. I truly recommend shadowing a range of healthcare professionals other than doctors. You can learn so much from nurses, occupational therapists and others.
>
> At the end of a placement day, it would be ideal to write a short reflection of situations encountered, emotions felt at the time and what you learnt from it to make improvements for future experiences. I've enjoyed using the reflective template provided in this chapter as I can print it and add it to my portfolio, but it's completely up to you and doesn't matter what you use as long as you do find time to reflect. Good luck!
>
> **Hey Gin, Medical School Applicant**

WHEN SHOULD YOU SEEK WORK EXPERIENCE?

It's never too early, but it may sometimes be too late!

Ideally, try to get some medical work experience as early as possible. The more exposure you have to the medical world, the better. It is common for students to look for opportunities post Advanced Subsidiary (AS) levels, but if you have the chance to have some work experience earlier on…take it! This would be beneficial for you.

HOW SHOULD YOU GET WORK EXPERIENCE?

1. Speak to your school and ask for any contacts they may have used for previous medical school applicants.
2. Use your personal contacts—write emails, make phone calls, ask any family, friends or relatives that you may have.
3. Contact your local hospital/clinic/general practice (GP)/medical trust and ask them if they have any opportunities.
4. Attend medical conferences and seminars. This is where you may meet clinicians with whom you can network. Send them your curriculum vitae (CV) if they seem interested in helping you.
5. You could also directly contact a doctor who works in a specialty that appeals to you. It helps if you read up on them and learn about the procedures you might see. This knowledge will help you build rapport with your mentors.
6. Speak to anyone you think could help secure you some work experience.
7. Use your 'Getting into medical school portfolio' and create a personal CV of your achievements. Build this up as you get more experience in the field, covering GPs, hospitals, care settings, etc. Send this CV around to those who may be able to help you secure some work experience.
8. Keep knocking and don't give up. If 10 people say no, keep going. If 20 people say no, keep going. Out of 50 people, one must say yes, and if not, keep going until you find that person!
9. If you're out of doors to knock on for opportunities, try to create a NEW door. By that I mean come up with the idea for a new role that you can have outside the existent shadowing or volunteering schemes within an institution.
10. Stay proactive and enthusiastic—consider all options including virtual work experience which can be equally valuable.

> I drew up a plan, made a spreadsheet of hospitals and doctors I knew and conferences and I made a checklist of all the potential places I could work and started contacting people. I started looking before my GCSEs. I may have started earlier than most but you don't need to panic, as it is never too late to start looking for any kind of medical experience.
>
> **Medical Student, Bristol Medical School**

Doctors have a vast network among themselves and most doctors are keen on helping prospective medical students, so hopefully after asking around, an opportunity will come your way.

> Doctors are busy people. They will want to help you but may not have the time and resources to do so, so they may have to decline taking you on as an observer. Do not take offence at this, and keep trying! There is bound to be someone who will accommodate you. It may not be in your first choice of specialty and may be a clinic or care home, but you must start somewhere.
>
> **Dr Zeshan Qureshi, Paediatric Registrar**

WHAT COUNTS AS 'WORK EXPERIENCE'?

WHAT ARE THE DIFFERENT TYPES OF WORK EXPERIENCE?

- GP placements
- Hospital placements
- Volunteering placements (national/international)
- Other placements
  - Hospices
  - Charities
  - Care homes
  - Research facilities
- Virtual work experience (including live and online courses)

GENERAL PRACTICE PLACEMENTS

GP, or primary care, is the principal way patients may contact the NHS. As a result, GP clinics can be very busy, with a range of patients coming in with different ailments.

Typically, you would sit in and observe the GP during consultations with their patients. The GP would ask their patient's permission for you to listen in on the consultation. Most often, patients have no issue with this, although some patients may express their discomfort with having someone else in the room. If this is the case, politely step out until the consultation is over. Hopefully the next patient will not mind.

Here are a few things that you can learn in a GP clinic:

- In a 10-minute window, GPs extract a large amount of information from the patient about their health issues without being abrupt and ensure enough information is available.
- How GPs assess the seriousness of symptoms and decide if the patient requires referral to a secondary healthcare service.
- How the members of the clinic—GPs, nurses, etc.—work as a unit to ensure the smooth running of the clinic.
- The GP's role in educating their patients on healthy lifestyles and management of chronic disease, as patients with long-term conditions like diabetes are very common in a primary healthcare setting.
- The continuity of care in a GP clinic, where patients have been coming to the same GP for years, and he/she has helped to manage their condition through the years.
- The GPs role as a listener—this is the emotional aspect of primary care, where patients often use GPs for emotional support.

HOSPITAL PLACEMENTS

Hospital placements will allow you to observe a doctor's work in a secondary care setting. You will also gain insight into how other healthcare professionals carry out their jobs and how doctors interact with nurses, lab technicians, radiology experts, etc., to treat a patient.

What you can learn in a hospital environment:

- Follow a doctor on a ward round—watch how the doctor sums up a patient's case and progress to members of the team.
- Sit in on a multidisciplinary team meeting—observe how healthcare professionals from different specialties work together to manage patients.
- Follow the work of a nurse/lab assistant/pharmacist—gain insight into how other healthcare professionals carry out their jobs.

VOLUNTEERING PLACEMENTS

Volunteering placements are invaluable in developing your skills to become a future doctor. Several students work at care homes or local charity organisations. Volunteering placements do not necessarily have to be medically related, and any experience in a caring role will be looked at in a favourable light. Wherever you obtain a placement, show consistency by attending over a long period, ideally a few months, as opposed to just doing a few days' work. Long-term volunteering allows you to build rapport with colleagues and patients, and the skills you develop from placements and your experiences will come across in your interview.

OTHER PLACEMENTS

Anything medically relevant or anything that can be applied in the medical domain can count as work experience. Hospices and care homes are often great places where you can make an actual difference for the people you look after. Having a chat with someone who feels lonely is a brilliant way to develop your empathy, communication and listening skills while also making their day more enjoyable.

The COVID-19 pandemic truly highlighted the importance of community health. Volunteering in your community (e.g. volunteering at a local vaccination clinic) can provide useful, transferable experiences for your application. Furthermore, designing your own community project that touches the lives of locals and is related to an issue you care deeply about can be one of the best forms of work experience for a career rooted in public service. As an example, two fantastic students in London were frustrated that COVID-19 information was not available in the Somali language, therefore making it inaccessible to their local community. They set on a goal to translate all public health campaigns related to the pandemic and launched a large social media campaign reaching hundreds of thousands of people in need. Now that's what we call proactive, enthusiastic and passionate applicants!

Another way of getting involved in work experience is through medical research. This can be especially appealing to those of you attracted more by the scientific side of medicine. This can allow you to stretch your prior scientific knowledge and satisfy your curiosity. Moreover, it can demonstrate your understanding of how multifaceted medicine is with both clinical and academic career routes.

Furthermore, some universities offer programmes that aid applicants in finding varied types of work experience. One such example that benefited me is the Pathways to Medicine programme organised by Imperial College London. These programmes may have specific criteria, though, so do your research to avoid disappointment!

VIRTUAL (ONLINE) WORK EXPERIENCE

The series of lockdowns, limited face-to-face interactions and periods of closure for public institutions during the COVID-19 pandemic have completely changed how medical schools see work experience. Whereas in the past, applicants would try their hardest to get experience in local GPs and hospitals (sometimes unsuccessfully), you can now engage in work experience from the comfort of your own home, at your own pace. The national Medical Schools Council (MSC) in the UK have said: *'Medical schools understand that it is difficult to get in person experience now. Many people have had to isolate and opportunities to gain experience in a healthcare environment may be limited. All medical schools are aware that the opportunities open to you have been affected and will take this into account'*.

As mentioned throughout this book, it is not about what you see or do during your work experience, but more so about your reflection points and how you use these throughout your application in your personal statement and during your medical school interview. All medical schools have now embraced virtual work experience and see it as valuable as in-person work experience if you can provide arguments and solid reflections based on what you've learned.

Examples of online work experience are extremely widespread and varied. National bodies such as The Royal College of GPs have designed specific, tailored online work experience programmes relating to their specialties. For example, ObserveGP allows you to engage in a range of scenarios unique to general practice, while learning techniques used by clinicians daily. Another infamous programme includes the Brighton and Sussex Virtual Work Experience, which takes you through specific scenarios that you can reflect on in your application. All relatively easy ways to access valuable work experience!

THE BIGGEST MISTAKE MADE BY APPLICANTS

A common mistake is to think that work experience is a simple box that can only be ticked if you shadow doctors in the hospital environment.

Several applicants had the opportunity to witness extensive surgeries and innovative patient care, but they couldn't explain what exactly they gained from it.

Why would admission tutors care if you've had the chance to drill a hole in somebody's knee while assisting the orthopaedic surgeons during a knee replacement procedure? The anatomy, the landmarks, the procedure, the equipment and everything else will be explained to you throughout medical school in lectures and tutorials. That's why you have at least 5 years to explore all medical specialties and learn anatomy and physiology.

It's not about assisting surgeons and trying to appear more knowledgeable than you are. You need to be able to show TRANSFERRABLE SKILLS. You need to have the building blocks—the foundation on which you can add through your time at the medical school.

> Unfortunately, I couldn't secure any hospital placements over the years. In the end, I worked for a UK charity called 'British Heart Foundation'. This was a voluntary role and it involved working in their charity shop, selling items, dealing with customers and raising funds during events. Over a 1-year period, I was part of several teams and held a leadership position during two fundraising events. When it came to the medical school application process, I realised that my voluntary work actually ticked all the boxes, even though it did not directly involve patient contact. I was part of a medical charity, raising funds for research and developing several transferrable skills including communication, listening, teamwork and leadership skills.
>
> It's honestly what you learn from it and how you put it to good use in your personal statement and interview. My friend got into UCL by making a connection between her job and the hospital environment. Sarah worked as a waitress in a busy café. In her personal statement and throughout the interview she used various examples of how her skills dealing with customers under pressure can also be applied in a busy emergency department. The interviewing panel loved it!
>
> **Tom B., Medical Student, Exeter Medical School**

HOW TO GET THE MOST OUT OF YOUR MEDICAL WORK EXPERIENCE

DURING YOUR WORK EXPERIENCE PLACEMENT

Below are five top tips for when you're on placement:

1. Dress smartly.
   Professionalism is at the core of being a good doctor. Dress up as if you are going to a job interview. Usually, the standard placement uniform is a white shirt and trousers or a knee-length skirt with smart formal black shoes. Make sure you look formal, professional and presentable. The hosting team will appreciate your effort and will be proud to introduce you to colleagues and patients.
2. Bring a notepad (not phone!).
   Using your phone can appear unprofessional especially for old-fashioned staff members who may be thinking you are surfing Instagram instead of paying attention and taking notes. Chances are you may be taking notes on your phone, but you may be wrongly judged by someone who doesn't know or understand your technical

skills and digital prowess. Bring a notepad and jot down everything you see—you would be surprised how much you can forget. This will come in handy when you need to reflect on your experiences for interviews and your personal statement.

3. Be polite and respectful of others.
   Remember, busy healthcare professionals are taking valuable time out of their day to support you and teach you. It's important to be respectful of their time, be polite and not interfere or disrupt tasks and activities unless directly involved by the hosting team. Be grateful for the opportunity and show your appreciation to the hosting team and institution by thanking them for having you. This will increase the chance of having a follow-up placement within the same team or as part of the broader institution.
4. Be proactive and don't hesitate asking questions.
   Your enthusiasm and curiosity to learn should be translated into a myriad of questions which you can ask on the day. As mentioned in our previous point, you have to be mindful not to interfere with patient activities, but chances are there will be plenty of time for questions during coffee breaks, lunch and much more. If prompted to do so, don't be afraid to ask questions or engage with patients.
5. Pre-read and prepare.
   Familiarising yourself beforehand with the topic or specialty you will be exploring can truly help you make the most of your work experience placement. This will enable you to learn the relevant jargon and understand deeper themes, allow you to ask insightful questions and empower you to build a better rapport with the placement providers.

FOLLOWING YOUR WORK EXPERIENCE PLACEMENT

Regardless of what work experience you do, it is crucial that you learn from it. It is not enough to merely go on placement; what is truly important is understanding what you took out of the experience.

Although it can be an arduous task after a long day on placement, it is crucial that you:

- Make notes about your experiences
- Reflect on them
- Revisit these experiences after a few weeks

What does it mean to reflect on your work experience? Here are a few points to consider when doing medical work experience:

- What exactly have I experienced today?
- What did the doctor do to manage this?
- How did the patient react to this?
- How did the doctor interact with colleagues/juniors/nurses?
- What may the doctor have done differently?
- How does the doctor learn this skill?
- Why was the action necessary?
- Was this a good example of medicine or a bad example of medicine?

To make things easier for you, we've put together a reflective template you can use after every single one of your work experience placements. Remember, **REFLECTION** is the key word here.

In fact, 'reflection' is something that will no doubt haunt you throughout medical school and your career as a doctor. As a medical student, you have to reflect at the end of the week on the patients you have seen in the hospital and what you have learned from your encounters. As a doctor, at the end of the year, you have to do an annual review of your practice and reflect upon your work. This is why getting good at this now will pay off in the long run and will also impress admission tutors during your interview.

Perhaps the most famous reflection model is the so-called 'Gibbs' Cycle' (Fig. 6.1). The cycle is made of six steps, starting with a description of the event itself and ending with a summary of the lessons you have learnt, and building an action plan in case you encounter this particular situation again in the future.

The good thing is that this cycle can be used for any work experience placement that you may be part of—be it voluntary work, hospital placements or even working as part of a team, any situation can be broken down using Gibbs' Cycle. An example is shown here.

Work Experience, Reflective Template

Title: Leadership Lesson for the future
Date: 10/05/2018
Activity: Bristol Fundraising Event
Description (What happened?)
Today I was the leader of a fundraising team, helping with a marathon in Bristol for Cancer Research UK, but half of my team called in sick, so we were lacking in numbers.
Feelings (What were you feeling/thinking)
At the time, I was frustrated, upset, felt incapable of achieving what I have planned initially.
Evaluation (What was good/bad about it)
Considering the bad aspects, I panicked, fell under pressure and didn't know what to do. However, I finally managed to gather myself and realised that I can still save what's left of this event. I delegated tasks, allocated people to different roles and changed what was initially planned—of course, things ran slowly, but we managed to cope under stress.
Analysis (What can you make of the situation?)
When I look back on my experience, I realise that I shouldn't have panicked and, in the future, I think I should consider my actions more carefully. Unexpected situations always happen, and you need to be prepared. My mistake was not checking the evening before to see who was still available and who wasn't. I should have also recruited more people than necessary, just in case something like this happened.
Conclusion (What else could you have done?)

After considering my experience further, I realised that I could have asked for help from my superior—maybe they had some available volunteers. This has been an important lesson that has allowed me to develop my leadership and teamwork skills.

Action Plan (In the future, what would you do?)

In the future, I will try to seek help early on and consider my actions more carefully. I should also plan ahead and gather more volunteers than required, as there is always the risk of someone calling in sick.

Note to self: Consider using this example in the future if asked anything related to leadership in an interview.

You can see how the previous example provided by Bogdan could also be the perfect answer in an interview setting to a question that may sound like this: *'Give an example of a time when you were the leader of a team and something went wrong. What would you do differently in the future?'*

HOW CAN THIS ENHANCE YOUR MEDICAL SCHOOL APPLICATION?

To help you stay organised and save precious time when it comes to personal statement writing and interview preparation, we developed the following template, which you can replicate in a plain Word document and use at the end of each day following your work experience placement. Write down quotes from those with whom you interacted, and reflect on your feelings and emotions.

Work Experience, Reflective Template

Title:

Date:

Activity:

Description (What happened?)

Feelings (What were you feeling/thinking at the time?)

Evaluation (What was good/bad about it?)

Analysis (What can you make of the situation?)

Action Plan (In the future, what would you do/what could you do differently?)

I know it is tempting to avoid doing this, but if you don't do it while the experience is fresh in your mind, you will soon forget everything, and all the time invested in that placement will go down the drain. Save yourself time by investing 20 minutes to document what you learnt at the end of each placement. Once you complete a reflective template, add it to your portfolio and watch it grow as days go by. As your folder grows bigger and bigger, you'll feel more motivated and confident that you are on the right track. Our brain loves it when we can measure our progress!

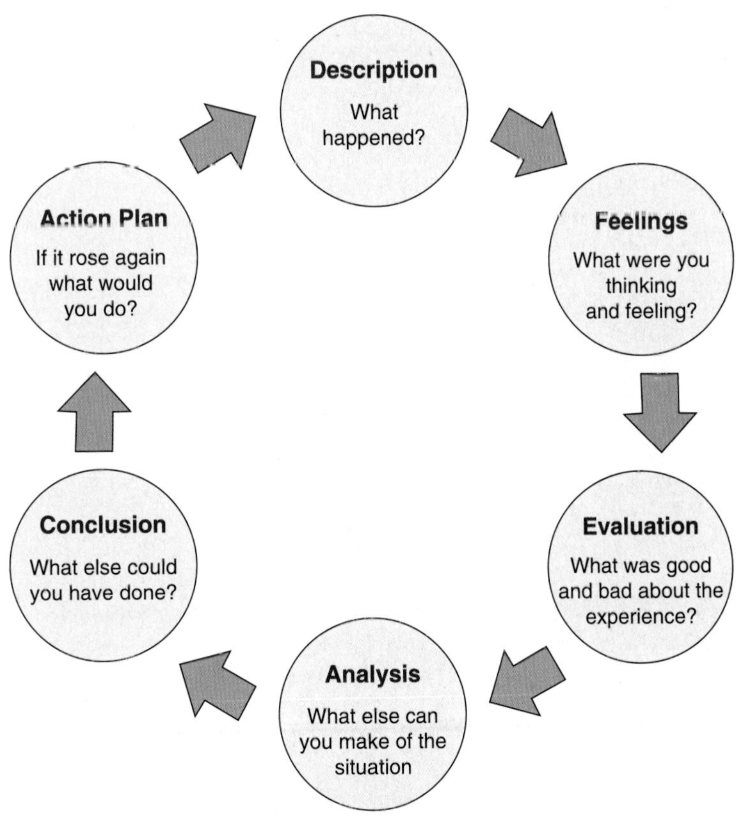

Fig. 6.1 Gibbs' reflective cycle.

During my work experience, I witnessed the sheer impact a doctor has on a patient, their family and the team they work with. There are certain experiences during shadowing that have stayed with me and will ultimately shape the doctor I hope to be. One that resounds with me is a doctor breaking the news to a patient that he had stage 3 pancreatic cancer. The quiet confidence of the doctor and the kindness he showed the patient are qualities I picked up on. He was kind without being patronising and his respect for the patient who wanted some time alone trumped his natural reflex to stay and comfort him. The doctor changed his communication style depending on how the patient reacted and what they needed at the time.

Medical Student, University of Bristol Medical School

Work experience showed me that communication is key when working with different types of caregivers. Doctors talk to one another, rely on reports or notes made by colleagues and work in partnership with nurses, anesthetists, radiologists and other medical personnel along with the patients and their families. It is essential to be dependable and trustworthy in caring for patients, as each part of the team depends on each other.

Medical Student, University of Cardiff Medical School

I thoroughly enjoyed my work experience; it helped me immerse myself in the medical field. I built relationships with some amazing people and ultimately enjoyed my time at a few hospitals so much that I didn't want to leave! The advice I received and what I learnt during my time shadowing has been invaluable. The doctors I learnt from will shape the doctor I hope to be.

Medical Student, University of Bristol

SUMMARY, TEST YOURSELF AND REFLECTION

What you do and see during your work experience will ultimately shape your perspective of medicine in your early medical school years.

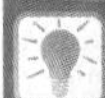

As We Reach the End of This Chapter, Please Remember To

- Apply early
- Talk to anyone and everyone who might have contacts, one contact could lead to another
- Be organised, have a plan
- Be persistent
- Accept whatever is offered to you—you can learn from anything!
- Find local charities/volunteering opportunities
- Make notes each day and reflect on what you have learnt and observed
- Read and research as much as possible to get the most out of your experience
- Dress appropriately
- Be polite, helpful and volunteer
- Ask questions when your mentor is available, and not in the middle of a consultation or during a busy time—remember, you're there to learn and observe, not disrupt their work!

Finally, confidentiality is key. As a potential medical student, you will be privy to private information about patients. As a result of this, you are obliged to keep all information about the work place in the work place.

A reflection box is provided for you to jot down any ideas or thoughts that you may have. Have you completed your work experience placements or are you still looking for one? Have you made a plan and a list of the people you can contact? How are you planning to make the most of your placement?

Test Yourself

- What are the different types of work experience placements?
- Does work experience only mean clinical placements?
- What is the Gibbs' Cycle?

Reflection and Notes

RESOURCES

Brighton and Sussex Medical School. Virtual work experience. Available at https://bsmsoutreach.thinkific.com/courses/VWE.

Gibbs cycle (Mind Tools) Explained: Available at https://www.mindtools.com/pages/article/reflective-cycle.htm.

Medical School Council. Medicine applications. Available at https://www.medschools.ac.uk/studying-medicine/applications.

The Student Room. Work experience. Available at https://www.thestudentroom.co.uk/jobs/work-experience/medicine-work-experience.

UCAS. Work experience. Available at https://www.ucas.com/connect/blogs/work-experience-important.

Royal College of General Practitioners. Observe GP work experience. Available at https://www.rcgp.org.uk/observegp.

7 Mastering Entrance Exams: The UCAT and BMAT

Rachel Howard, Dupinderjit Rye and Gareth Lau

Chapter Outline

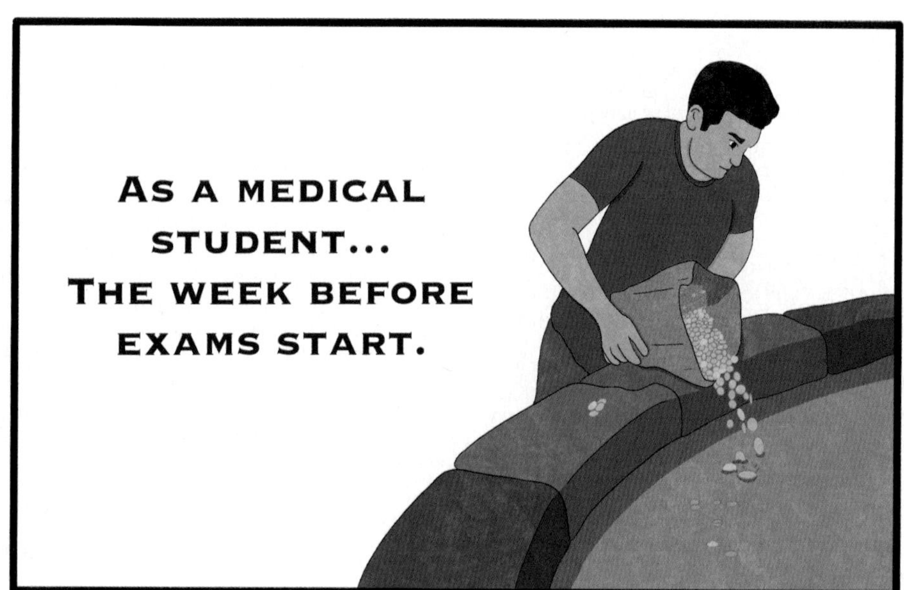

AS A MEDICAL STUDENT...
THE WEEK BEFORE EXAMS START.

THE THEORY OF LEARNING—ACING ANY EXAM

Before we talk about the rather boring medical school entrance exams, let us focus on a couple of studying and exam preparation hacks, all based on science and used by successful medical school applicants and students worldwide.

APPLYING THE SCIENCE OF LEARNING

As any respectable scientist would do, let's look for evidence-based answers and not base our opinions on assumptions any longer. A lot of research has been done on learning and studying theories over the years. The following common question emerged: How many hours of practice do you have to put in to be good at something?

10,000 Hours

Perhaps one of the most widely known theories for acing a particular subject is the '10,000-hour rule'. Some of you may already be familiar with this concept, as it has received a lot of attention over the years. Ten thousand hours to learn something new? That's quite discouraging, isn't it? That's years and years of deliberate practice in one particular area, or approximately 3 hours a day for 10 years to be more specific! This must be false; otherwise, we'd never learn anything new for the rest of our lives.

Here's the catch. The 10,000-hour rule was first introduced by Anders Ericsson, a professor at the University of Colorado. According to professor Ericsson, 'If you want to master a subject area, you need to spend 10,000 hours of work and practice in that particular area'. This theory was based on data from **expert-level** individuals in various fields. Ericsson was studying world-class champions, not people who just wanted to ace the University Clinical Aptitude Test (UCAT)! People misinterpreted Ericsson's theory over the years and concluded that 10,000 hours is all it takes to get 'good' at something. Further misinterpretation eventually led to people stating that 10,000 hours is what it takes to learn something new—which is completely ridiculous, to say the least.

20 Hours

Luckily, you won't have to spend 10,000 hours to get ready for the UCAT and Biomedical Admission Test (BMAT). Famous psychologist Josh Kaufman researched the science behind learning and acquiring new skills. His research demonstrates that you can learn anything if you focus on individual skills for as little as 20 hours. To understand how this works, and put it into context, we've created a graph illustrating the science behind learning (Fig. 7.1).

Let's take the learning curve and dissect it a little bit.

1. **Initial frustration**

   How many of you have tried learning to play an instrument or anything similar? Do you remember those first few days when all you wanted to do was throw the instrument away and get on with your life? In those moments, all you feel is utter frustration because you can't play the ukulele, especially when there's a YouTube video of a 5-year-old kid who can!

   Whatever you plan on learning—be it a language, swimming or the UCAT—the initial phase is one of utter frustration. We don't like feeling stupid at all, do we? You see, our brain has two hemispheres. The left side is the logical, serious side, while the right side is the one jumping around feeling emotional, being creative and having fun. When you learn something new, your left hemisphere tries supressing your right hemisphere, because you're doing a crap job and making yourself look bad (especially when neighbours have screamed at your parents in despair three times already over the phone because you're playing the drums again). The duration of the frustration curve differs depending on what you plan on learning, but it's been roughly estimated to last for around 5 to 6 hours of focused practice.

> When frustrated about learning ANYTHING new, the secret is to look back at all the things you've learnt in the past. Reflect, and take some time to observe how, after a bit of practice, you started getting the hang of that particular skill and your initial frustration was replaced by joy. Skiing, swimming, writing and driving have become second nature for you because you've pushed through the initial phase of frustration.

2. **Logarithmic growth**

   The magic happens during the second phase of the learning curve. As you can see on the graph, what occurs after around 5 to 6 hours of practice is that you rapidly climb up and experience a logarithmic increase in knowledge. This is because of the few core skills that you focused on during the initial learning phase. Instead of just strumming the guitar, you start playing actual chords. The transition is very smooth from your perspective, however, to the point that you may not even notice how good you get over time. It's the same with aging. You age a bit every single day and the only ones who notice are your old friends who haven't seen you for a year or more. In comparison, you see yourself every day in the mirror and so the transition is too smooth to be noticed. In our case, you play for 30 minutes every day, improving little by

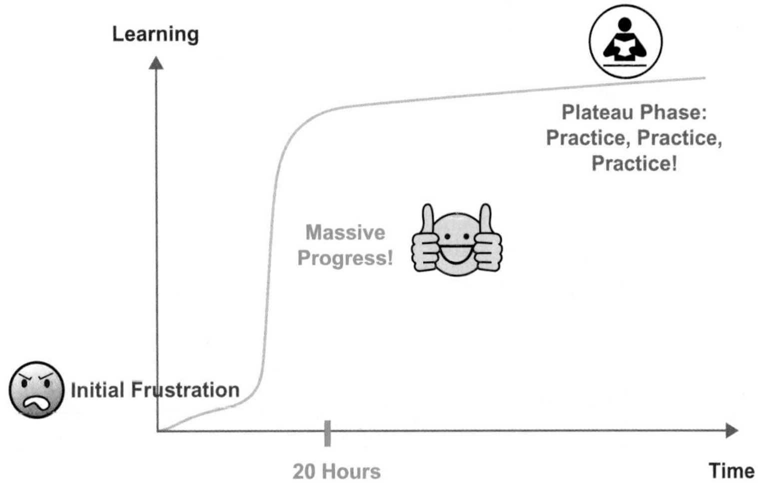

Fig. 7.1 Learning curve.

little until one day you are fairly good, but it didn't happen overnight; it took day after day of deliberate and consistent practice.

3. **Plateau**

Moving on to the third and final phase of the learning curve, once you've set the bases, you can build on them from there and become fairly good in around 20 hours of deliberate practice. Of course, that is 20 hours broken down in daily, focused practice, not spending an all-nighter to put in 10 hours in one go. I am sure you already know why that won't work, since most of you are doing biology and have heard about synapse regeneration and memory formation during sleep. It also has to do with habitual learning. Do it often enough and it becomes a part of you—how many times do you have to think before you put socks on in the morning before going to school? You've done it so many times over the years that you got used to doing it; it feels normal and appropriate. Same with brushing your teeth.

This final phase of the learning curve is also known as the plateau curve. You've already learnt the basics. You are generally good at what you're doing and improving further is slow and steady, as you are now working towards an expert level. This is where the 10,000-hour rule comes in. However, the question is—why do you want to learn something? Do you want to drive because you want to have a car and it would make your life easier, or do you want to be a Formula 1 racing driver? Do you want to play the violin as a hobby or do you want to compete? Do you want to prepare for the UCAT just enough, so you can be better than other applicants and get a place in medical school, or do you want to write a book about the UCAT and start creating questions? The answer to these questions will provide a guide to how many hours you have to put in to achieve your goal.

In his book 'The First 20 Hours', Kaufman describes some of the issues with modern culture and learning. Nowadays we take learning very 'academically'. We look at it as a chore, a task and try to squeeze as many things at once into our brains, without taking note of the various small skills that could be learnt by having a bit of fun.

Take for example the UCAT. Most applicants are tempted to do practice questions until they get the hang of it, without investing time in spotting what kind of skills are tested on the exam and WHY examiners use this test. We are all human, and understanding why admission tutors have chosen the UCAT to differentiate between applicants will help you focus on the exact skills that they are looking for, one at a time, until you excel in each section. To put this into context even further, the UCAT is a time-based test and efficiency is very important. Not only do you need to focus, but you also need to learn how to skim and speed read, for example.

Kaufman created a couple of steps to follow when putting the 20-hour rule into practice, as shown in Fig. 7.2.

1. **Decide what you want.**

First, you have to set a goal. What is it exactly that you want to achieve? What is the desired level of performance? Can you be specific about this?

2. **Deconstruct the skill.**

Second, everything that we do, each skill that we try to learn, can be broken down into sets of subskills. Let's take driving, for example. You don't just hop into the car and off you go, right? Before you do that, you need to learn the theory and rules around driving, you need to get a good instructor and then practice your motor skills and attention while driving.

The key here is to **practice the most important subskill first**. In other words, what is it that would give you the biggest boost in terms of learning? What can you do first to significantly improve? In our case with the UCAT or BMAT, that may be first understanding the format of each exam, and perhaps only later moving on to speed reading. However, these are person specific and differ from one student to another—you roughly know what you're good or bad at. For example, if you're an international student and your first language isn't English, it may possibly be the case that you need to strengthen your English skills first, as that would give you the biggest learning boost.

3. **Research your skill.**

Before you jump blindly into a topic, Josh says in his book that you need to learn just enough so you can spot the times when you're wrong and self-correct from there. By researching a skill, you also find out more about its subskills and

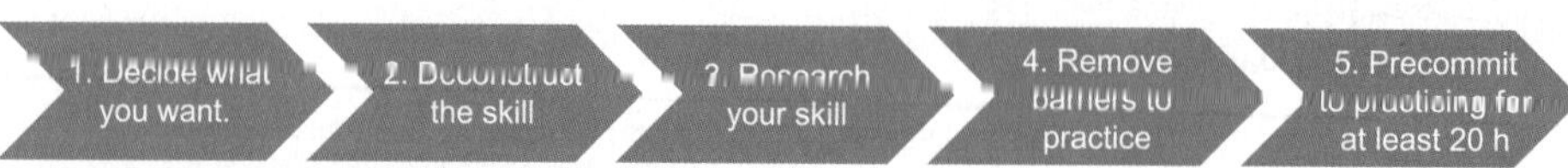

Fig. 7.2 Putting the 20-hour rule into practice.

this is helpful when choosing what to focus on first. This is why students who simply jump into practice questions from the start often fail to achieve greatness in the UCAT.

The trap here is spending all your valuable time on researching the skill and learning more about it without practicing. This is when researching your skill can become a barrier to practicing and, therefore, learning. Don't exaggerate—for example, with the UCAT, all you need is a good introduction to the subject and to the different sets of subskills that are being tested through this admission test. Once you know what's being tested, you can take each subskill one by one and work on it.

4. **Remove barriers to practice.**

Procrastination is a student's biggest enemy. Before you start practicing, remove anything that could distract you. The 20-hour rule only applies if you spend FOCUSED work, not shallow work while multitasking and checking your newsfeed. We'll discuss this further in our section regarding the importance of building a studying sanctuary.

5. **Precommit to practicing for at least 20 hours.**

We humans have a way of writing all our goals at the beginning of a new year, but within a maximum of 2 weeks' time we're back to old habits once all motivation has disappeared. To avoid giving up when things feel uncomfortable—and they will feel uncomfortable as demonstrated by the learning curve—you need something to keep you pushing through this pain. Some may say that this is what parental figures are there for, to push you when you would have given up already, but when parents aren't around, you need to make a deal with yourself. You need to remind yourself about your dream of studying medicine, about the oath that you took in the beginning of this book. A strong WHY will always find a HOW.

Right now you may ask, 'All right genius, but how do you adapt the 20-hour rule to the UCAT?' Statistics show that this test is the biggest predictor for students receiving an interview invitation from UK medical schools. No pressure, right? Before we dive in to the nitty gritty of studying for UCAT or BMAT and adapting the 20-hour rule, it is essential to have the correct study environment established.

STUDY HACKS

Creating a Studying Sanctuary

How many times have you started studying and after 3 minutes felt the need to eat, go to the toilet or the classic example of picking up your phone and checking Facebook or Instagram or calling a friend?

Before we even mention any other study tips, we need to make sure our study environment is 'healthy'. The reason behind this is that your brain is very powerful, and you can trick it into doing powerful things. Let's take eating, for example. When we eat, we chew the food, but we don't really think about it. It's the same when you're in class and the teacher asks everyone a question—everybody puts their hand up, but if the teacher asked you personally a question, you wouldn't put your hand up, correct?

The previous scenarios are examples of 'habitual learning', a fancy term for 'you do it so many times that you begin to do it automatically without even realising'. Does that mean we can trick our brain into staying focused and triggering our desire to study automatically? The answer is yes, and all you need to do is to create a study space.

For example, only study in a quiet area, at your desk or in the library. Arrange your study materials in a certain way and always start your study sessions in the same manner so that your brain gets used to it. By that I mean really OCD style—red pen always on the left, black pen always on the right, two books at the top of the desk and one white sheet of paper to take notes in front of your laptop—whatever works for you, but this has to be repeated daily so that you associate these surroundings with the need to start studying. The more you do it, the easier it will become. Most importantly (I know you've probably heard this a hundred times already), turn off your phone and get rid of any other distractions.

Study Less, Study Smarter!

You might think that the more you study, the smarter and more knowledgeable you will become, right? For example, if you study for 5 hours straight, surely you will retain all the information and excel in that subject, correct? Well, that's not quite right. Science shows that our brain can only focus for 30 minutes at a time. This means that after 30 minutes, your brain shuts down. Yes, you can still keep on reading or listening to your teacher, but what you hear goes in one ear and out the other.

There's a secret though—want to know how to hack your brain into staying focused and refreshed so you can keep studying for long periods? It's fairly easy. All you need to do is take a 5-minute break every 30 minutes. During these 5 minutes, do something fun—listen to a song, go for a quick walk, get a snack or dance around for a bit!

Once your brain is fully relaxed and 5 minutes have passed, get back to studying for another 30 minutes, then take another 5-minute break, dance around, then study for another 30 minutes and so on.

Careful though, don't do anything that could distract you completely, such as playing video games or watching Netflix. Let's be honest, that would take more

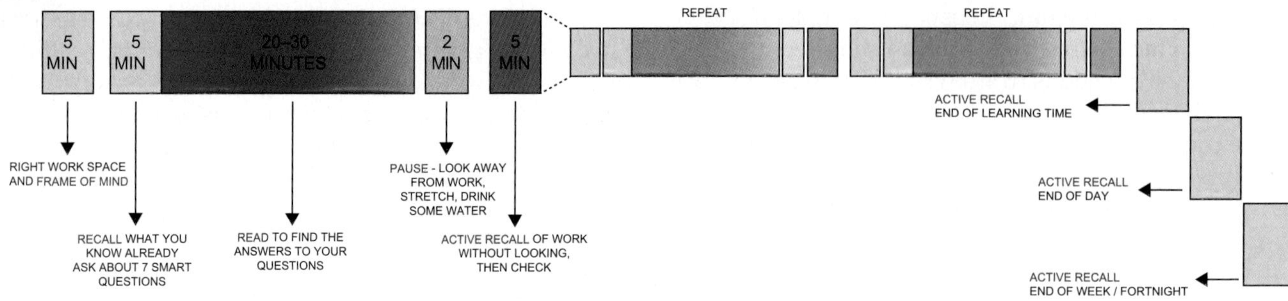

Fig. 7.3 An effective learning strategy.

than 5 minutes, and you could end up binge-watching a whole season of 'Game of Thrones' in no time! At the end of your study session, plan something fun that can serve as a reward—watch a film with your friends, play some sports, games or anything that makes you happy. You'll feel productive and enjoy yourself to the maximum, knowing that you've worked hard and stayed focused all day long.

When preparing for exams that require a lot of memorisation (A-level stuff or even the BMAT), the following technique may help. It's essentially what we've just talked about, 30 minutes of studying followed by a 5-minute break, but it also takes a few minutes to ACTIVELY RECALL what you studied before the break. This way you'll force your brain to recall and reinforce previous information. Science suggests that this is the best way to study and it makes your learning effective (Fig. 7.3).

Active Studying

How many of you highlight what you consider 'key facts' while studying? Well, I am about to tell you why that doesn't work and you should stop. You see, our brain does two things when you're studying: recalling and recognising.

Recollection has to do with something that you will remember and will be brought forward by the brain in an exam situation, whereas recognising something has more to do with patterns, not with the whole concept—meaning that although you'll recognise the word, you won't necessarily know its definition.

When you are highlighting something and you later come back to review what you've highlighted, your brain may trick you into thinking that you can fully recall that concept, when in fact you just recognise it because you've highlighted it in the past.

For this reason, you must study and learn actively. You need to quiz yourself, you need to draw, write down key words and think about the potential styles of questions that could come up on exams. Practice questions are a great way to study if you have access to any previous papers.

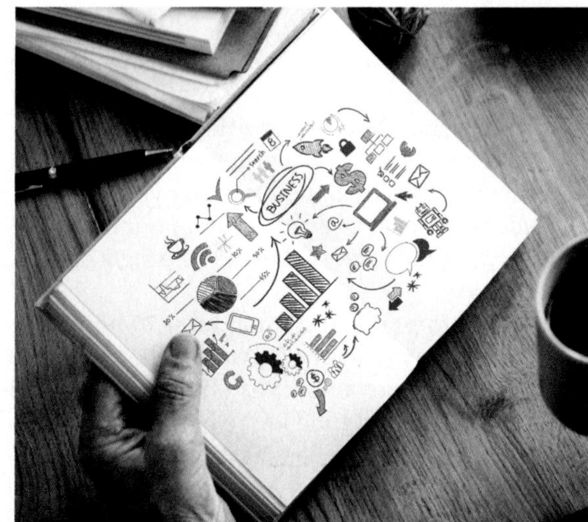

Fig. 7.4 A mind map.

Famous psychologist Marty Lobdell says, 'The more active you are in your learning, the more effective you'll be'.

Other ways of active studying include:

- Using flash cards
- Using mind maps (Fig. 7.4)
- Using funny analogies
- Using visual/auditory learning materials

Let us now jump straight into the UCAT and its various subsections. If you want to find out more about the science of learning, further reading, materials and resources can be found later.

REFORMS TO ADMISSION TESTING FROM 2024

In 2023, the Cambridge Assessment Admissions Testing announced that there will be changes to a series of university entrance exams with effect in academic year 2024/25. The proposed changes involve the removal of the BMAT exam from the medical school application process in this year.

For the academic year 2024/25 onwards, the seven UK medical schools that use BMAT tests as part of their admissions process (Brighton and Sussex, Imperial, Lancaster,

UCL, Cambridge, Leeds and Oxford) as well as medical and healthcare schools in other countries will put alternative arrangements in place.

Cambridge Assessment Admissions Testing

At the time of writing this book, there is no further information available as to what will replace the BMAT exam. It is therefore vital to make sure you check the BMAT section of the Cambridge Assessment Admissions Testing website regularly if this will affect you: https://www.admissionstesting.org/for-test-takers/bmat/.

Several universities across the world are likely to continue using the BMAT as a method of assessment. For this reason, we have decided to include the BMAT as a core section of our book, should you consider applying internationally to universities where BMAT is still being considered an entry requirement.

HOW TO ACE THE UNIVERSITY CLINICAL APTITUDE TEST (UCAT)

When you are initially familiarising yourself with the exam format and questions, you may think, 'This may be the most unique (or crazy) exam I've seen so far!' You may also wonder, 'What is the purpose of this exam?' and 'Why do I need to take it?' Well, you're not alone. At some point, we have all wondered why this exam exists.

The first concept I would like to convey is that, by trying to undertake this exam, you must change your thought process to become more 'doctor-like'. Things are not always done the same way in the real world compared to the medical world. For example, doctors need to assess a patient to ensure they get better. In order to do so, they must employ a specific set of skills. This exam is meant to, in its own unique way, test that skill set to determine if you have the potential to not only be a good doctor, but also an efficient one. Therefore, it is important to start thinking accordingly. This will ensure that you and the exam are working together, and not against each other.

Second, this is not an exam you can excel at by memorising and regurgitating information, as you may have done for your previous exams. In order to do well, you must understand the common principles and theories behind a question and apply them appropriately. Therefore, the most common theme in this book (even when discussing technique application) is to practice, practice and PRACTICE!

Hopefully, this chapter will help you develop strategies for approaching the exam. Each section has an example that applies the strategies to aid familiarisation. However, as there is only so much a comprehensive guide to medical school applications can cover, it will be up to you, the candidates, to identify a suitable dedicated UCAT practice database. This will prove very useful when applying the strategies mentioned. Before you practice, you need to understand HOW to practice well; otherwise, anyone could answer thousands of questions and ace the UCAT. Online UCAT question databases are recommended, as they will familiarise you with the computer-based format of the exam. Free mock exams can be found on the official UCAT website. Use these to apply the techniques and strategies demonstrated in this chapter.

WHAT IS THE UCAT? WHAT DOES IT INVOLVE?

UCAT is a 2-hour computer-based multiple-choice test. Fortunately for everyone, it is not negatively marked, so you *don't* lose marks if you get a question wrong. The UCAT is a series of sections that test different aspects of your cognitive abilities, from reading and comprehension, problem-solving skills, pattern recognition and cognitive reasoning (thinking logically) to situational reasoning (thinking morally). Surprisingly enough, the last time you most likely did questions similar to the UCAT was in primary school! (Although these aren't as easy, unfortunately.)

There is an argument for the presence of natural talent in some of these sections, with some students able to understand abstract reasoning patterns from day one. However, I personally believe, based on my students, that this natural talent can be replicated by practicing the correct techniques. In fact, I believe that if you can completely explain to me the reasoning behind your answer instead of stating, 'My brain works that way', you are in a better position to tackle challenging questions than students who practice according to 'natural talent'. This is not to take away from those who understand abstract questions from day one, as they can also learn the material and improve their techniques further to achieve the same effect.

The exam itself is composed of five different sections which must be answered in order (left to right) (Fig. 7.5). They are explained further in the appropriate subsections.

Each of the subtests (except situational judgment (SJ)) is scored from 300 to 900, out of a total of 3600 points. Each of the items in the respective subtests is worth the same amount of marks, i.e. the hard questions and the easy questions are worth the same. The scores are calculated on the computer system as soon as you submit your exam. They will be available for you in the form of a printout before you leave the building, usually from the reception area of the exam site.

> As soon as you get your UCAT printout sheet, take a picture of it with your phone (or photocopy it) and keep the printout safe. It costs a premium fee to replace that piece of paper if you lose it.

Now, you must be wondering, if the five sections are scored out of 900, how is the SJ section scored? The situational judgement section scores don't have

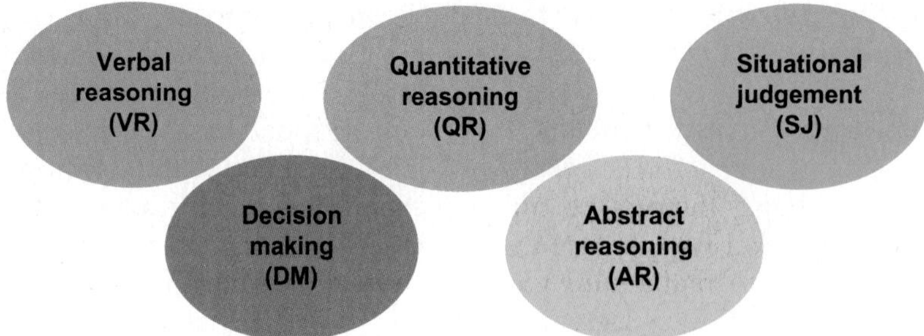

Fig. 7.5 Composition of the UCAT.

a numerical value attached to them; instead, candidates are grouped into bands 1–4. The SJ section is marked according to how closely your answers match the answers of an expert panel (the 'ideal' answers). If most of your answers matched theirs, then you will be in band 1. If some matched, with a few partially correct (correct but not ideal answers), then you will be in band 2. The same progression follows for band 3 and 4 ratings.

WHY IS THE EXAM IMPORTANT FOR YOU?

First and foremost, getting into medical/dental school.

A majority of medical schools in the UK use the UCAT as a baseline for determining who they would like to interview. Some medical schools place more emphasis on the UCAT and therefore rank students according to scores, while others place less emphasis on the exam and use a specific score as a cut-off value. Either way, most medical schools will use your score, to some degree, to determine if they would like to interview you.

So, in extremely basic terms: The higher your UCAT score, the higher your chance of securing an interview (considering you are competing with thousands of other students applying for the same courses). Therefore, I would argue that this exam is extremely important and could be the factor that gets you an interview or stops you at the door.

WHAT IS A GOOD SCORE? WHAT CAN YOU DO TO ACHIEVE IT?

For the past 3 years, around 35,000 students have sat the UCAT each year with an average score of around 2500. From year to year, the average score remains roughly the same. You may be thinking, that's all well and good, but I want to score higher than average! If this is you, perhaps you would like to achieve a score in the top 20% (≈2700) or even the top 10% (≈2850). To find out how to achieve these scores, keep reading.

Preparation Before the Exam

Registering for the exam/having a date in mind

You are a keen student, and you're getting hyped to take this test because you think it will help expand your boundaries and more (insert inspiration here). However, before you proceed any further, you need to have a deadline in your head. You can do this by registering your exam date on the UCAT website as soon as booking opens. It is important to remember that your test date can be moved if you decide you are not prepared come test day or perhaps you are prepared earlier than expected and want to get it over with, so don't be shy about booking a date so far in advance!

> The dates go very quickly. Personally, I recommend booking an exam date beforehand, preferably 2 months in advance.

From the experiences of my students and myself, I have learnt that having a deadline helps you envision your goal. This date will be the zombie apocalypse for which you can be either extremely prepared or absolutely daunted.

Setting Up a Study Schedule

Now that you've set the date, you need to determine how much time is left until your big day. I ask you to do this because you may want to set up your own study timetable, which is tailored specifically to you. This may be the next most important thing to do (aside from practice), as it allows you to systematically approach the UCAT to maximise your practice efficiency and your end score.

How much or how little time you invest in preparing for the UCAT is completely up to you. For those of you who feel ambitious and are able to spend more time practicing for the UCAT, I have illustrated in my personal 6-week plan for acing the UCAT later in the chapter. This is just a guide, subject to adjustment based on your personal commitments and estimated UCAT performance. This timetable may seem a bit intense so feel free to adjust based on your progress. In fact, some of you may naturally excel with little practice. That definitely wasn't the case for me, however. I had to work hard. Very hard.

I recommend using this timetable if you've started planning early. If you don't have much time, the 4-week study schedule provided later in the chapter is the minimum recommended to perform well in the UCAT exam.

Previously in the chapter, we learnt all about Kaufman's '20-hour rule'. Let's see if we can put these steps into action and build our own '20-hour rule' for UCAT.

1. **Decide what you want.**

   To get a decent score on the UCAT. Of course, this is your goal and it's up to you what level you want to achieve, but here we focus on a plan that will make you 'good'.

2. **Deconstruct the skill.**

   The UCAT, as you will read later on, has five different sections that all utilise different types of skills. For example, abstract reasoning assesses your ability to draw a hypothesis from a series of data, whereas situational judgement assesses the morality of your behaviour in certain situations. Both of these topics utilise unique skills but in a different way from daily life. Therefore, each section requires a dedicated period of time to familiarise yourself with it. Use the approaches described in the UCAT chapter. Some aspects can be easier to grasp and some harder. Break down each of the approaches into a specific subset of skills and focus on the less proficient skill.

   > Adjust the 20 hours you spend on each section to be more or less focused on certain subskills depending on your adeptness. For example, you are good at graph-type questions in quantitative reasoning but not so good with tables. In this case, spend the time focusing a greater proportion on graphs and less on tables (e.g. 6:4). Recognising your strengths and weaknesses is key.

   Additionally, it would be wise to use the first 1 or 2 weeks to do untimed practice, where you are specifically trying to apply the skills required to succeed when answering the question. In order to succeed after initial practice, you must begin focusing on these skills under time constraints and simulated exam conditions. This allows you to fine tune these skills and utilise them much faster, something a lot of students struggle with.

3. **Research your skill.**

   Read about the UCAT in this chapter, including the theory behind each section. Try to be critical of what skills you are good at, and which need improvement. Use the weekly structure.

4. **Remove barriers to practice: Stay focused!**

   By focused practice, I REALLY mean focused. As I am writing this chapter, the guy next to me in the library is listening to an anatomy lecture on his headphones, but at the same time he is smiling and texting a mate on his phone. I can assure you that he isn't smiling because of the anatomy landmarks he's hearing about on his headphones; he's probably having fun with his mate via text. By focus, I mean completely the opposite of what he's doing. Not only will he not remember what he's listening to, he will also go home with a false sense of having been through that lesson. When the exam comes up, he'll only remember, 'What do you call a doctor fixing websites? A URLogist' because that's what his friend texted him, and although relevant to the medical field (I guess), it's not relevant to his current exam (unless the question is URLogy related!).

5. **Precommit to practicing for at least 20 hours.**

   Make a plan and stick with it. Here's what you can do. Because the UCAT tests multiple skills, each section will require 20 hours of work. For the purposes of getting a good UCAT score, this will help you schedule your studies.

   The following weekly structure is based on a conventional 9-hour schedule, purely because most applicants start practicing during their summer holiday. Of course, you can adapt the timetable to suit your daily activities.

   The following timetable allows you to effectively cover the range of subjects used in the exam. This is a basic structure that allows you to focus on one section at a time, with multiple sections covered in the day. The idea is to maintain focus and get used to switching between the topics (like the actual exam). However, this is only a plan, and it can be adjusted based on your sleep schedule and personal life.

   Now, from experience, we know that what works for one applicant may not work for another. Over the past 2 years, we've tested this theory on hundreds of applicants just like you. So based on your feedback, we've created two versions.

   The first version (Table 7.1) spans 4 weeks and is dedicated to those of you who are short of time and don't have much left until the UCAT. This may also apply to those of you who prefer a less intense study schedule.

   The second version (recommended) spans 6 weeks (Table 7.2). This is what we recommend as you give your brain enough time to consolidate all information and get enough practice for each skill.

   As mentioned before, the plan is subject to change depending on your personal life, events and your motivation and progress. Not everyone can provide the same level of dedication; therefore, please adjust the timetable to be more or less intensive depending on how you study and progress with the exam. Some of you may also have a natural talent for such exams, in which case you'll get along very well with little preparation. For most of us, however, hard work is the only key to success.

   Take it step by step, do your first practice hours with us by using the information from this

Table 7.1 Four-Week Plan

TIME BEFORE EXAM (MINIMUM)	TYPE OF REVISION	SECTIONS PRACTICED	TIME SPENT
4 weeks	Mix of timed and untimed practice	All sections every day (1 hour per scored section, 1 hour SJ) 2 full mocks per week	30 minutes untimed, 30 minutes timed per section, SJ all untimed Total = 5 hours daily (excluding mocks)
3 weeks	Mix of timed and untimed practice	All sections every day (1 hour per scored section, 1 hour SJ) 3 full mocks per week	30 minutes untimed, 30 minutes timed all sections Total = 5 hours daily (excluding mocks)
2 weeks	Mix of timed and untimed practice	All sections every day (1 hour each) 4 full mocks per week	15 minutes untimed, 45 minutes timed per section, SJ all timed Total = 5 hours daily (excluding mocks)
1 week	Mix of timed and untimed practice	All sections every day (1 hour each) 5 full mocks per week	1 hour timed all sections Total = 5 hours daily (excluding mocks)
Day before	**Untimed practice only**	All sections	However long gives you confidence for the big day. It is important not to overdo it the day before. You need to be well rested and feeling confident when you start the exam.

SJ, situational judgment.

Table 7.2 Six-Week Plan

TIME BEFORE EXAM (MINIMUM)	TYPE OF REVISION	SECTIONS PRACTICED	TIME SPENT
6 weeks	Mix of timed and untimed practice	All sections every day (1.5 hours per scored section, 1 hour SJ) 2 full mocks per week	1 hour untimed, 30 minutes timed per section, SJ all untimed Total = 7 hours daily (excluding mocks)
4 weeks	Mix of timed and untimed practice	All sections every day (1.5 hours per scored section, 1 hour SJ) 3 full mocks per week	30 minutes untimed, 1 hour timed per section, SJ 30 minutes timed, 30 minutes untimed Total = 7 hours daily (excluding mocks)
2 weeks	Mix of timed and untimed practice	All sections every day (1 hour each) 4 full mocks per week	15 minutes untimed, 45 minutes timed per section, SJ all timed Total = 5 hours daily (excluding mocks)
1 week	Mix of timed and untimed practice	All sections every day (1 hour each) 5 full mocks per week	1 hour timed per section, SJ all timed Total = 5 hours daily (excluding mocks)
Day before	**Untimed practice only**	All sections	However long gives you confidence for the big day. It is important not to overdo it the day before. You need to be well rested and feeling confident when you start the exam.

SJ, situational judgment.

chapter, and once you get the hang of all the practice techniques, spend the rest of your time on mock UCAT tests. Simulate test conditions as best as you can: time constraint, environment, earplugs, etc. Essentially, we're here to support you through the frustrating part of the learning curve. You'll then rapidly climb up the learning curve and become better than you thought at the UCAT.

Is 20 Hours All It Takes for Me to Get Over 700 in the UCAT? Achieving Greatness

Now you may say—well, you told me I'd be good if I put in 20 hours of focused practice for each section of the UCAT, does this mean I'm ready to ace it? No, you're not. Twenty hours on each section spread out over a month will get you good, better than some applicants, but not excellent. As Voltaire once said, 'The best is the enemy of good'. To put this into context, if you want to become better than other applicants, you need to keep practicing daily on top of these hours. We've provided a starting point for you. It's your turn to focus on your weaknesses and practice until you fill all the gaps. It's your turn to work towards the 10,000-hour target. Obviously, that's not the aim, but the more you practice, the better you will do on your exam.

> For me, the worst thing about the UCAT is how mentally draining it is so you have to train yourself to stay alert for the whole 2 hours—that's why mocks were the biggest part of my revision and I'd do one every day at the same time as my exam.
>
> **Amy Downes, UCAT 3330, Medical School Applicant 2022–2023**

You must remember that sometimes it isn't about how much time you spend on a task; it is about the quality of work that you do for that task. Sure, you can say you've practiced for the UCAT for 10 hours today, but let's be honest, in reality, 6 of these hours were spent staring out the window, chatting to friends over the phone and complaining about how hard it is to work on the UCAT, scrolling down your newsfeed on Facebook, going to the bathroom at least five times in 1 hour and snacking on anything you can find!

Read Through UCAT Techniques and PRACTICE

Utilise the subsections in this book to master techniques for taking the UCAT. Although this book will help you to pass your exam, it will not broaden your horizons or necessarily help you obtain the highest score. There are multiple dedicated UCAT books on the market to help determine which techniques fit you best (according to your previous practices and thought processes). In addition, I recommend using a book or an online database of UCAT questions to refine your techniques. This will give you an ample amount of practice so you are completely prepared for the exam and don't pass out from nervousness.

During the UCAT

Generally speaking, there are a few tips, some of which are disseminated across the chapters, which can help you with the UCAT and improve your overall performance across all subsets. First and foremost, my advice is to remain calm. It has been shown that your performance can be affected if you are not in a relaxed state of mind, leading to a lower score than what you are capable of, especially in a high pressure exam environment like the UCAT. Avoiding nervousness is a skill. Whenever you try to practice, do so under exam conditions: in a quiet room, at a desk, sticking exactly to the timing and style of the UCAT. Second, although it sounds very cliché, attempt some breathing exercises and power poses before the exam. This can help you to combat nervousness and enter the most optimal exam state for you (the so-called 'zone').

Now that you have become one with the exam, it's probably a good idea to read over the instructions they provide, just so you are aware of the exam's rules and structure, which you may or may not have already known. Reading the instructions does not take away from your question answering time (please confirm this yourself with current UCAT guidelines). It can serve as a good break between the different sections.

What to Do When Stuck

If during the exam you find yourself facing an extremely hard question, don't panic and keep an eye on the time. If you find that you are spending the majority of the allocated time per question simply trying to figure out what the question is asking, and time is running out (essentially when you reach the point when you should be determining an answer but are still stuck on the question), then pick a 'best guess' answer and use the flagging option to return to that question when you have time at the end. This is very unofficial advice, only to be used in situations where the question is completely outside of your capabilities and it is starting to burn into the time. **Remember, every question is worth the same amount of marks.** You won't get more marks for spending more time on a harder question; you will simply miss out on the remaining easier marks and end up with a lower score.

At the same time, you may think it sounds terrible, not to mention unprofessional, to say 'pick a random answer'. However, this can be broken down a bit further, so let me clarify.

Sometimes, due to time constraints, it is hard to calculate an exact answer or arrive at the correct answer with a thorough explanation. In these cases, it can be more appropriate to make an educated guess. This involves eliminating two to four answers you are sure cannot be the correct answer, as their reasoning or their values are too far from the 'correct answer'. This will leave you with one or two answers to choose from. You can then go on a bit further to deduce the correct answer or, if you are running out of time, pick one of the two and then move on.

Again, use this method very carefully. Excessive guessing can lead to a lower final score. Ideally, this method should only be used for the very few questions which leave you completely baffled, despite months of practice.

After the Exam

Go home with your score to look at which universities will accept your UCAT score (both the average score as well as the sub-sectional scores). Be very careful. Make sure you have checked the UCAT cut-offs for all of your university choices.

If after the exam you find that you have missed the mark, or failed to live up to your own expectations, there are a couple of options for you:

1. Have a go at BMAT.

2. Apply to universities that traditionally accept lower UCAT scores.
3. Re-sit UCAT the next academic year and try again.

You will have to take the UCAT exam again if you choose to reapply the following year. The UCAT is only valid for 1 academic year; i.e. if you take it in summer 2022, it is only valid for 2022/23 applications. So make sure to always keep your books (they can come in handy whether you are retaking the exam or giving them away to your siblings/friends).

The UCAT is hard! It takes a lot of time and dedication to score well. If, however, you can get your score into the top 10%, you have opened the door to a lot of universities. Even years later I credit my UCAT score for allowing me to achieve four medical school offers.

Dan, Top 10% UCAT Scorer, Medical School Applicant 2019-2020

SECTION 1: VERBAL REASONING

This is the first section of the exam and, for most people including myself, the most difficult section. It may seem like the examination board are being horrible by including this section, but they are also testing some very valuable skills transferrable to your future practice as a doctor. Verbal reasoning (VR) is fundamentally testing your reading and comprehension abilities, with particular emphasis on cross-reference and inference skills. The questions may seem extremely lacklustre from a student's viewpoint. However, when you are a doctor, it is very important to understand information quickly, interpret it and apply it to the patient in front of you. So, it makes sense that they would like students to have a basic understanding of these concepts before applying to medical school.

Overview

In this section, you will be given 11 passages to read, and each passage will be accompanied by four questions. The entire section allows for 21 minutes, with an additional minute for instructions. Therefore, you will have less than 2 minutes for each passage and its four questions (roughly 28 seconds per question).

But before we get to what you need to do and how you do it, let me tell you a bit more about what types of questions come up and what this means for you.

There are **two types of questions** you will encounter in VR:

1. **True/False/Can't tell questions**
2. **Reading comprehension questions**

Both types of questions utilise a similar kind of text passage consisting of random topics ranging from historical figures to economical concepts. These passages will generally be two to three paragraphs (totalling approximately up to 400 words). Essentially, the topics can range from anything to everything, including the most controversial and obscure topics.

True/False/Can't tell questions will provide you with a statement, usually just one sentence long, and asks you whether the statement is:

Type	Meaning
True	Supported by the passage
False	Completely contradicts the passage or the message derived from the passage
Can't tell	Unable to conclude due to insufficient/vague information

The other type of VR question, as mentioned earlier, revolves around reading comprehension questions. These questions provide you with a question at the beginning and four statements below it. It will be up to you to determine which of the statements is correct. The question could ask you to identify which of the statements is supported by the passage, which holds true or, in more uncommon cases, which statement contradicts the information in the passage. As a result of this structure, it is possible to treat some of the harder comprehensive statements as mini True/False/Can't tell.

The majority of questions you will see on test day are the reading comprehension questions. It is very important to get familiar with reading through passages and extracting key points as well as the overall theme of the passage. Therefore, it is very important that you **familiarise yourself with the language used in the UCAT**, especially if English is not your first language. This will help you interpret information easier in a shorter time period.

General Tips

I suggest finding a reading resource (e.g. a news website such as BBC News or a short book/novel) and practicing reading over the information provided, as quickly as possible, to improve your proficiency. At the end, summarise the information and see if the principles you've extracted from the article are the same as those it states in the summary. Conversely, it is also possible to download a few speed-reading applications (on your phone or computer) to enhance your reading ability.

Don't bring outside knowledge and opinions into the exam. **It is fatal to bring 'outside UCAT knowledge' into the exam.** This will be a recurring piece of advice in any section that utilises information with which you may be familiar. It is important in medicine to always make evidence-based decisions. This is reflected in the exam, and they expect you to base all of your answers on the information provided in the passage or the data.

Verbal reasoning was the part that I didn't perform well on at all, as you have got a long passage with questions that were not easily spotted. Thus, it comes down to practice and more practice. If you believe that you might not be a quick reader and sometimes struggle with comprehensive reading, I definitely suggest you do lots of verbal reasoning exercises online, under time pressure. Practice on a computer screen as well—you may find that reading on a screen is even more difficult and definitely more exhausting. I started practicing around 1 month before I took the test by doing as many online exercises as I could. It helps massively—it's my top tip.

Ryan, Medical School Applicant

Now to the bulk of the issue: How to approach the VR section.

Basic Approach to Verbal Reasoning

VR is not a new section of the UCAT. Therefore, there have been multiple years of discovering and refining techniques to find the most efficient and successful. However, these techniques are only guides. You are encouraged to modify and adapt these approaches to make them more suitable for you. An approach is shown in Fig. 7.6.

Practice is important for getting into the correct mindset and mastering the skill. Learning the skill of 'scanning', in other words just finding the keywords, is crucial for maximising your score in this section.

Frederick, Top 3% UCAT Scorer, Medical School Applicant 2022–2023

Things to Consider

Earlier in the chapter, there was mention of understanding the language used in the UCAT. Although this will mainly come from growing accustomed to the passages used and understanding their structure, there are some aspects you can actively consider. Match the language of the statement and the passage. Specifically, the use of terms, are they firm and specific terms or uncertain terms (will vs could)? This can be a very effective method of eliminating options that don't match.

Similarly, when looking at language, ensure that you do not jump to conclusions. Be thorough with examining the information found and try not to come to conclusions easily.

Tips for Harder Questions

The strategy suggested in Fig. 7.6 can be applied across the entirety of the VR section. However, in recent years, they have increased the difficulty of some of the questions, making reading comprehension harder.

The newer reading comprehension format can sometimes feel a lot more time-consuming and, generally, harder than the older format. However, the core principles are still the same. Remember to use those keywords to find the relevant sentences, understand what they say, deconstruct their argument and conclude. Sometimes, this may not lead you to a firm answer, but don't panic and pick the most appropriate answer (sometimes the most appropriate answer is the 'least ambiguous' choice).

SECTION 2: DECISION-MAKING

As one of the more unique sections, decision-making is relatively unexplored territory. As with the previous sections, decision-making explores aspects of your cognitive processes, with a heavy emphasis on logical thought progression and how they form a good foundation for a doctor.

Overview

Decision-making will provide you with 29 items/questions, with a total of 31 minutes for the questions and 1 minute for instruction, leaving approximately 1 minute to answer each item/question and another minute at the end for any leftover (harder) questions. This is by far the most relaxed section in the exam, so take your time thinking through the arguments and making your thoughts as logically progressive as possible.

The section will require you to have prior understanding of probabilities (very important to understand, especially for dice rolls and genetic probabilities), basic mathematical knowledge and the ability to interpret diagrams (most commonly Venn diagrams, so re-familiarise yourself with them before the exam). It will also test aspects of your logical reasoning, i.e. interpreting information and drawing conclusions. The information can be presented in multiple formats such as statistics, as described earlier, or in the form of puzzles, most popularly Einstein puzzles.

General Tips

Decision-making is not as time pressured as the other sections of the exam; therefore, you have some breathing room to work things out. It is highly recommended that you utilise the whiteboard and pen when determining the answer. This allows you to keep the correct order and leaves less room for recall error. It also helps when referring back to the text and trying to determine the logical flow of the question.

However, just because you have more breathing room does not mean you can become lazy or inefficient. In this section, you must always understand the information that the question is asking you to examine and solve the question for those specific pieces of information. Trying to solve the entire question may end up burning more of your time and bringing you back into a more time pressured environment (not ideal when you have to organise your thoughts).

Another tip is to pay very close attention to wording, as it can change the entire meaning of a sentence. These include terms that can turn a fact into an assumption, and vice versa. For example:

Read the question first. Avoid reading the passage at the beginning as it can waste a lot of your time, leaving you with no time to answer the actual questions. Determine what the question is saying and how it is phrasing the language.

Step 1

Determine what keywords are being used in the question. What subject is the question revolving around and what is the action being suggested. This is a very basic method of finding the keyword in a question, and works in the majority of cases. Example:

'Once the law banning marijuana use was repealed in 1968, most Amsterdam shops opened on Saturday'.

The question has a subject. The subject is usually key dates, people, places or events which have occurred. The action is the proposed consequence of that subject. In the example above, the subject was the 'law repealment' in 1968 and the following action was most shops opening on Saturdays. Therefore, the keywords can be chosen from the subject and the action. When approaching the text, a possible approach would be to choose the date 1968, confirm the corresponding subject of the date in the passage as you read through it and also confirm the proposed action against the dates in the passage.

Step 2

Scan the passage. Once you have found the sentences corresponding to your chosen keywords, it is important to gain context to the sentences you have identified. Therefore, **read the sentences before and after those which contain your keywords**. You may think this is a waste of time, but there is a reason behind every move.

Avoiding the common trap: Most examiners will implement specific strategies to counter standard VR techniques. One such strategy is including counter statements within the same section of text. So what does this mean? Sometimes, the examiner can use sentences, before or after the sentence with the key words, containing information which invalidates the original sentence you have found. Therefore, be aware of the context with which your sentence was proposed to ensure it is not made irrelevant (essentially giving you better evidence with which to answer your question).

Step 3

Keep scanning for keywords throughout the passage to ensure you have collected all the valid information. Be careful not to settle for the first term you see and assume the answer without consulting the rest of the text. Make sure you have reached a point where the answer is extremely clear. If they are being exceptionally horrible, you may have to piece the information together from different parts of the passage (simply because they have distributed the relevant information across the entire length of text).

Step 4

Fig. 7.6 Approaching verbal reasoning questions.

a) Will/Must: **Firm language** indicating an event will definitely occur.
b) Could/Might: **Uncertain language** indicating an event has a possibility, but no guarantee, of occurring.

Attention to this is extremely important, as some puzzles or syllogisms require you to equate different pieces of information or rank them in order, and attention to the language helps you determine the specifics of the question.

So we have discussed what types of skills they are testing, but we haven't really explored how they test these skills or how you can improve your own skills doing them. The information further in this chapter dissects the question format and gives you a basis for evaluating the different types of questions. Therefore, as always, they can provide a good foundation for understanding the UCAT, but in the end you need to practice their application to truly be the very best.

> Decision-making is the only part of the exam you can finish early. I strongly recommend finishing 5 minutes early. Why? Because there are a lot of logical questions and puzzles. It is very likely you will get stuck on some questions the first time but will have no problem solving them when you come back a second time, once you've finished the other questions in the section. Take advantage of the timing, finish early and go back to maximise your score.
>
> **Dan, Medical School Applicant**

How to Evaluate Arguments

If you read the BMAT section, then this will not be new to you. If you haven't, then fret not; let's borrow some basic literature analysis skills required for the BMAT. Most of this will follow as common sense or you will realise you have been doing this subconsciously, but it is also good to be aware of the process.

Before we learn the evaluation of an argument, we must define what constitutes an argument. An argument is a reason or set of reasons given in support of an idea, action or theory. This reason can be derived from a particular statement or proposition (premise) within a set of information to reach the conclusion (theory, idea or action). **A premise is evidence used to support the conclusion**.

When drawing arguments from decision-making questions, it is always important to base them on conclusions from the evidence found in the information given. It is very easy to make assumptions regarding some of the information to support a conclusion. In this case, the conclusion can be unreliable because even though it is supported by evidence, it is also based on a series of assumptions, some of which may never occur. Therefore, a strong argument or conclusion in the decision-making section should be directly connected to the information provided and not contain any personal or 'outside UCAT' information/values/bias; i.e. it should be strongly **based on** the evidence provided in the question (this may also be applied to the VR content).

It is important to make sure your logic flows from one fact to another, i.e. **directly**, as indirect or irrelevant information regarding the subject can lead to very weak arguments, especially if they are also based on assumptions.

Therefore, applying this principle is quite simple. In the exam, you will be presented with a series of arguments in the choices for the answers. When analysing the arguments, you can eliminate those without a strong basis, i.e. those based on certain assumptions or those that reach a conclusion indirectly (without complete support from the premise/information).

You will have 1 minute to read the information and answer the questions, so take your time to dissect the information and extract the core 'points' (these will help you when you look for the correct answer or eliminate the incorrect answers).

How to Logically Deduce

To deduce is to conclusively arrive at a fact by logical reasoning. This can be based on a set of provided statements or premises that are presumed to be true. In the exam, this can involve using multiple statements to infer sequential pieces of information, eventually arriving at a conclusion. To demonstrate very basically, a question states that $d = e$ and $e = f$, therefore from this you can infer that $d = f$.

As hinted at the beginning, deduction in the decision-making section of the UCAT has multiple question types. One such type, Einstein puzzles, provides you with information as a set of parameters. It can be in multiple forms, most commonly text, but also tables and pictures. They will be presented in a complex manner but all link together in one correct way. It is up to you to sort them out in the order of value suggested to arrive at the correct answer. The values can be either single parameter or multi-parameter.

The following example is of multiple parameters, the more common of the two in the exam.

Question

Lewis, Jay, Amy, Becca and Bartholomew visit a field and take one flower each. The flowers are red, pink or white.
There are two types of flowers, roses and petunias.
Three flowers are roses and the rest are petunias.
All the petunias are white. Roses are either pink or red.
Bartholomew and Lewis do not have roses.
Among Jay, Amy and Becca, only Amy has a pink flower.

Run Through

In either scenario, the best way is the old-fashioned way, whiteboard and pen. Now is the opportune time to use that piece of paper they give you in the exam.
Read the information (don't skip any of the text in these questions). The initial text will set the tone for the questions and let you know the parameters involved.
Now use the pen and paper to physically rank them in order.
Establish a grid or a table on your piece of paper with the parameters at the top (in this case, individual, flower and colour) and along the side the specific independent variable (in this case the names of the individuals).
Use the information provided in the statements to fill the grid/table. You should end up with:

Name	Flower	Colour
Lewis	Petunia	White
Jay	Rose	Red
Amy	Rose	Pink
Becca	Rose	Red
Bartholomew	Petunia	White

(Continued)

This table method should allow you to logically organise the information, giving you plenty of material to deduce the answer. After a while, the physical aspect of the technique may become unnecessary, and this type of question will become more of a mental exercise. During the exam, abbreviate the parameters to save time when writing (L = Lewis or Be = Becca).

Always try to rule out the other statements before arriving at a final answer.

Similarly, questions that evaluate a conclusion through inference can also be approached very logically. You are expected to equate pieces of information from different statements with a link to come to a logical conclusion. It's much easier to explain through a simple example.

Question

All goldfish are orange. All carp are brown. This fish is either a goldfish or a carp.

Which of the following conclusions follow? (Yes if follow, no if not.)

Conclusion	Yes	No
This fish is brown or a goldfish.		
This fish is orange or a goldfish.		
If not a goldfish, this is a carp.		
This fish is orange or a carp.		
This fish is brown or gold.		

Run Through

For these types of questions, it is important to understand the subject of the question (what it is talking about) and nuances of the passage (how it is saying them).

The passage will always provide you with definite terms and terms that are dependent on other items. It is important to identify these terms in each instance. Therefore, attention to language is very important; 'most', 'all', 'many', 'partly', 'must' and 'only' are a few examples of terms you should look out for. They are very important in determining the correct conclusions.

In the previous example, if we approach each individual conclusion, we can break them down and **rationalise them against the information in the passage.**

1. The passage explicitly states that the fish can be either a goldfish or a carp. As carps are brown, we can substitute brown with carp and therefore conclude that the fish is either a goldfish or a carp. The use of definitive language suggests that there are no exceptions. Therefore, this conclusion follows and is true.
2. This option describes the fish as either a goldfish or orange (i.e. a goldfish), therefore implying that the fish **definitely** belongs to the goldfish category. As a result, this answer does not follow.
3. **Only look for the information the question is asking about.** As the fish can only belong to the two types, if we exclude one of the types from the answer, then it logically follows the fish can only be the remaining type. Therefore, yes, it follows.
4. Similar to the previous explanations, a simple substitution of terms will allow you to understand that this conclusion follows. This is because the colour orange implies the fish can be a goldfish. Once substituted into the conclusion, we can see that this follows the original statement.
5. This conclusion draws on information sources not in the passage. There is no mention of the colour gold or which type of fish may be this colour. Therefore, neither the goldfish nor the carp can qualify to be this colour. As a result, this conclusion does not follow the information in the statement, and the conclusion is false.

How to Interpret Venn Diagrams and Probabilities

Venn diagrams are a brilliant method of presenting multiple sets of data to demonstrate their similarities and differences. The diagrams are made of circles. These circles are groups of data. When a data value is inside one of these circles, it is within that data set. When a value is inside two circles, the data in the overlapping section occur in both data sets (Fig. 7.7).

When dealing with numbers, it is important to always account for the overlapping number and the original number in the circle, add them, to get the total data for that set. This is a **common trap** as people assume that the number in the circle is the total value of the data set without accounting for the number that was separated to be placed into the overlap.

The only advice available for Venn diagrams is to learn what parameters place a data value into a circle and what data values remain outside the circles. Always double check.

Interpreting Probabilities

These types of questions are the very basic of the statistics modules you may have done in school or are currently attempting at maths A-Level. You will be presented with a very short passage containing statistical information and asked to select the best response to the question. It may be better to demonstrate.

Question

A coin is flipped twice. For Julie to be successful she must flip heads consecutively.

Is the probability that she will succeed ¾?

- Yes, it is ¾ as there are four combinations in all, three of the combinations include heads.
- Yes, it is ¾ as flipping two tails is only one possible combination from a number of coin flips.
- No, it is ¼ as the second flip is equally likely to be heads or tails.
- No, it is as there are three combinations that flip head at least once and one combination that includes all head flips.

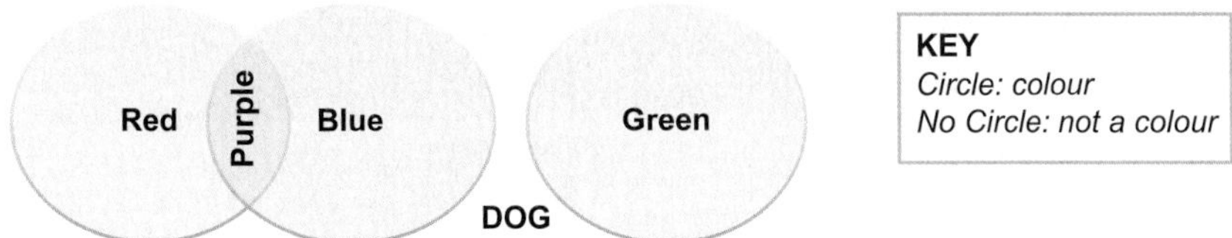

Fig. 7.7 An example Venn diagram.

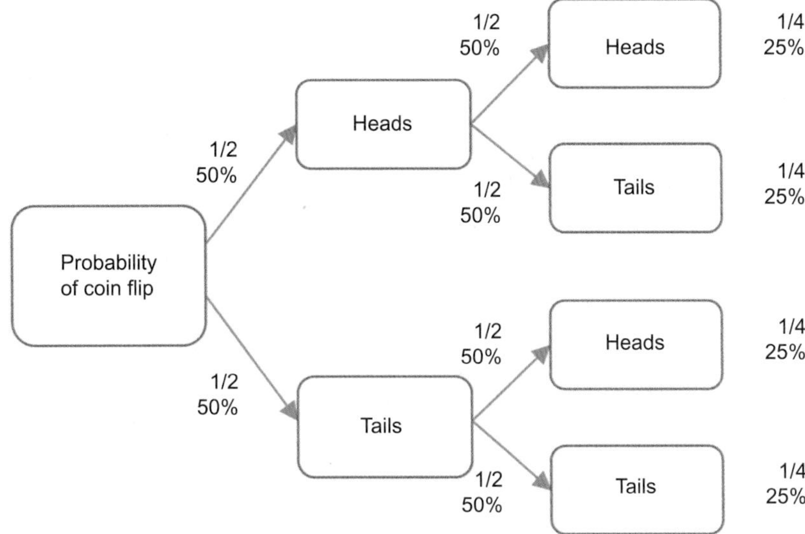

Fig. 7.8 Probability tree diagram.

Run Through

For probability questions similar to this one, it can be very useful to draw out the probability tree diagram (Fig. 7.8). For example, in the previous case, simply understanding that the first flip will definitely be a head flip and the second flip is equally likely to be a heads or tails, as shown, will let you come to a solid conclusion. This can also be done by multiplying the probabilities of one branch and the subsequent branch to show the total probability of that event occurring.

SECTION 3: QUANTITATIVE REASONING

This is known widely as the mathematical section. However, don't be fooled as this section is slightly different from your traditional form of mathematics. The section is very time pressured, and you are expected to answer questions using sophisticated mathematical analysis and logical reasoning.

Depending on which branch of medicine you embark upon, mathematics can play a small or a large role in your practice. A basic understanding allows you to perform drug calculations based on patient weight, age, etc., while advanced usage involves the ability to interpret, critique and apply results in the form of complex statistics in medical/dental research. Either way, at an entry level, you are expected to understand the basic calculations, and recall and execute them promptly.

Overview

This section will give you nine scenarios, each with four multiple-choice questions (MCQs) (similar to the VR format), for a total of 36 questions. You are expected to complete this section in 25 minutes, with 1 minute for instructions and 24 for questions, allowing 40 seconds for each question. This can be fast or slow depending on your ability and prior exposure to similar calculations. Not to worry, there is always room to improve.

The information provided in the questions can be given in multiple forms. However, it is important to not be dumbfounded by all the information and look specifically for the data's context. The specific focus of the calculation will depend upon the nature of the respective question.

The questions will revolve around the basic principles of maths, which you should have exposure to from primary school through to college. These include, but are not limited to, basic arithmetic (remember BODMAS (B—brackets, O—order of powers or roots, D—division, M—multiplication A—addition and S—subtraction)), percentages (both calculation and percentage increase), averages (mean, mode and median), ratios and fractions (calculation and how to convert), common formulae and geometric formulae (working out the area and volume of different shapes, also shown later).

Specific Mathematical Formulae

You must be aware of some common and recurring formulas for the UCAT. It is best to keep these at the

Percentages	$\left(\frac{\text{Part}}{\text{Whole}}\right)\times 100$
Percentage changes	$\left(\frac{\textit{Difference}}{\text{Original}}\right)\times 100$
Mean	$\frac{\text{Sum of all the data values}}{\text{Number of data items}}$
Mode	The most frequently occurring data value
Median	1. List data in numerical order 2. Locate the data value within the middle of the data set
Determining speed	$\textit{Speed} = \frac{\textit{Distance}}{\textit{Time}}$ Remember: Racers get (ST)Ds

Fig. 7.9 Key definitions.

Circle	Area: Circumference: Cylindrical volume:	$A = \pi r^2$ (r = radius) $C = 2\pi r$ $V = \pi r^2 h$ (h = height/length)
Square	Area	$A = a^2$ (a = one side)
Cube	Volume Surface area	$V = a^3$ (a = length of one edge) $A = 6a^2$
Triangle	Area	$\frac{(\textit{Base} \times \textit{Height})}{2}$
	Triangular prism Volume	Area of the cross section (area of a triangle) multiplied by the length of the prism.

Fig. 7.10 Geometric formulae.

forefront of your mind so you can use them promptly and confidently. Practice lots of questions with these formulas to the point that you can passively recall them, although I'm sure you already know most, if not all, of them from school and college mathematics (Fig. 7.9).

Common Geometric Formulae

These formulas are also good to be aware of as they can come up frequently (Fig. 7.10). The basic types are listed later.

General Tips

Don't be thrown off by the amount of data/maths; it is actually a series of simple mathematics. The trick behind quantitative reasoning is understanding what information to use, manipulating the formulae and doing it within the specified amount of time. One technique for improving your timing is getting familiar with the on-screen calculator. Use the UCAT practice questions online and bring up the calculator. Whenever you attempt questions on any database, paper or online, use the practice website calculator to get extremely familiar with it. I recommend trying both the number pad and the mouse to see what works best for you. At the same time, don't become reliant on the calculator; try to minimise usage with simple mental maths (i.e. you don't need to add 10 plus 10 with a calculator to know it's 20).

On the contrary, if you are extremely familiar with the calculator and fast with your fingers, then see which method is faster for you. Always personalise the tips we provide, as something that worked for others may not work for you.

Approaching a Question

Now that you've seen the basic formulas often used in the UCAT, it's time to learn how to approach a question to apply them efficiently.

The first step is to take a step back. Questions may present you with a massive amount of information but you have to remember you only have 40 seconds per question. Therefore, take a step back and try not to read all of the text first, as much of the text and data can be irrelevant. It is important to examine the most important aspects (the core of the data) to understand what the data are presenting. This is usually accomplished by looking at the pictorial representation (diagram, table, graph, etc.) first.

For the next step, **read the question and read it properly**. You must accurately interpret what the question is asking, as you don't have time to repeat your calculations in the exam. So read the question and pick up on the data points it is asking you to analyse. Now return to your pictorial representation and refer only to these data points (the rest will only serve to distract you and waste your time).

Some students prefer to reverse the order and read the question first, then apply data analysis. Other students prefer to understand the data, and then apply it to the question. Try both methods and feel which one is more suited to your individual style.

The calculation itself will depend on the questions and it is unlikely that any quantitative reasoning (QR) strategy will also involve dealing with every specific calculation. The best advice I can give here is to understand the formulas provided earlier and estimate the remainder. Understanding the formula will allow you to determine how to reach the answer, but sometimes estimation is required to efficiently move past the questions with more calculation steps (as inputting everything into the calculator can slow you down).

Therefore, try **rounding the numbers** to the 'nicest closest' number and use that number in the calculations, e.g. the 'nicest closest' number to 95 is 100. This will not give you an exact answer but will usually lead you to a range between two answers.

When estimating and rounding, always remember to keep the magnitude of the numbers in check, as this will help if you are stuck between two choices. When rounding, you can either round up or down. It is a good idea to note how much a figure was rounded either up or down. This will help you determine if your final estimate was either under or over the actual value. So when you are stuck between choices, knowing if it's an underestimate or an overestimate, you can choose the bigger or smaller answer, respectively. Try to minimise the maths, to maximise your time efficiency.

Basic Data Analysis

When you interpret a graph to understand the subsequent questions, it is important to **extract some vital information**. This is the same basic approach as a mathematics question in school exams:

1. The **type of data** presented and how the data links, i.e. reading the table's title, then reading the headings of the columns and the rows to understand what the type of data or scenario is being presented, e.g. the columns' headings showing different bus numbers and the row titles displaying where they stop.
2. **Labels and units**. It is very common to fall into the 'units trap' even in school exams, so make sure to read the units and use the correct/same units as the question is asking. Otherwise, it can often lead to the wrong answer.
3. **Brief understanding of the accompanied text/data** (use some of those VR fast reading skills). Usually, the text provided before the pictorial representation is not very relevant and can be a waste of everyone's time. However, sometimes the textual information can be used to supplement the information in the picture, so it is always best to run over the information. Particularly, **keep an eye out for specific numbers or circumstantial data** that may pop up in the text.

Serendipity. What does this even mean? Well, it's a fancy way of saying calculated gambling. Professional poker players win more often than amateurs, not because they are 'lucky', but because they gamble in a more calculated way. They don't know for sure what they will get, but they know more or less what could happen (i.e. 80% probability of winning, 20% probability of losing and so on).

You want to use this skill with every single question you don't know or are not sure how to answer. You make a calculated guess and hope that it's the right choice. In my opinion, the difference between good and great results is the use of this practical skill. For example, if you solve 70% of the questions 100% correctly and the rest you throw absolutely at random, on average, you would get 77.5% of the questions correct. If you use serendipity, you solve 60% of the questions 100% correctly, and the rest you throw at random and hit 50% to 75% depending on your ability, you would get between 80% and 90% of the questions correct. The goal is obviously not to gamble at all but most likely you will have to.

IF you decide to gamble, you have to gamble smart. You have to improve your chances of hitting the answer at random, and try to work faster to get as many 100% questions as you would get without 'smart gambling'.

Dan, Medical School Applicant

SECTION 4: ABSTRACT REASONING

The first time you encounter abstract reasoning, you may be unable to make sense of what is happening in this section. As someone who has also taken the UCAT and experienced its growing pains, I can assure you that most people feel the exact same way when they encounter abstract reasoning. Let's see if we can break that down a bit further so it all makes sense, and hopefully you will see the method in their madness.

Abstract reasoning is a section that assesses your ability to synthesise, modify and apply hypotheses in a time-pressured environment. This helps you in practical medicine when you are dealing with an emergency situation and need to determine the cause of the patient's presentation (the diagnosis) based on the clues they give you in the history and examination. Therefore, it makes sense to test this particular set of skills.

Overview

The abstract reasoning section gives you a total of 13 minutes, with 1 minute for instructions and 12 minutes for 50 items, giving you a total of roughly 14 seconds per sub-question. This will be the rapid-fire section, so it's very important to get familiarised with the questions and techniques so that you can be as efficient as possible. In order to do this: PRACTICE (practice until you see patterns everywhere, even in your curtains).

Abstract reasoning has four different types of questions:

(Illustrated examples follow in the chapter)

1. **Type 1**: Two sets of shapes are shown. You will be asked to determine if the test shape belongs to Set A, Set B or neither.
2. **Type 2**: You will be shown a series of shapes and you must determine how they are changing. You will be asked to pick which shape is next in the sequence from a series of test shapes.
3. **Type 3**: You will be presented with two rows of two boxes each. The first row will show you the transition between two boxes. The second will ask you to theorise what the fourth box will look like based on the third box and the principles of change from the first row.
4. **Sets Type 4**: Two sets of shapes are shown. You will be asked to pick a shape from the series of test shapes that falls into a particular set.

Start familiarising yourself with these questions as soon as possible. This will help your brain pick up pattern types and recognise basic patterns without even thinking about them—the so-called 'I can just see them when I answer'.

However, even if you are able to see the patterns, sometimes you may encounter an advanced, unrecognisable shape. At this point, we need to go back to basics and systematically approach the question. So, let's see how!

Specific Strategies

Step 1: Keep it simple

It is very easy to be overwhelmed by the sheer number or complexity of the patterns. Therefore, it is important to take a step back and pick the simplest box, or the one that looks the nicest to you. Usually, this means the box with fewer shapes or the least complex of the series. This helps you to focus on the core patterns/rules that occur in that set, and focus on establishing those rules. Once you feel you have established a set of rules (usually two for most questions and three or more in harder, complex questions), try to cross-reference them against another simple box to see if your rules hold true for that box. If they do, then continue onto the next box and repeat until you have compared your rules against all six boxes in a set. Sometimes, you may encounter a situation where you have established a set of rules from box one but only one or two rules hold true after comparison. Stick with these rules and see how far they take you.

Step 2: Keep it basic

If you stare at a box long enough, you will be able to establish a ridiculously large number of rules (which may or may not hold true against the other boxes). However, during the exam, you will have approximately 14 seconds for each sub-question, so keep it simple. You don't need to establish 20 rules in those 14 seconds. Gather a few simple rules. Apply them consistently, and within the time limit, to maximise your efficiency. If you're still not convinced, then let's look at it another way. The examiner knows that you are pressed for time, so (for most questions) they will not establish a complex set of rules that take you 30 seconds to find. Instead, they will make a few core rules to assess the consistency with which you can establish and test your own rules. This means start simple. If simple doesn't lead you to the answer, then utilise a few more uncommon/complex rules to elicit the answer.

Step 2.5: 'Common pattern screen' when stuck

Once you start revising for abstract reasoning full time, you will find that there are a series of recurring patterns (some types keep being reused), because there is a finite pool of patterns they can pick from. Therefore, if you learn to screen for some of the common patterns when you're stuck, the majority of the time, you will be able to interpret at least one rule and have some ability to answer the question.

These are differently phrased in every book you may read, but when I took the UCAT, I found that it's easier to categorise them into two sections:

- Shape
- Relationship

Shape involves checking for features and signs of one particular aspect of the box.

Relationship involves seeing how one aspect and another (if the question involves multiple features) link to each other.

> First sit back, and look at ALL squares: is there anything that is recurrent? Remember, it doesn't have to be even ALL on left or right; it could be ALL on top or bottom. Think about relative positions, shading, etc. Then, if you got a pattern, use 10 seconds to see if you can figure out a more complex pattern. If not, then just answer with what you have. If this doesn't work after 10–20 seconds, focus on the simplest square and start from there. If there is no pattern after ~30 seconds, just guess the most 'reasonable' pattern. (You might be able to figure that out in 2 minutes, but why sacrifice two sets for this maybe particularly difficult one?)
>
> **Frederick, Top 3% UCAT Scorer, Medical School Applicant 2022–2023**

Table 7.3 outlines a basic approach to the types of patterns you could think about when you are stuck. Give it a read, and if it's useful, use it. When approaching difficult questions consider the following approach:

Step 1: Try to locate the simplest box and describe it to yourself in as much detail as possible. What specific shapes are there, what colour are the shapes, what size are they, how are they positioned within the box or relative to each other?

Step 2: Look at what is common to the simplest box identified in step 1. For example, does that triangle appear in both boxes? (If so, how?) (If not, can you exclude this from the pattern? Is it a distractor?)

Step 3: Do all boxes in that set have that same quality? If yes, great, you have worked out your pattern. If not, either flag and move on or look back at the boxes identified in steps 2 and 3 and see what else they have in common.

This can also be represented in a mind map (Fig. 7.11). Use the blank spaces between the boxes below to add more arrows and patterns to personalise the screen for yourself.

Table 7.3 Approaching Difficult Questions

SCREEN TYPE	WHAT TO LOOK FOR
Shape 1	Type of shape
Shape 2	Colour/pattern/fill of shape
Shape 3	Size of the shape
Shape 4	Number of shapes
Shape 5	Number/types of angles/sides of a shape (odd or even number, 90° angles, acute vs obtuse angles, etc.)
Relation 1	**Position of the shape relative to the box (top left corner, touching one particular side, etc.)**
Relation 2	Position of the shape relative to another shape (above/below)
Relation 3	Position of the shape relative to angles (perpendicular/ tangential)
Relation 4	**Position of the shape relative to direction (Shape facing left/right)**
Relation 5	Position of the shape relative to its symmetry (rotational symmetry)

> There are many more patterns to consider if you want to do a full screen, but this should help you get started when approaching a difficult question. Hopefully at least one aspect will stick, allowing you to answer the question.

> Always remember to look for multiple patterns and combinations of shapes and relations. They may not always be used in isolation.

A lot of the time, if you cannot find a pattern in a particular set, e.g. Set A, it's in your best interest to move onto Set B, as they are usually linked together. Most of the time, the rule you find for one set utilises a common aspect but proposes it in a slightly different, usually opposite, manner for the second set. For example, look at Fig. 7.12.

It is possible to use these small rule changes between different sets anytime you are stuck on a particular set. Draw inspiration from the other set and apply it back onto the original set.

Type 2 Questions. Follow one specific shape and see how it changes. There will commonly be two elements to the question, so follow the changes in both those elements and you will arrive at how they are changing. For example, look at Fig. 7.13.

Type 3 Questions. The questions will show a box with one picture and ask how it relates to the second box. The best approach is to substitute and correlate shapes between the two different rows, i.e. pick one object/ position in the first box and see how that object has transitioned or the position has changed in the second box. Apply it to the remaining shapes/positions in Box 1 and their corresponding Box 2 counterparts, and see if the change is consistent. Then apply this rule you've found to Box 3 and you can determine what Box 4 will look like. For example, look at Fig. 7.14.

Step 3: Don't kill the time

I feel like I may be repeating myself again. But, nevertheless, this is a very time-pressured section. If you

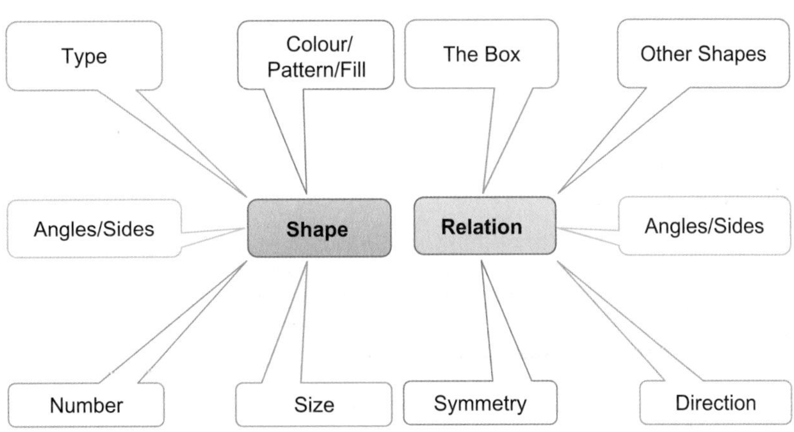

Fig. 7.11 Mind map on assessing shape/relationship.

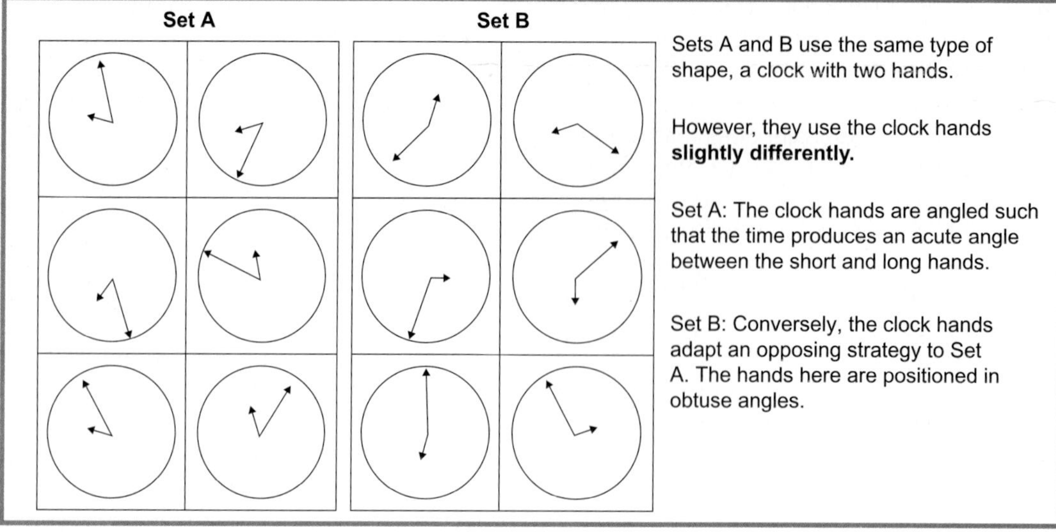

Set A
Set B
Sets A and B use the same type of shape, a clock with two hands.
However, they use the clock hands **slightly differently.**
Set A: The clock hands are angled such that the time produces an acute angle between the short and long hands.
Set B: Conversely, the clock hands adapt an opposing strategy to Set A. The hands here are positioned in obtuse angles.

Fig. 7.12 Analysing Set A and Set B.

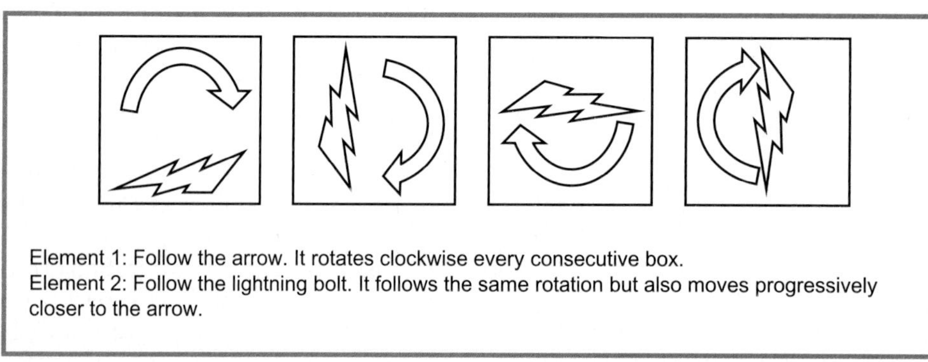

Element 1: Follow the arrow. It rotates clockwise every consecutive box.
Element 2: Follow the lightning bolt. It follows the same rotation but also moves progressively closer to the arrow.

Fig. 7.13 Type 2 question example.

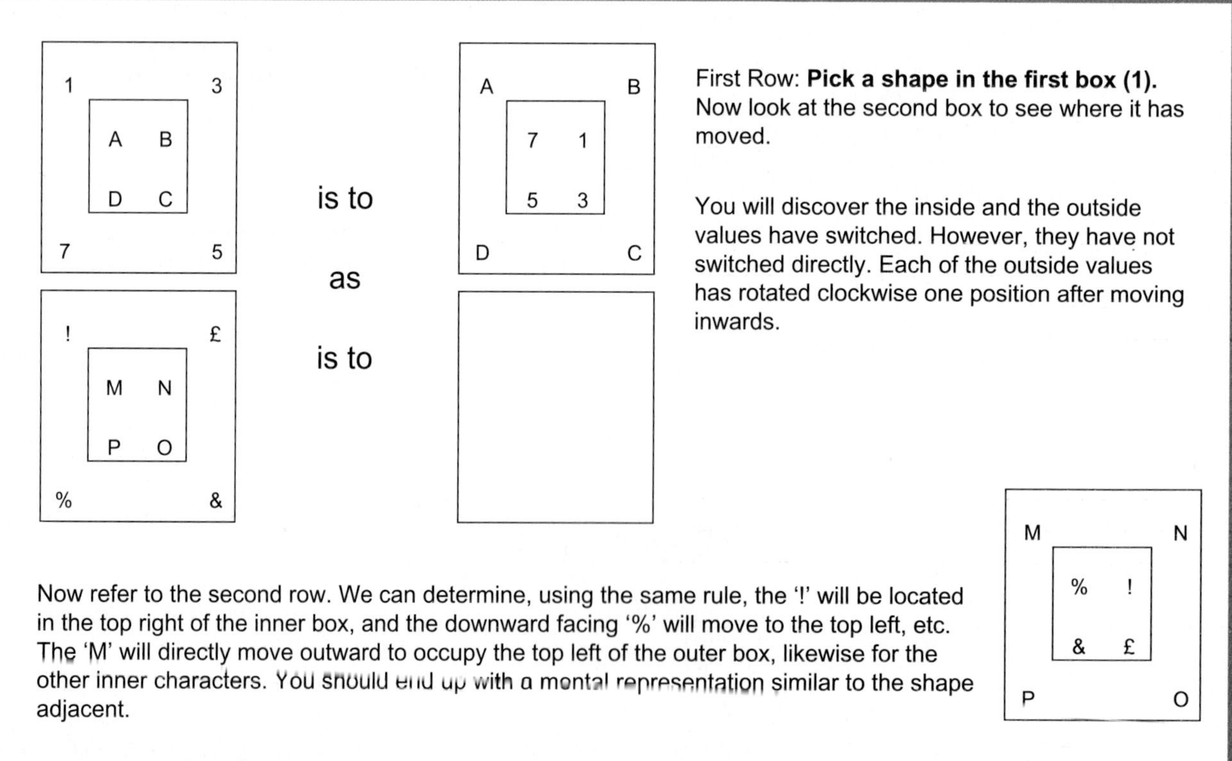

1 3 A B D C 7 5
is to
A B 7 1 5 3 D C
as
! £ M N P O % &
is to
First Row: **Pick a shape in the first box (1).** Now look at the second box to see where it has moved.
You will discover the inside and the outside values have switched. However, they have not switched directly. Each of the outside values has rotated clockwise one position after moving inwards.
M N % ! & £ P O
Now refer to the second row. We can determine, using the same rule, the '!' will be located in the top right of the inner box, and the downward facing '%' will move to the top left, etc. The 'M' will directly move outward to occupy the top left of the outer box, likewise for the other inner characters. You should end up with a mental representation similar to the shape adjacent.

Fig. 7.14 Type 3 question example.

are not able to answer a question in the 14 seconds, despite screening for basic patterns, then it is time to move on to the next question. Don't take time away from your other questions (which you could be getting right) just to get the satisfaction of answering a hard question. This can be difficult to adjust to when you are transitioning from school exams to the UCAT, but it is important to move on when you have run out of time. Remember, you can always **flag the tough questions and come back to them** at the end with fresh eyes.

Final step: Practice

Although not really a strategic step for use in the actual exam, practice is the one thing that will not let you down. This section is all about grasping the different types of patterns and allowing your brain to understand and apply them consistently. The best way to accomplish this is by practicing until you are able to understand the patterns as soon as they come up.

> Abstract Reasoning was definitely the section I struggled with the most since pattern recognition isn't a commonly taught skill so I found it handy to have a list of all the patterns I've seen so that I have a mental list of the ones to look for when I get stuck on a question.
>
> **Amy Downes, UCAT 3330, Medical School Applicant 2022–2023**

SECTION 5: SITUATIONAL JUDGMENT

Nearly there! This is the fifth and final section of the exam, but I wouldn't relax just yet. Situational judgement is a recurring exam throughout medicine, and you will encounter it when you are finishing medical school, before applying to certain medical specialities and, now, before you apply to medicine. The goal is to expose you to situations that could occur during your time studying medicine and even further along, as an actual doctor.

Again, similar to the other sections, the examiners are testing traits they think would make you an empathetic doctor who is able to express some of the core attributes of patient–doctor relationships: honesty, integrity, perspective taking, teamwork and, due to the nature of the exam, adaptability. Therefore, whenever you answer these questions, you must consider how a doctor or medical student would respond in those particular scenarios.

Overview

You will be presented with 66 questions associated with scenarios (each scenario can have up to six questions associated with it). It is important to point out that this section is testing noncognitive thinking, i.e. does not require medical or procedural knowledge, just requires your ethical and moral values. The entire section allows for 27 minutes, 1 minute for instructions and 26 for answering the questions, allowing you roughly 22–23 seconds per item.

The section, as described before, is not marked out of 900. Instead, your answers are matched against the answers of an expert panel. Depending on how large the proportion of answers match/are partially correct will determine what band you are placed into, with band 1 being the highest and band 4 the lowest.

The questions themselves are divided into two different types:

1. Appropriateness questions: These questions will ask you to determine how appropriate a particular response is to a scenario. They make up the majority of the questions.

Response	Indication
Very appropriate	It will address at least one aspect (not necessarily all aspects) of the situation, **i.e. the action is only/very positive**
Appropriate, but not ideal	**Could be done, but is not necessarily a very good thing to do, i.e. the option is generally positive but with a negative component**
Inappropriate, but not awful	Should not really be done, but would not be terrible, **i.e. generally negative but with a positive component**
Very inappropriate	Should definitely not be done and would make the situation worse, **i.e. the action is very/only negative**

2. Importance questions: These questions ask you to rate the importance of a series of options in response to the scenario. These will make up the remainder of the section, so it is good to know how to deal with them.

Response	Indication
Very important	Something that is vital to take into account
Important	Something that is important but not vital to take into account
Of minor importance	Something that could be taken into account, but it does not matter if it is considered or not
Not important at all	Something that should definitely not be taken into account

General Tips

The most important tip, which should define your thinking for this section, is 'How would the examiner answer this question?' and 'What is the BEST action to take here?' If you can differentiate between a negative and a positive answer, then you can narrow your choices down to two. However, when determining the answer, it is important to remember that the best answer may not be the most immediate one (so don't be tricked by the time frame). The question could be hinting at the best option overall (immediate action vs. most appropriate action). This is not to say, however, that the immediate option can't be the most appropriate, so take it case by case.

One overall tip to live by in the whole situational judgment section:

- *Appropriateness questions: You need to* ***be aware of the negative or positive-ness*** *of the action to determine the answer*
- *Importance questions: You need to* ***be aware of language*** *used to determine how absolute the action is.*

For nonmedical people, or those not related to medics, this section can seem daunting, especially if you haven't had the same level of life experience as other people. Personally, I experienced something similar and wasn't sure how to approach the section.

My best tip would be to get exposure to as many questions as possible to understand how certain situations should be approached. After a while, you will see the pattern of behaviour behind similar types of dilemmas and automatically pick the correct (or partially correct) answer.

Lucy, Medical School Applicant

How to Approach the Situational Judgement Test (SJT)

Pillars of medical ethics

As outlined in Chapter 5, the pillars of medical ethics are important principles to convey and could help you determine what actions are positive or negative in your SJT, especially if you are having trouble deciding what is appropriate and its degree of appropriateness. Therefore, the pillars of medical ethics can be a good starting point when you are determining how to interpret the core issues of the scenario.

There are four 'pillars' of ethics as shown in the following table.

Autonomy	Respect for the patient's right to self-determination
Beneficence	The duty to 'do good'
Nonmaleficence	The duty to 'do no harm'
Justice	To treat all people equally and equitably

As a recap, let's look at an overview and understand how they can be used to understand if the scenarios pose a positive or a negative implication.

Autonomy. Autonomy essentially means respecting the patient's wishes and decisions. It is important to understand that a patient is also a person, and therefore, you cannot simply push your ideals onto them and act without their consent. If, in the exam, you find that there are scenarios that are compromising the patient's choices (such as medical paternalism), they are very likely to be inappropriate choices. The only exception to this would be if the patient's safety is compromised and they do not have the capacity to make a decision (capacity is determined by the patient's ability to understand and make an informed decision based on the relevant information, e.g. severe learning difficulty, brain damage or confusion/loss of consciousness).

Beneficence. To always do good. Take it as literally as it comes. In the exam, if you are not the nicest person in the world, always helping the old lady cross the street, then you are doing something wrong. This is a good principle, similar but distinctly different to nonmaleficence, which can help you rule out some of the answers and give you a good indication of whether the action is positive or not. If the action suggested is not helpful to, or in the best interest of, the intended individual/group in the question, then it is unlikely upholding this principle and could therefore be inappropriate. **This will help you determine what is a positive action.**

Nonmaleficence. Do no harm. This is distinctly different from beneficence. With nonmaleficence, the principle idea is to do no harm, i.e. don't be bad. However, this does not imply always being good, as you could also remain neutral without harming someone. Again, it may seem like I am repeating myself, but this should be a very obvious point in your exam. If there is a choice that compromises patient safety, especially as a result of your actions (directly or indirectly), then it is highly inappropriate to initiate/continue the action. **This will help you determine what is a negative action.**

In the real world, causing harm to a patient is a very serious offense, and consequences can be as severe as your medical licence being revoked (not to mention harming someone can also lead to severe consequences through the criminal justice system).

Justice. Treat everyone the same. Offer everyone the same options, regardless of their socio-economic background (esp. in the UK where the system is public rather than private, allowing everyone to access the same level of care at the point of need). This will show you are taking everyone into consideration and not ignoring one group of people for the sake of another. An answer may suggest only helping one group of people over another, although dependent on the circumstances, discriminating between people who have the same circumstances is a definite 'no go'. This is **another method to determine if an answer is negative in the exam.**

When the four pillars fail

If the situation does not seem to fit the four pillars of ethics, then it may be more appropriate to utilise some of the core values of a doctor, as described by the General Medical Council (GMC) within 'Good

Medical Practice'. In the following text I have tried to summarise concisely how you can apply them to the SJT. It must be noted that this is not a comprehensive list of the GMC's good medical practice document. In order to gain a complete understanding of how to behave as a medical professional, I highly suggest reading it online before your UCAT. This will help you understand some of the minutiae of medical professionalism and what is expected of you as a medical/doctor/healthcare professional. Some of the core principles follow.

Professionalism. Integrity as a doctor, which embodies how you behave, interact and portray yourself, is crucial to understanding situational judgment. As budding doctors, you must be able to envision yourself as a doctor and, using this mindset, be able to answer the questions. Always maintain honesty with patients and colleagues. Consider the wider perspective of every situation, taking everybody's perspective and feelings into account before making a decision. Understand the consequences of your actions and take routes (in the exam especially) that have better outcomes. Establish yourself as the moral compass of the team; this is the mindset needed for the exam. **Dishonest or illegal actions that show a lack of morality will always be deemed only negative (very inappropriate or not important)**.

Confidentiality. This is another important aspect of every healthcare professional, regardless of whether they are a doctor. If anybody discloses something to you in confidentiality, unless there is evidence that withholding that information will cause harm to the public or the individual, you must keep it confidential. A common scenario is a family member asking for information on the patient's condition. In this scenario, if the patient has not told you that they are happy for the family to know, you cannot disclose any information regarding the patient (doesn't matter how close the family member says they are). It is not recommended to assume family dynamics without the patient's input.

Confidentiality can be quite weird for someone who is encountering it for the first time, especially when the patient's family is involved. However, I would recommend thinking from another perspective. A doctor is also a human being and should therefore be respectful of the patient's wishes (especially the concept around family).

Communication. Communication is an essential part of working in an efficient and well-oiled machine called a team. This is one quality that is tested throughout your medical career, from your time as a first year medical student until you are an 80-year-old senior consultant looking forward to finally retiring. Therefore, communication skills are emphasised throughout medical entry and actively sought out in interviews. Putting communication type scenarios into the situational judgment section would hence make sense.

There are also some important aspects of communication, between healthcare professionals, which some of the students find harder to interpret, most likely due to the lack of contact with the medical profession/National Health Service (NHS). **Everyone on the team is equal**. In the current NHS (especially in this exam, with a heavy emphasis on teamwork), everybody on the team has the same level of input into the patient's care, particularly when patient safety is compromised, and they can intervene if they feel something inappropriate is occurring. If there are any discrepancies between different team members, then they are expected to calmly talk things through, outside of the patient's view (to maintain professionalism). If the issue is not resolved between the two members, then they can escalate it further to one hierarchal level higher (this is especially true for issues between students, but be careful when judging what level of hierarchy is appropriate).

In every communication scenario just consider the very basic values of interaction/dialogue: *empathy, approachability, confidence and reciprocating communication*. **Essentially, be a nice person who has the other individual's best interests at heart**.

'To be virtuous, one must act as a virtuous person would act'

– Aristotle

HOW TO ACE THE BIOMEDICAL ADMISSION TEST (BMAT)

WHAT IS THE BMAT? WHAT DOES IT INVOLVE?

The BMAT can undoubtedly be a daunting test—I know because I've taken it as well, and trust me, I was very nervous waiting outside the examination hall. Some of you might share the same perspective, and that's perfectly fine. It is good that you are worried about the test. The fact that you're reading this chapter shows your desire to succeed. Hopefully this chapter will provide you with some tips on how to study for the BMAT and help you to jump one of the biggest hurdles standing between you and medical school.

First, let's briefly outline some important messages. Keep in mind that different medical schools in the UK require different tests, such as the UCAT. The ones that require BMAT, as of 2022–23, are listed in Table 7.4.

The format itself is quite simple. It would be wise to **visit the official BMAT website** if you haven't already.

Essentially, there are a total of three sections, each testing different skills. The first two sections involve answering MCQs (Aptitude and Skills, Scientific Knowledge and Application), with the final section (Writing Task) consisting of a writing task.

The BMAT itself is a **written test**, and not a computerised test like the UCAT.

Table 7.4 UK Universities That Use BMAT

Brighton and Sussex Medical School	Imperial College London	University of Cambridge
Keele University (only 'overseas for fees' applicants)	University of Manchester Medical School (for some groups of international applicants only)	University of Oxford
University College London	Lancaster University	University of Leeds

WHY IS THE EXAM IMPORTANT FOR YOU?

Like any other admissions test, your scores on the test will be collated and judged against other candidates. Universities will often have a cut-off score to separate out higher-scoring candidates. Different universities will prioritise candidates according to different aspects of their application, such as their personal statement or predicted grades. These are taken into consideration when determining who is invited to interview. The BMAT score is no exception. Assuming that your grades meet the university standards and your personal statement is decent, your BMAT score could just **secure you a place for interview**.

You may be wondering then, how well must you do in order to have any sense of safety—don't worry, that question will be answered later.

GENERAL TIPS

If you're going to get anything out of this chapter, let it be this: **Practice makes perfect**. I feel like a parent lecturing my child when I say that, but you can't deny that it holds true. Here are some general tips that may again sound trivial, but don't overlook their importance. It is a basic lesson in good exam technique. A large percentage of this, if not all, can be applied to tests that you may come across in medical school—of which you will have plenty.

Read the Question

I'm not sure if you were taught this at sixth form, but this was something that my biology, chemistry and physics teachers recited to our cohort like sermon.

Interpret it as you will, but for the purposes of this book, it stands for **Read the Full Question**. Speed-reading can be a useful tool when using the least amount of time to read through a passage and simultaneously absorb large blocks of information, but test writers can easily catch you out if you carelessly misread the question. It is, after all, what matters ultimately. There's no point in reading a passage or block of data thoroughly but then accidentally skipping a line when reading the prompt. Read it twice, three times or more than that if you really need to, to avoid dropping the simplest of marks.

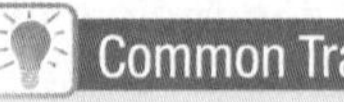

Common Traps

- Some questions may require you to **choose all answers that apply.** It is extremely easy to lose marks if you automatically assume that there's just one correct answer.
- There may be some questions that want you to express a numerical value a certain way. It is important to always use **the correct units.**

Attempt ALL the Questions

As I mentioned before, there's no negative marking. **Try EVERY SINGLE question** in the first two sections. You may inevitably leave some questions blank and move on to another question. First, **REMEMBER** or make a note to yourself that you have left a question blank so that you know to come back to it. As each section is timed separately, you will not have the full 2 hours to complete the test in an order that you personally prefer. This means that, yes, you are tight on time, which also means that you will have to guess if you are completely unsure. Who knows? Maybe you'll end up guessing some answers correctly.

Eliminate and Guess

Playing the guessing game is another aspect of the multiple-choice sections. You may come across some incredibly tough questions that the BMAT committee expect only the top of the food chain to answer correctly. Don't panic! Eliminate some blatantly incorrect answers. If you're on the fence about some of them, think through the answers logically. Although this may take up some time, with enough practice you can learn to use your rationale to swiftly cross out red herrings. Personally, my rule in test taking at medical school is to eliminate at least two or three answers. In a question with five choices, this gives you at least a third or half of a chance to guess correctly. It doesn't sound like much, but I would take 50% over 20%, or 0%, any day.

Bubble Properly

If you have taken the American Scholastic Assessment Test (SAT) or American College Testing (ACT) like I have, you may be familiar with this type of marking system (if you haven't, don't worry about it) (Fig. 7.15).

This is the so-called 'bubble answer sheet'. It doesn't take Stephen Hawking to know that in order to answer a question, you fill in the circle that corresponds to the correct answer on the test paper. These will be the answer sheets for sections 1 and 2. They will be scanned through a computer to determine which circles you've filled in. **Do me a favour: Please don't half-ass your circling**. If you are going to answer a question, then fill in the entire circle—don't scribble lightly. You'll be using a pencil to do it, so you can erase it if you want to change your answer later on. However, you must

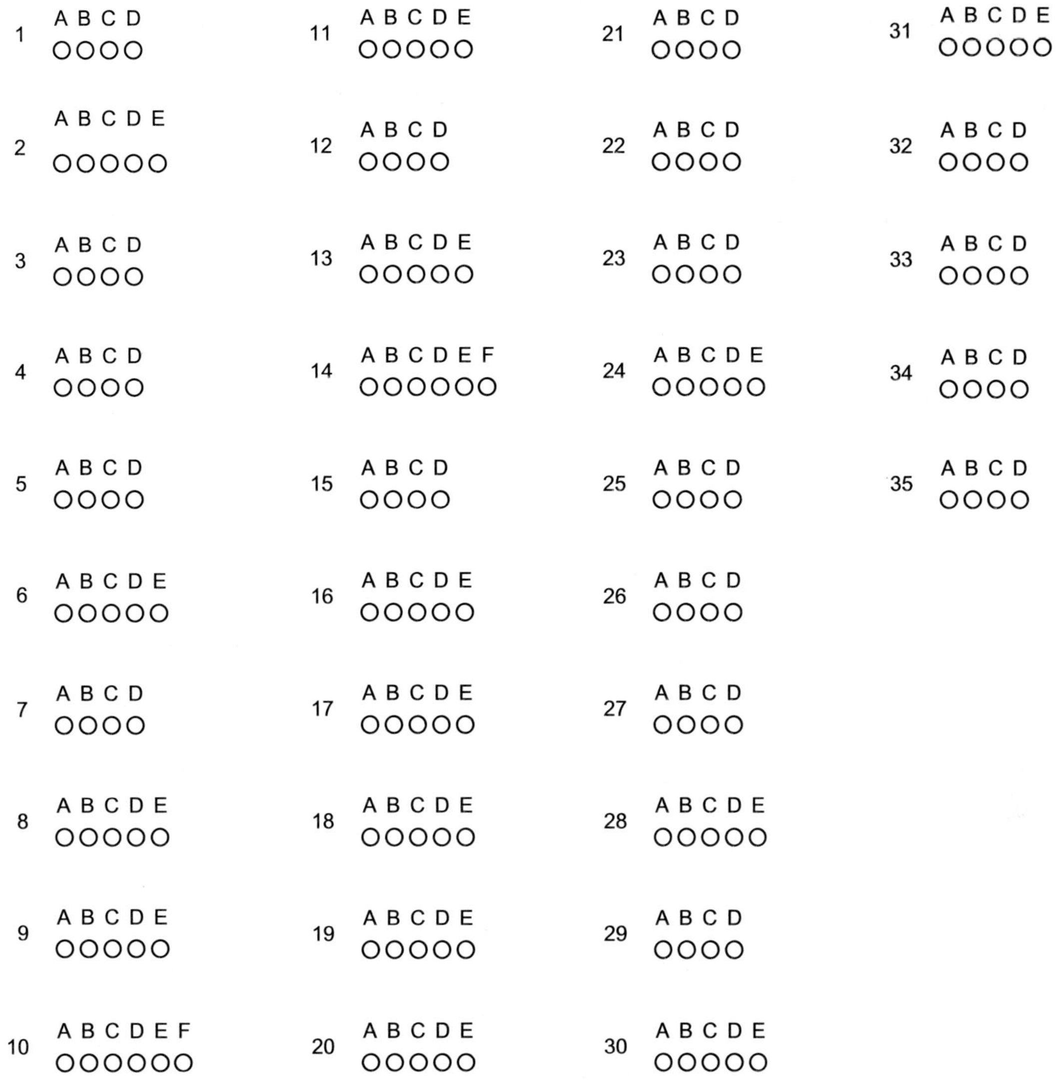

1	A B C D ○○○○	11	A B C D E ○○○○○	21	A B C D ○○○○	31	A B C D E ○○○○○
2	A B C D E ○○○○○	12	A B C D ○○○○	22	A B C D ○○○○	32	A B C D ○○○○
3	A B C D ○○○○	13	A B C D E ○○○○○	23	A B C D ○○○○	33	A B C D ○○○○
4	A B C D ○○○○	14	A B C D E F ○○○○○○	24	A B C D E ○○○○○	34	A B C D ○○○○
5	A B C D ○○○○	15	A B C D ○○○○	25	A B C D ○○○○	35	A B C D ○○○○
6	A B C D E ○○○○○	16	A B C D E ○○○○○	26	A B C D ○○○○		
7	A B C D ○○○○	17	A B C D E ○○○○○	27	A B C D ○○○○		
8	A B C D E ○○○○○	18	A B C D E ○○○○○	28	A B C D E ○○○○○		
9	A B C D E ○○○○○	19	A B C D E ○○○○○	29	A B C D ○○○○		
10	A B C D E F ○○○○○○	20	A B C D E ○○○○○	30	A B C D E ○○○○○		

Fig. 7.15 Bubble answer sheet.

erase it completely, or you will not get a mark for that question. On that note, also bring a pencil sharpener.

Practice Tests Might Not Be the Same

Although the format of the test is static, the questions are not. All the keen beans out there would have done every single past paper available as well as practice questions out of every practice book. However, don't expect the style of the questions to be the same. As of this moment, all practice material that you have encountered can only give you an idea of what will appear on test day. Therefore, be prepared for the worst, and expect the unexpected.

Do You Even Know Your Candidate Number?

Double check, triple check and quadruple check that you've filled this in correctly at the top of each section (Fig. 7.16).

The last thing you want is to come out of the examination hall with your head held high, feeling like you completely aced that BMAT, and then come to find on results day that you've somehow not gotten a score for any section. Tears will flow.

Handwriting

Finally, can anyone currently read your handwriting? Your English might be impeccable and your ideas out of this world, but what's the use in writing a supposedly compelling essay that isn't legible?

You will be given scratch paper to mind map with, so feel free to scribble as much as you want on that. Think through how you're going to write your essay very thoroughly, and write it out neatly in the space given. You want to make sure that the examiners can interpret your genius easily and not compel them to use the Rosetta Stone to decipher your hieroglyphs.

Timing

For all sections of the BMAT, you should be practicing thoroughly. This means that you should be **practicing each section timed and untimed**. However, for every marathon there needs to be a warm-up. Do your first

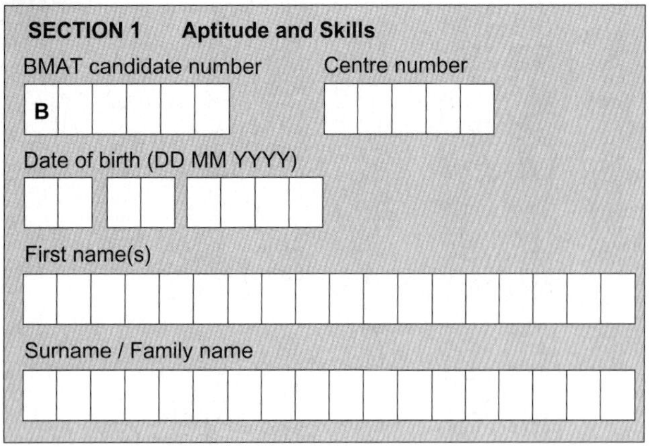

SECTION 1 Aptitude and Skills

BMAT candidate number Centre number

B

Date of birth (DD MM YYYY)

First name(s)

Surname / Family name

Fig. 7.16 Filling in details.

practice without time pressure so you can introduce yourself to the format of the test and format of the questions. Be careful not to become too comfortable about time constraints, and make sure you do an appropriate amount of **practice tests or sections under timed conditions**. It may be useful to print out all practice tests available, and label which ones you will be attempting timed and untimed so that you don't end up wasting whole papers. There are only a limited number available, so **treat them valuably**.

If you think past papers aren't that important—think again or you'll regret it! It is SO important to practice answering various questions while also timing yourself. Don't do what I did—I misread the time I had left and ended up writing only 30% of my essay. Try to skim through the questions quickly and answer the easy ones first, then work your way through the hard ones. I repeat, practicing under timed conditions helps massively.

Reem H., Medical School Applicant

It's a test that will play a big part in deciding your future, which is an undeniable fact, so it's okay to be nervous on the day. This mission, should you choose to accept it, will help you realise that everyone is in the same boat. If you have slaved through hours upon hours of preparation, then you can be sure that you will have no guilt going into the exam. Waiting outside the examination hall can be **nerve wracking**, but I chose to combat this by **talking to other candidates** about how they're feeling. Knowing how other people feel can really put you at ease. You may also choose to do some **breathing exercises** or **power poses** for some emergency confidence.

SCORING OF THE BMAT

You may be wondering at this point, how does the scoring system work, and, more likely, how high must I score on the test in order to guarantee a good chance of getting into medical school? To begin, I will address the first question.

Table 7.5 Score on Content

Description of scores relating to quality of content	
1	An answer that somewhat relates to the question but doesn't tackle it in the way expected. It is unclear and unfocused.
2	An answer that takes into account most of the question's components and is structured in a sensible way. Some components of the argument may however be muddled. Some aspects of the main proposal or counterargument may be unconvincing.
3	The essay presents a reasonably well-argued and rational answer that takes into account all aspects of the question. A reasonable counter argument is made. Some elements of the argument may be weak or overlooked.
4	The essay presents a good answer with little weakness, again taking into account all aspects of the question. The main proposal and counter-argument are strong, rational and well balanced. Ideas are coherent.
5	The essay presents an excellent answer with no apparent weaknesses. On top of addressing all aspects of the question, everything argued is logical and considers a wide variety of pertinent points that lead to a fascinating diagnosis.

Scoring System

The scoring system of the BMAT is quite simple (Tables 7.5 and 7.6). Note that there is **no negative marking** in the multiple-choice sections (i.e. you will not lose any marks for getting a question wrong), so you should **try every single question** to the best of your ability!

All MCQs are worth one mark each. These marks are totalled up and translated into the BMAT's own special system, ranging from a score of 1.0 to 9.0, with 9.0 being the highest possible score. These scores are to one decimal place only.

The main concern for most candidates regarding scoring usually pertains to the writing task. Two examiners will mark your essay, and they will award their marks individually. The final mark for your essay will be the average of the two given scores. This is where it gets a little more complex. The format of your given mark will look a little something like this:

3.5 B

You might think, what on earth does that mean? Examiners will mainly assess two aspects of your essay:

- **Numerical Value: Quality of the essay content.** This is marked on a scale of 1.0–5.0, with 5.0 being the highest mark.
- **Adjacent Letter: Quality of the English used in the essay**. Scoring letters range from A to E, with A being the highest mark.

Table 7.6 Score on English

Description of scores relating to quality of English			
A	*Good use of English*	a)	Fluent
		b)	Good sentence structure
		c)	Good use of vocabulary
		d)	Sound use of grammar
		e)	Good spelling and punctuation
		f)	Few slips or errors
C	*Reasonably clear use of English. There may be some weakness in the effectiveness of the English*	a)	**Reasonably fluent/ not difficult to read**
		b)	Simple/unambiguous sentence structure
		c)	Fair range and appropriate use of vocabulary
		d)	Acceptable grammar
		e)	Reasonable spelling and punctuation
		f)	Some slips/errors
E	*Weak use of English*	a)	Hesitant fluency/not easy to follow at times
		b)	Some flawed sentence structure/ paragraphing
		c)	Limited range of vocabulary
		d)	Faulty grammar
		e)	Frequent spelling/ punctuation errors
		f)	Regular and frequent slips or errors
X	*Anything below the standard of a mark of E*		

Examiners are allowed to give integer scores for essay content, and letter scores of A, C and E for the standard of English. For example, if your two scores were 3A and 4C, your average score would be 3.5B, as seen earlier.

As essay marking is a bit fussier than marking MCQs (which are objectively either right or wrong), there are lists of criteria that help examiners determine what score your essay deserves. After examiners have read your essay and before they finalise your score, they are asked to consider these things:

- Has the candidate addressed the question in the way demanded?
- Have they organised their thoughts clearly?
- Have they used their general knowledge and opinions appropriately?

As two examiners mark the essay, a large discrepancy between marks given by both examiners warrants a remark. This remark is final and will be checked by the BMAT Assessment Manager.

How Well Do You Have to Do?

Entry marks for universities vary. There is no way of saying exactly how well you must perform in order to land yourself a place in medical school. Long story short, **do the best you can** (since there's no pass or fail mark).

However, there are some things that you can do yourself to get an idea of the range of scores achieved worldwide, both before and after the test.

Before the test, you can access the BMAT website and have a look at their statistics, presented graphically in easy-to-find links. Scores are designed so the majority of candidates will score around 5.0 in sections 1 and 2. Relatively few candidates score higher than a 6.0 on either section, which is generally regarded as a high score. The crème de la crème score is 7.0 or higher. In section 3, 2021 around 60% candidates scored a 3.0 or 3.5 for quality of content, and upwards of 75% of candidates scored an A for their quality of English.

After the test, it may be useful to access student discussion forums, especially ones like 'The Student Room'. You are bound to find a page discussing how everyone thought the BMAT went and, after the release of results, how everyone else did relative to you. Moreover, there are separate pages for the individual universities that require the BMAT. Not only can you find other applicants discussing their scores, but there may be useful information regarding predicted grades, interviews, etc., that you may feed off of to give yourself a better picture of what the applicant cohort is like.

SECTION 1: APTITUDE AND SKILLS (32 QUESTIONS, 60 MINUTES)

This section tests general skills such as problem solving, understanding arguments, data analysis and inference. It will typically ask you questions from a finite selection of blatantly obvious themes. As this section is 1-hour long, you will have, on average, less than 2 minutes to complete each question. Therefore, it is important to wisely allocate your time when answering each question.

Argument Comprehension

You will be expected to break down arguments and use your analysis to answer a question about the text. Arguments usually consist of a short paragraph. You may be asked to identify the argument, or what assumptions have been made, considering the information given. You may also be asked questions regarding what statements (given in the answer choices) strengthen or weaken the presented argument.

These types of questions that come up in the first section are notorious for being the most challenging ones. The question stem, as discussed before, is usually a short scenario. It is up to you to identify and distinguish between the facts and the assumptions brought forward in the text, and determine whether the argument has a fundamental flaw. You may also be asked to pick out, within the choices given, which statements best weaken or strengthen the argument.

One thing that you must keep in mind is that you have to assume everything provided to you in the question is 100% true. For example, consider the following.

Patrick gave his son thirty pounds for his birthday. His son said thank you.

Patrick gave his son £30. Not £3, not £300, THIRTY. Therefore, even if it doesn't make sense to you, you can only **analyse how one event leads to another, and not the events themselves**.

Strengthening an argument means that the outcome of the argument will have an increased likelihood of being true. For instance, if one of the options said, 'Patrick's son was well mannered', that would make it more likely for him to thank his father for the birthday money. On the flip side, weakening an argument would make the outcome of the argument have a lesser likelihood of being true. This doesn't mean that the statement has to entirely refute it. If 'Patrick's son was a newborn', for example, this would make it less likely he would be able to thank his father. Essentially, all it takes to weaken the argument is a statement that reduces the impact of the assumption that supports the argument/conclusion.

However, the previous concept would only apply if the assumption supported the final argument/conclusion. **Undermining an assumption that has a positive effect upon the conclusion would ultimately weaken the argument, whereas undermining an assumption that has a negative effect would ultimately strengthen it**. Thus, if the assumption made were against the conclusion, then diminishing that assumption would strengthen the argument.

Other times, questions may test your ability to analyse and identify the assumptions made in an argument. Paraphrased, 'an assumption is anything that does not require any proof in order to be believed or recognised as the truth'. This means that in order for the author of the paragraph to have made some conclusion from the facts provided, the assumption must have been an 'invisible bridge or pillar' linking the two factors. Without this connection, the argument would not logically follow. It is, in other words, a keystone to the basis of the argument. Take this, for instance.

Paul is saving up for his dream car and has been doing so for the past several years. In a year's time he will be able to afford it.

There are so many assumptions constructed from this argument, and here are just five of them:

a) Paul's financial situation is reliable enough to the point where he won't lose a large sum of money anytime soon.
b) He will not lose interest in buying his dream car in the next year.
c) The car will still be on sale by the time he saves up enough money.
d) The price of the car will not increase within a year.
e) He will still be alive in a year's time.

So, you can see here that if a statement in the MCQ options contradicts any of these assumptions, it would automatically diminish the strength of the argument's conclusion. If Paul suddenly acquired a life-threatening illness and died, then he wouldn't even be alive to buy the car, would he?

Again, notice how these assumptions are basically prerequisites for the conclusion to take place. Statements that appear like assumptions, but are not, can be identified by comparing the outcomes of the argument with and without that particular assumption. See the following example.

Paul is working a high-paying job.

Work that into the argument as if it were an assumption. Yes, it bolsters the argument by saying that his high salary could be the key to the success of one day owning his dream car. However, taking it out of the equation does not change much. For all we know, Paul could be working a low-paying job but saving 90% of what he earns to get his dream car. We can therefore conclude that this statement isn't an important assumption, because Paul doesn't absolutely require a high-paying job in order to save up for his dream car.

Problem Solving

How good are you at identifying red herrings in questions? Often times in medicine, it is important to distinguish between what information is useful and what is not. In the case of the BMAT, it may sometimes present itself in the form of large blocks of text, complex graphs with many data points or a combination of both. This tests your ability to utilise the data given to compare and contrast information to find trends and solve problems.

Drawing Conclusions From Data

In terms of what these questions test for, it shares a lot with problem solving. You will again be met with chunks of data that examine your ability to deal with large amounts of information and make a reasonable conclusion based on it.

General Tips

I really do feel like I'm beginning to repeat myself, but this section is simple in the sense that you don't have to flip through pages upon pages of textbooks to prepare for it. Factual knowledge is not required at this stage of the test. Instead, you can think of these questions as tasks that are, when you take a step back to observe them, fundamentally easy. However, they are difficult in the sense that they are a set of simple calculations or observations that you must compute in a certain order to end up at the correct answer, for example, picking out relevant values from a vignette, converting them individually into the desired units and putting them into the correct formula. Still sounds relatively trivial, right? Your biggest obstacle won't be the complexity of the questions, but instead the time that you are given to finish them. You should therefore work as methodically as possible.

Some specific things you may want to practice doing quickly include:

- Percentages
- Time differences
- Simple calculations including addition, subtraction, division, multiplication and exponents (practice doing quick calculations with big numbers and decimals)

Cumulatively, being able to plug numbers into a simple calculation can add up to a lot of time saved, possibly enough for you to spend some of that time on more challenging questions.

Often times, you may stare long and hard at a question wondering how on earth you're going to solve it in the given amount of time. Sometimes, the perceived workload of a question may seem like walking from one end of the Great Wall of China and back—too much work. It may be useful though to have an eye for these questions, as there is usually an easier way to solve them with clear, logical thinking. For example, review the following question.

Example

What date is the third Wednesday in June, if May 3rd falls on a Wednesday?

a) June 7th
b) June 14th
c) June 21st
d) June 28th

Run Through

I used to hate these questions because, in my mind, I needed a calendar to count each day, one by one, until I reached the correct date. Stupid, to say the least, because it was a waste of time, when in reality, I could have just eliminated the answers if I bothered to think:

June 7th can be eliminated because 7 days isn't enough to yield even two Wednesdays. June 14th wouldn't be right either, because if we tried to make it the third Wednesday, we would have to make May 31st land on a Wednesday. This contradicts the fact that if we scaled it back, May 3rd would no longer be a Wednesday, and June 14th would only manage to be the second Wednesday at most. Furthermore, there are simply too many days between the first day of the month and June 28th for that date to be the third Wednesday, as 28 days would infer 4 weeks. Twenty-first June is therefore the right answer.

Superficially, some questions may appear easily solvable, and in truth they very well might be. However, don't take your mind for granted—it is not a TI-84 calculator, meaning it is not completely error proof. Once in a while you'll make a careless mistake, and we don't want that to happen here. You're given extra blank mind mapping paper for a reason, so that you can scribble on it. Not only is it a good tool for planning your essay, but also if you're used to doing most problems in your head, it could be beneficial for you to illustrate your thought process. Sure, you could have memorised the equation to calculate the wavelength of electromagnetic radiation, but let's be honest, you're bound to mix up the numbers at least once or twice in your lifetime. In addition, it might help you organise your thoughts into a list logical enough for you to make sense of the question should you be confused.

SECTION 2: SCIENTIFIC KNOWLEDGE AND APPLICATION (27 QUESTIONS, 30 MINUTES)

You will have a little more time per question on this section, around a minute for each one. As the title of this section suggests, you will be required to have general science knowledge, namely physics, biology and chemistry. In addition, there will be some mathematics questions.

Knowing, however, is only half of the picture. As a healthcare provider, there is no use in obtaining specific knowledge you cannot apply to clinical situations. Furthermore, as a medical student, you will find that many topics can overlap. Being able to pick out patterns can help you utilise concepts and principles inferred in one subject and apply them to another.

As per BMAT official specifications, there will generally be more scientific questions (biology, chemistry and physics) than mathematical questions (Table 7.7).

You are expected to draw from previous knowledge of these four subjects, taught in school by the age of 16, i.e. at approximately GCSE/International General Certificate of Secondary Education (IGCSE) level (Table 7.8). Be aware, **they may also touch upon some principles developed though the first year of A-Levels**. However, if you are unsure or worried about what specific topics may come up, it can be useful to look at the appendix of the BMAT specifications document itself, which can be found online. This may serve as a practical guide to touch up on subjects you may have problems with. Obviously, don't just stick to this like a bible. Most students also

Table 7.7 Question Breakdown in Section 2

SUBJECT	QUESTIONS	APPROXIMATE TIME
Biology	6–8	8 minutes
Chemistry	6–8	8 minutes
Physics	6–8	8 minutes
Mathematics	5–7	6 minutes

Table 7.8 Generic Overview of Topics Covered in Each Subject

SUBJECT	TOPICS
Biology	Cells Movement across membranes Cell division and sex determination Inheritance DNA Gene technologies Variation Enzymes Animal physiology Environment
Chemistry	Atomic structure The Periodic Table Chemical reactions and equations Quantitative chemistry Oxidation, reduction and redox Chemical bonding, structure and properties Group chemistry Separation techniques Acids, bases and salts Rates of reaction Energetics Electrolysis Organic chemistry
Physics	Electricity Motion and energy Thermal physics Waves Electromagnetic spectrum Radioactivity
Mathematics	Numbers Algebra Geometry Measures Statistics Probability

find it beneficial to cover topics outside of what the specification expects (which can aid you in obtaining some of the more obscure marks). School textbooks are a perfect place to start.

> Get enough sleep. Your sleep schedule may be completely desynchronised like mine, but if you don't get the adequate amount of sleep that you usually do in a regular day, then it's important that your body acclimatises to a healthy schedule in the days before the exam. Start sleeping earlier and waking earlier if it suits you, and **make sure you get enough hours.**

There's no hugely successful secret strategy to doing well in this section. Since it is all based on facts found in your school textbooks, and I've given a rather comprehensive (hopefully) guide to what can come up, you either know it or you don't. As discussed previously, this section is about both knowing the knowledge and applying that knowledge. What separates excellent candidates from good ones is the ability to use what they know to solve problems with similar themes. Therefore, read...everything.

Other than that, the best tips that I can provide are all on good exam technique, which are essentially the tips from Chapter 3.

SECTION 3: WRITING TASK (30 MINUTES)

Yes, the BMAT will require you to write an essay (insert groan here). Within half an hour, you must select the topic of your choice from a list of three choices. In previous years, you were given four, but from 2017 onwards, you are given one less topic. These topics can be generic, medical or scientific and may ask you to discuss things that are potentially controversial in the realm of medicine, or express your views on some current events. Although mind mapping on scrap paper is permitted, the final essay must be written on the piece of paper given to you. This consists of 30 lines on a piece of A4 paper. **You must not exceed the given limit.**

This section mainly tests your abilities to understand a topic's different aspects and how they may come about. You may deal with contradictions in clinical practice and will be required to consider different sides of arguments, particularly when high-risk patients are involved. Therefore, you must show your ability to write a **cohesive, concise and persuasive argument** for your chosen topic and, more importantly, put those arguments down in written form.

The recommended structure of your essay would hence follow a similar pattern to Fig. 7.17.

It is also important to remember what you've written! This last section of the BMAT may be given to university admission panels to look at, separate from your other BMAT scores in Sections 1 and 2. This means, in the interview, they could bring a copy of your essay, deconstruct it and then question you (i.e. grill you on it). By keeping a note of your written content, you can keep track of or do further research on your topic to prepare for interview. Be certain that you can not only write a persuasive argument but also back yourself up in person. 'Knowledge itself is power.'—Sir Francis Bacon, *Meditationes Sacrae* (1597).

If my genius tells me correctly, then this probably isn't your first time writing an essay. In regards to how to score well in this section, I refer you to the information previously presented in 'the structure of the BMAT' and 'BMAT scoring'. I will elaborate on the mark scheme, preparatory work and mind mapping.

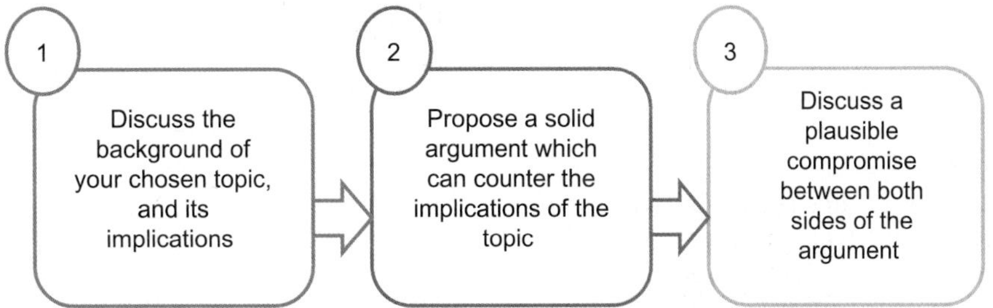

Fig. 7.17 Typical pattern to essay.

Satisfying the Mark Scheme

First and foremost, for any test, it is safe to say that satisfying the mark scheme will get you full, if not high, marks. These tips pertain to both good use of English and good content. Both the mark scheme and the examiners want an 'excellent' answer. What exactly is that?

Your answer must paint a complete picture and, most of all, satisfy all components of the question vignette. If the question asks you to analyse and discuss a quote, and afterwards present an argument that counters it, you need to do all of those things. If even one of these components is missing from your final product, don't expect to score very highly. It is your responsibility to outline all parts of the essay in the mind map and reread it again after writing to ensure you've covered everything.

Your answer must also be organised and presented in a well thought out order. It is easier than you think to fill out 30 lines on paper. If you happen to have any spontaneous epiphanies midway through your paragraph that make you think, 'Actually, that would have fit better in the beginning', you probably should have spent a little more time planning your essay out.

Paragraphing is the easiest way to organise your thoughts, as each individual body of text groups together a bunch of relevant arguments. If the examiner is looking specifically for a particular point they feel is essential to your argument, they can quickly scan through the appropriate paragraph to find it. Don't forget, it is also acceptable to use bullet points to list out information.

Your points must be focused. Whatever you do, do not write a paragraph with arguments that go around in circles or with points that stray too far away from the question stem. Often, explaining a point in unnecessary detail diminishes the argument itself and may allow the reader's mind to wander, especially if the unnecessary detail begins to digress. Practically speaking, it also uses up more space on your paper, so you will have less space to work with when writing the rest of your essay. An essay with an imbalance in the strengths of argument and counterargument can hurt your final score.

A useful skill that can sometimes enhance the quality of your essay is the ability to step into another perspective and present arguments from a different viewpoint. It is even better if you can consider multiple perspectives at a time but, of course, essay length would be a limitation. Going through this process allows you to logically analyse the points from each perspective and decide on a balanced conclusion. Portraying only your perspective can be interpreted as narrow-minded—a very bad impression to give the examiner.

Finally, use proper conventions. The conventions of written English are comprised of mechanics, usage and sentence formation. Mechanics are essentially aspects of English that aren't used in spoken English. This includes capitalisation, punctuation, spelling and paragraphing. Usage refers to components such as word order and verb tenses. This may be especially important in multilingual individuals, where certain languages have rules about word order that don't apply in English. Sentence formation relates to the methodology in using words, phrases or clauses to construct basic or elaborate sentences. For instance, run-on and fragmented sentences should be avoided, and parallelism should be maintained.

> Don't forget to bring your tools. Pens? Pencils? Rubber? Bottle of water? Make a checklist of things that you want to bring on the day. It's all right to forget a bottle of water, provided you don't get very thirsty, but you won't want to be that guy who's asking around, 'Can I borrow a pen?'

It is worth mentioning that some examiners won't actually sit down with a mark scheme to scrutinise every tiny bit that you've got wrong and are actually quite open-minded when it comes to marking essays. Sometimes, all it takes is original ideas being presented well.

Preparations

If I had a magical glass orb that told me what the next set of BMAT essay questions were, trust me, I would gladly tell you… The bad news is that I don't have one. The good(ish) news is that there are plenty of past papers that you can look through online to get an idea of what might come up. It is important to build a good foundation for yourself when it comes to knowing what to write in one of these essays, so doing some regular reading on current events and developments in scientific and medical subjects may benefit you.

However, I would like to stress that **you shouldn't read articles solely for the sake of doing well on the BMAT**. Sure, you can start reading scientific magazines like 'New Scientist' now, then stop right after your exam, but don't forget what you've read. Medicine encourages a passion for science and its endeavours, so having any affinity for reading these articles might well be a predictor for whether you'll find medical school enjoyable on an academic basis.

Essay titles are usually quite philosophical and can be very ethically based:

- Should doctors be allowed to strike?
- Should euthanasia be banned in the UK?
- Should abortion be legal?
- Should we allow doctors to work more hours to cover more patients?

Some titles can be vague or very generic, making them quite open ended. These can be:

- Define empathy.
- What is meant by altruism?
- What is the purpose of science?

Other times, the question is a quote from a book, movie or person.

Being around many opinions at once can nurture a mind capable of good critical analysis. Furthermore, by sharing your personal ideas, you can get a taste of how others perceive the same issue differently. Hence, by reading up such issues, you can form a mind palace containing all these examples to draw from. Access:

- Opinion sections in newspaper articles/magazines, especially those that deal with ethical issues
- Medically related TV programmes (would recommend '24 hours in A&E' on Channel 4)
- Internet forums for debates (Reddit is a great place to start)

The last week/3 days should be for casual studying. You may have done an incredible amount of preparation leading up to the final days before the exam already, so the last thing you want to do is stress yourself out even more by doing hard-core studying. If you're disciplined and stuck to the timetable you made for yourself, you would have done enough studying to do well. The last several days should be just for flipping through your completed past papers, and making a mental note of what you've made mistakes on and what you've done well on.

Planning

Now is the time to actually plan out how you're going to write your essay. For starters, you can save precious time by experimenting with writing short essays about topics with which you feel comfortable. Do this untimed first, then time yourself to see how long you need to plan each paragraph out, and to see how quickly you can write in a given time span. This will prepare you well enough to not tear your hair out on the day.

Table 7.9 Scheduling Time for Written Tasks

STAGE	TIME
Choose question	1–2 minutes
Mind map	7–8 minutes
Writing	15–20 minutes
Proofread	2–3 minutes

With half an hour at your disposal, it might help to make a schedule for yourself (Table 7.9). First, read through all the questions to pick out which one will help you write the best essay. This should take only a minute or two. When writing out your ideas on scrap paper to mind map, you should only write down keywords and phrases in bullet point form that accurately summarise the gist of each paragraph. Write further bullet points underneath the main keyword or phrase to list ideas that expand on the argument you will make. Do not write full sentences at this stage or you will lose out on time. This should take around 10 minutes. The rest of the time should be allocated to writing the full essay. At the end, some dedicated time should be allocated for proofreading for errors.

This can serve as a general outline; you don't have to follow this religiously. Shape it as you like to fit your requirements.

With the adequate preparatory work, you may still end up with a set of questions that you don't feel confident deciding between. That's a truth that can be hard to swallow when you suddenly find yourself flashbacking to all those hours of research boiling down to one moment of sheer anxiety. That's all right, as plenty of other candidates will also be in a similar position. The most important thing is to keep your calm and reason yourself through each question.

Remember that your essay may be taken to your interview by the interview panel of the university to which you applied. Hence, it may be useful to pick an essay topic in which you have an interest. You don't want to write an essay that doesn't reflect any personal curiosity towards a subject. You will make it a lot easier on yourself in the interview when you're asked to talk about it, because naturally you will come across as passionate about what you've written. Being passionate and confident about your area of interest usually leaves a very positive impression on the interviewer.

For some people, it can be hard to think of things to write about on the spot for some topics. Do not fret, as you can think your way around it. If it's an ethical dilemma, then you can think about different perspectives of the general population on that issue. It's important that you also state your perspective, compare them and follow with a logical conclusion to your arguments. If it's a question asking you to discuss relevant current developments, think about the past, present and future. Compare and contrast what there was, is and will be in the near future regarding the development. Don't be afraid to add what you and society have to say about it. If you don't feel optimistic about being able to target every part of the question and discuss each component to a thorough but concise extent, then it may be a good idea to leave it, as your essay will only be able to score a maximum of two points.

This brings me to our next fact. As the BMAT is for both medical and veterinary students, there may be a topic targeting the latter (e.g. questions about animal cruelty). However, each question can be answered well, depending on how one goes about doing so. Medical students can answer veterinary questions, and veterinary students can do medical questions. As long as you can write a compelling argument, you're safe.

Your mind mapping process should not only be a time for creativity, but also a time for organising your thoughts well onto paper (Fig. 7.18). Spider web-structured mind mapping is probably the most standard method.

It is a good method of connecting your thoughts to the main topic as they come in. Use different types of arrows to connect ideas to one another if you have ideas that are relevant. This can help make your essay flow. Alternatively, you may choose to use other methods of mind mapping, but this is my go-to.

After you're done with that, try organising your ideas into bullet point form, with each one under a larger heading that summarises the goal of each paragraph. This gives you a sense of how the essay will flow, and you want it to flow in a logical manner. It also doesn't hurt to give a very brief recap of what is being sought in the question, so you make yourself and the reader more aware of your starting point. For example, if the topic is something about euthanasia, your ideal outline would be as shown in Fig. 7.19.

Your bullet points would go under each heading.

When you finally get around to writing your essay, keep in mind that you aren't permitted much space. Depending on your handwriting, your words might take up either the entire line or a microscopic portion of it. Therefore, try to picture how your essay will physically appear on the lined sheet of paper. You only have one sheet, so brevity is encouraged when it comes to explanations. If you can, try to write a bit smaller than usual; every extra line helps.

As your standard of English will also be assessed, make sure that you understand how to write an argumentative essay. It may be useful to look up online how these are written, as structural composition, keywords and forming a logical conclusion are all important aspects of a good argument. Other types of writing, like descriptive writing, won't help you much in this section. A wide vocabulary may not be accessible to all candidates, but if you do happen to take advantage of yours, it may magnify the power and impact of your arguments greatly.

Make yourself a revision or study timetable. If you already have one for yourself, good on you! If you usually find random free moments throughout the day to do work (like me), then you may find it useful to make yourself a timetable. This allows you to see how many hours you are willing to commit to practicing BMAT questions. Tailor your schedule to your lifestyle and other commitments, and try to do at least 2 to 3 hours each day, 2 or 3 months from the exam. It sounds excessive, but better safe than sorry.

Don't just practice one section for a certain time period. There's a chance you might forget the strategy or skill that you used to answer questions in each section. Instead, do a little bit of each section leading up to the final day.

Do you remember the 20-hour rule discussed at the beginning of this chapter? Apply the same principle to create your own timetable and schedule protected time slots each day for the BMAT.

GOOD LUCK!

May the exams be ever in your favour.

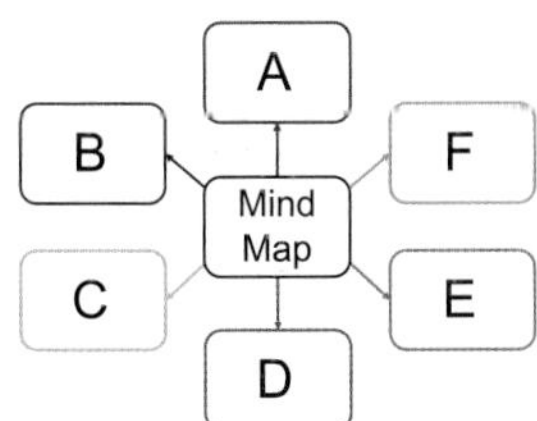

Fig. 7.18 Mind map.

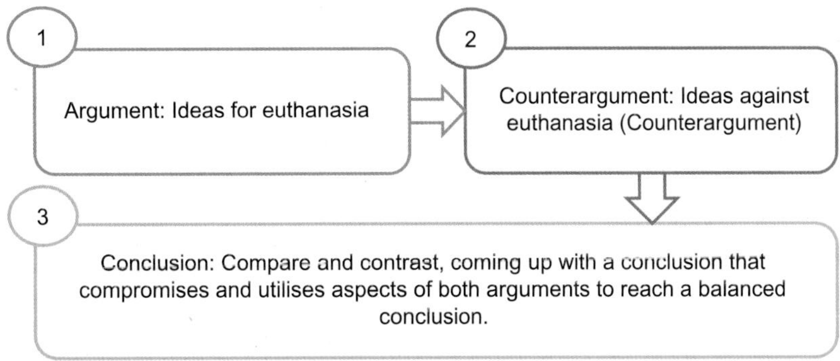

Fig. 7.19 Outline of essay on euthanasia.

SUMMARY, TEST YOURSELF AND REFLECTION

Huh, now that was heavy. Well done for getting through this chapter. All applicants know the entrance exams are the trickiest part of the medical school application process. Oddly enough, with a bit of practice you'll begin to enjoy working for the UCAT and BMAT, as this is one aspect of the application that you are in control of. We also want to remind you that your UCAT score is known as one of the biggest predictors for receiving an interview at medical school and many medical schools have a cut-off score for rejection.

Your Luck Is in Your Own Hands, so Remember To

- Start as early as possible to get used to the format of the questions.
- Practice as much as possible using simulated exam conditions.
- Make a studying schedule and stick to it religiously.

Now that you know what the entrance exams are and how to tackle each of them, we've provided a reflection box for you to jot down any thoughts or ideas that you may have. What steps are you going to take to ensure you ace the UCAT and/or BMAT? What ideas are you going to put in action from this chapter moving forward? What are your weaknesses and what should you improve on?

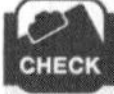

Test Yourself

- Use the online mock tests for UCAT and BMAT to test your current knowledge. Attempt the tests under strict exam conditions and stick to real test timing to ensure accuracy of results. These can be found on the official pages for UCAT and BMAT: http://practice.ucat.ac.uk/ (UCAT) and http://www.admissionstesting.org/for-test-takers/bmat/preparing-for-bmat/practice-papers/ (BMAT).

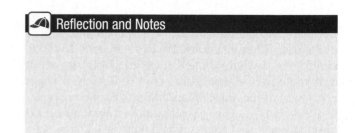

Reflection and Notes

RESOURCES

BMAT. Available at http://www.admissionstesting.org/for-test-takers/bmat.

Cambridge Assessment Admissions Testing. BMAT practice papers. Available at http://www.admissionstesting.org/for-test-takers/bmat/preparing-for-bmat/practice-papers.

Medify. UCAT/BMAT preparation. Available at https://www.medify.co.uk.

Gladwell, M., 2008. Outliers: The Story of Success. Hachette UK.

Kaufman, J., 2013. The First 20 Hours: How to Learn Anything… Fast. Penguin.

Lobdell, M. Study less, study smart. Available at https://www.youtube.com/watch?v=IlU-zDU6aQ0.

Medical Schools Council. Applying to medicine. Available at https://www.medschools.ac.uk/studying-medicine/making-an-application.

The Medic Portal. Free online UCAT questions. Available at https://www.themedicportal.com/e-learning/ucat.

UCAT. https://www.ucat.ac.uk.

UCAT. Practice tests and question banks. Available at http://practice.ucat.ac.uk.

UCAT and BMAT mentoring. Available at https://www.medefine.net/tutoring.

Dissecting the Perfect Medical School Personal Statement

8

Charlotte Stoll, Bogdan Chiva Giurca and Akanksha Subramanian

Chapter Outline

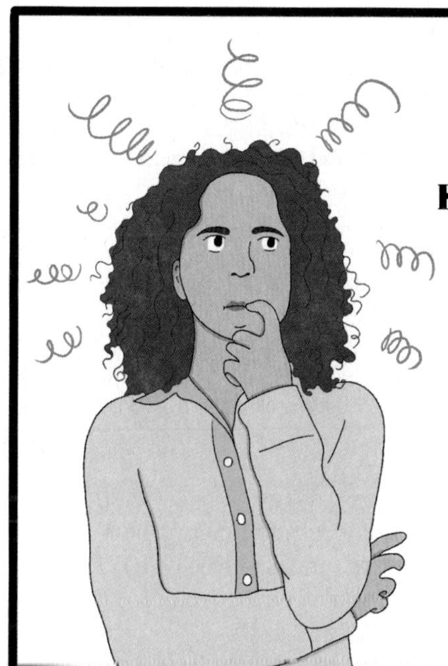

WHEN THE PROFESSOR ASKS HOW I SLEPT BEFORE FINALS...

"GREAT, I GOT A FULL 40 MINUTES!"

INTRODUCING THE PERSONAL STATEMENT

EXPECTED CHANGES TO UK-BASED MEDICAL SCHOOL APPLICATIONS

Over the past few years, there have been several proposals to replace the personal statement section of the application process for UK-based medical school applications. Students and teachers felt that the personal statement offered an opportunity for applicants to promote themselves, but unfortunately favoured students who had access to high-quality advice and family support and, therefore, widening the inequality gap. The latest proposal has been introducing a series of short-answer structured questions.

Given the likely scenario that personal statements will be transformed into short-answer questions, the Universities and Colleges Admissions Service (UCAS) has outlined six areas in particular that such questions will be focusing on. Although these are likely to change and differ from one university to another, we have provided an informative list of likely scenarios in Table 8.1.

Table 8.1 Potential Topics and Questions Replacing the Personal Statement

TOPIC	QUESTION
Motivation for course	Why do you want to study these courses?
Preparedness for course	How has your learning so far helped you to be ready to succeed on these courses?
Preparation through other experiences	What else have you done to help you prepare, and why are these experiences useful?
Extenuating circumstances	Is there anything that the universities and colleges need to know about, to help them put your achievements and experiences so far into context?
Preparedness for study	What have you done to prepare yourself for student life?
Preferred learning styles	Which learning and assessment styles best suit you—how do your course choices match that?

Nevertheless, whether the university you are applying to is using a personal statement or a series of short-answer questions, the following chapter provides key real-life examples and excerpts from successful students of the past. We encourage you to check the latest guidelines and up-to-date entry requirements for each university you are applying to as these can change from one year to another.

Now, let's delve deep into the broader topic, especially as several universities across the world may still decide to use personal statements. To put it simply, the personal statement is a 4000-character (approximately 500-words) essay that should not exceed 47 lines. Yes, it's that specific. Four thousand characters (including spaces!) to cover all your achievements to date, together with your reasons for applying to medical school. As you can clearly gather from the word limit, they are looking for QUALITY, not quantity. As mentioned previously, however, many universities are replacing the personal statement with a series of short-answer questions. We encourage our readers to please check the UCAS and university-specific websites prior to applying.

> Don't think about the word count when you start. In fact, try to ignore it if you can. You will revise your essay at least 20 times before you submit your final draft!

I'm afraid you cannot escape the personal statement (or short-answer questions), as it is a compulsory step of the application process. To highlight its importance, admission tutors often call the personal statement 'your passport for the interview'. Don't blame us; we didn't make the rules, the UCAS did. By the way, if you're not familiar with UCAS yet, this is the perfect time to visit their website and understand how they work (www.ucas.com). UCAS works like a dating app: You apply to universities through their platform, then wait to hear back depending on whether they offer you a place or not. We've decided not to add further information here as everything is self-explanatory and readily available on the UCAS website.

> Research each medical school entry criteria carefully. How much emphasis is put on the personal statement differs significantly between universities. Carefully select the medical school that best fits your criteria. For example, Bristol Medical School and Brighton and Sussex do not use personal statements in their assessment criteria and prioritise the University Clinical Aptitude Test (UCAT) when shortlisting candidates. On the other hand, King's College London takes into consideration the personal statement and Oxford and Leeds' medical schools use the personal statement to form some of the interview questions. It is important that you are aware of the following:
>
> - Do your medical school choices consider the personal statement?
> - Will your personal statement be used to form interview questions?
> - Is your personal statement required to show a specific skill? For example, Leeds Medical School want students to display their enthusiasm and motivation.

A few years ago, I was in the same position as you. I clearly remember my personal statement (or at least, the first and last line of it). This statement might, rightly so, make you cringe; let me take this opportunity to explain myself.

Applying to university is stressful for everyone, and no matter how many times you sing Miley Cyrus's 'The Climb' to yourself, it never seems to start being about the uphill battle as you're forever wondering what's on the other side. This, plus the added elements of the medical application process, can feel like you're hiking a mountain alongside your peers, except you have an obstacle every 100 m and have to reach the top in half the time. You're swamped with exam prep, research essays, extracurricular activities, last-minute coursework, keeping up with your grades (and the Kardashians), entrance exams, more exam prep—now add to this trying to maintain a social life, self-care and spending time with your family. I think I'm forgetting something... oh yes, the application process. At this point in time, the uncertainty that arises from this monstrous pressure makes all of the above disorienting, scary and, quite frankly, seemingly impossible.

Going from a life where you know exactly what subject you have on your timetable at 10 AM 3 months from now—probably dreaded chemistry with Mrs Malini—to not having the slightest idea what you will be doing 3 months after you graduate can be extremely daunting. For the control freaks among us, this uncertainty can feel like the end of the world.

While attempting to fit 17 years of my academic life and personality into the small boxes and tight word limits of tedious application forms, I found myself questioning my value and abilities in a place where more was asked about my grades than myself.

This is where the personal statement (I later found it to be my personal cheerleader) easily got buried under my Everest-sized mountain of work. I'm hoping that by the end of this chapter, you love these 4000 characters the way that I grew to love them and they grew to love me.

How on earth do you fit your whole life on one page, you may ask? In this chapter, we're going to be interactive. So grab a pen (and take a deep breath or two)—it's time to get down to business. Let us take it at our own pace, shall we?

UNDERSTANDING THE PERSONAL STATEMENT

First, it is important to understand the style in which personal statements are written, by various people, for the multitude of courses across the UK. There are several different types of medical school applicants, so the more statements you read, the more you will understand what is expected from you. When you read personal statements, you not only grasp the essential components required and omitted from the 4000 characters, but you also develop a taste for these essays. You notice what you like about someone's essay and what you'd like to see in your own, while you get a feel for things that are distasteful in your opinion.

To help you develop this taste and understand how to write a medical personal statement, we have included personal statement snippets throughout this chapter for you to read and analyse. You will notice that the snippets have been left blank—this is to give you the chance to think about (and annotate if you'd like), your thoughts on the paragraph, e.g. noteworthy likes, dislikes, any changes you would make, etc. Then, on the following page, you will find the same example paragraphs annotated to give you a breakdown of what we think about these successful personal statements. Use a highlighter or a pen and take notes. Be as proactive as you can. The more you put in, the more you get out of it.

DIFFERENT MEDICAL SCHOOLS, DIFFERENT VALUES

Similarly to the differing emphasis that medical schools place on the various components of the application process, they also place varying emphasis on core values and beliefs that they are looking for. It is necessary to be aware of this in order to tailor your personal statement to fit the medical school. This may sound a little confusing, so we have provided some examples in Table 8.2 to help you out.

Table 8.2 UK Medical School Curriculums

CURRICULUM	EXAMPLE	CORE VALUES/BELIEFS
Traditional	Oxford/ Cambridge	Traditional universities tend to prioritise research, critical thinking and academic passion
Integrated	Leeds/Exeter Medical School	Integrated courses combine lecture-based learning and problem-solving-group-work, resulting in an emphasis on both academic pursuit as well as communication skills, empathy, reflection, listening skills, compassion, etc.
Problem/ case-based learning	Manchester Medical School	Although the majority of courses tend to be integrated, there are still medical schools with a primary focus on case-based problem solving and teamwork. These medical schools require communication skills, teamwork, listening skills, empathy, flexibility, adaptability, etc.

When choosing your medical schools, it can be helpful to understand the type of course you want to study (there are online quizzes to help work out which you are best suited to) in order to write a personal statement that fits the core values and beliefs of all your chosen medical schools.

To help you understand this better, we have included examples of how one scenario can be adapted to suit the three different styles of medical schools.

How to Adapt Your Reflection Depending on the University

Now that you understand the core values and beliefs that traditional, integrated and PBL medical schools are looking for, you can begin to consider how this may influence the reflections you include in your personal statement.

Generally speaking, all medical schools will want you to demonstrate academic prowess, commitment to medicine, good interpersonal skills and intrinsic motivation. However, it is the ratio of each of these that makes a difference depending on the type of medical school you're applying to. Take a look at the following examples of how you would adapt one scenario to suit the three course styles (*italics* represent the more academic examples and reflections, while ***bold with italics*** reflects the more interpersonal).

Scenario: You're an aspiring medical student who has taken part in a research project looking at the extent to which young adults are more inclined to seek out alternative forms of stress management than pharmaceutical medicines.

Traditional

To support this research, I extended my interest from A-level Biology on how drugs affect neurotransmitters to a neuroscience MOOC [Massive Open Online Courses], *which taught me the importance of critical thinking to medics. While science suggests drugs cure patients through altering action potentials in postsynaptic neurons, a journal article by Bushnell G.A.* et al. *'Treating Pediatric Anxiety' suggests long-term efficacy of these medications has not been sufficiently studied, raising concern over potential harm. This is a challenge I've been inspired to pursue, prompting me to write a TEDx talk on the less positive side of the pharmaceutical industry. This experience honed my analytical skills, relevant to diagnosing and treating patients appropriately.* ***I have been fortunate enough to witness the application of these skills in a multidisciplinary team meeting, discussing a patient reluctant to have a surgery for a stoma bag. Through collaboration and shared-decision making, a management plan was formulated that balanced the patient's physical and mental health.***

Integrated

To support this research, I extended my interest from A-level biology on how drugs affect neurotransmitters to a neuroscience MOOC, which highlighted the need for continuous scientific advancement and taught me the importance of critical thinking when managing a patient as contradictions such as whether or not depression is linked to serotonin levels exist in all areas of medicine. ***This inspired me to pursue a work experience in a psychology clinic, where I was able to discuss the wide range of treatments available for patients with mental health conditions, such as depression. I truly understood the importance of trusting relationships between healthcare professionals and patients as well as skillful communication skills upon learning that CBT can be more effective than medication.***

Problem-based Learning

To support this research, I extended my interest from A-level biology on how drugs affect neurotransmitters to a neuroscience MOOC, which taught me the importance of intrinsic motivation to a lifelong education. Upon completion of my research and MOOC, ***I presented my findings to my peers and engaged in discussions and debate throughout. This honed my presentation skills and ability to share my thoughts coherently; traits relevant to partaking in multidisciplinary team meetings. I have been fortunate enough to witness an MDT discussing a treatment plan for a young woman with a stoma. Her career as a fashion influencer made her reluctant for surgery, however, through shared-decision making with the patient and other healthcare professionals, the surgeon was able to reach a decision that would protect her physical and mental health, mitigating her concerns. This experience demonstrated the necessity of good communication skills, empathy and viewing patients as people not conditions.***

What Does All This Mean?

From earlier paragraphs, you will notice that they all began from the same scenario of a research project; however, the proportion of the paragraph taken up by academic reflection vs work experience and soft skills reflection differs. In the traditional paragraph, almost all of the links are academic, with a shorter mention of a multidisciplinary team meeting (MDT) at the end. In the integrated paragraph, there is a fairly equal split between academic links and work experience/soft skills. Contrasting the traditional paragraph, the problem-based learning paragraph is primarily focused on work experience and soft skill reflections.

> If you remember one thing, please remember that DIFFERENT medical schools have DIFFERENT values and teaching styles.

At the end of this chapter, we have included five personal statements for you to read. This will help you understand the entire personal statement and evaluate the essay as a whole, while the example snippets included throughout this chapter will give you a sense of appreciation for the individual components of the personal statement.

To help you in your conquest of dissecting these essays, we have created a checklist of questions outlined in Fig. 8.1 that you can go through when reading each personal statement. The checklist is followed up by three reflective questions you should consider for each personal statement.

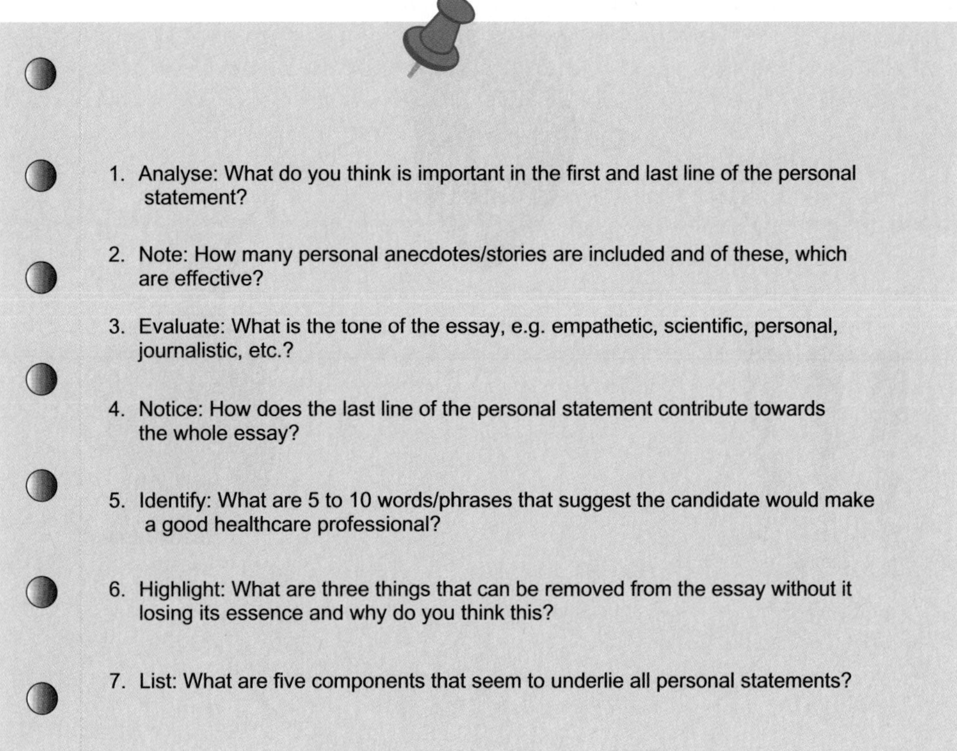

1. Analyse: What do you think is important in the first and last line of the personal statement?
2. Note: How many personal anecdotes/stories are included and of these, which are effective?
3. Evaluate: What is the tone of the essay, e.g. empathetic, scientific, personal, journalistic, etc.?
4. Notice: How does the last line of the personal statement contribute towards the whole essay?
5. Identify: What are 5 to 10 words/phrases that suggest the candidate would make a good healthcare professional?
6. Highlight: What are three things that can be removed from the essay without it losing its essence and why do you think this?
7. List: What are five components that seem to underlie all personal statements?

Fig. 8.1 Seven-point checklist—how to dissect personal statements.

THREE REFLECTIVE QUESTIONS TO ASK YOURSELF

1. What stands out most to **you** in this personal statement?
2. What do **you** least enjoy in this personal statement?
3. What one thing are **you** going to adopt from this personal statement?

THE ANATOMY OF A PERSONAL STATEMENT

Is there one winning formula to structure the perfect personal statement or one specific recipe to produce the most tasteful reflections? In short, no. Think about it, what are formulas and recipes used for? In maths and physics, we use formulas to turn unique numbers into an expected solution. When cooking and baking, we use unique ingredients to produce an expected outcome. The secret to a great personal statement is using unique elements to reach a unique essay that sets you apart from your competition. The admissions team is expecting the unexpected!

There are several structures that you can use; however, most of our successful applicants enjoyed using the human body as an analogy (Fig. 8.2). Welcome to our own autopsy lab. You'll need some scrubs and a scalpel for this one!

The heart: All personal statements begin with a personal story of the 'aha!' moment when you realised, 'You know what? I think I like the idea of medicine'. The heart represents your **why**, your passion and reason for pursuing medicine. This could be when you read a book, saw someone injured, met a nurse—or anything that really got that fire burning in you.

The head: Once you've established your interest, you must evidence your interests with other supporting activities, further backing this personality that you've depicted in your story. The head represents **what** you have done in school and outside it in terms of academic and intellectual pursuits, as well as the relevant clinical work experience relevant to a career in medicine. Therefore, the head can include coming up with a list of experiments to conduct at your chemistry club, winning a biology competition or even a research paper or essay that you have written from scratch as part of your A-Level or IB. It may have been watching the blastocyst dividing at your shadowing experience, which then caused you to take a course on embryology, or it could have been breaking your leg that interested you in the structure of bones and understanding muscular atrophy in the elderly community. It might have been that 4-month general practice placement where you learnt that medicine is a combination of art and science, and soft skills such as communication and empathy are as important as hard facts.

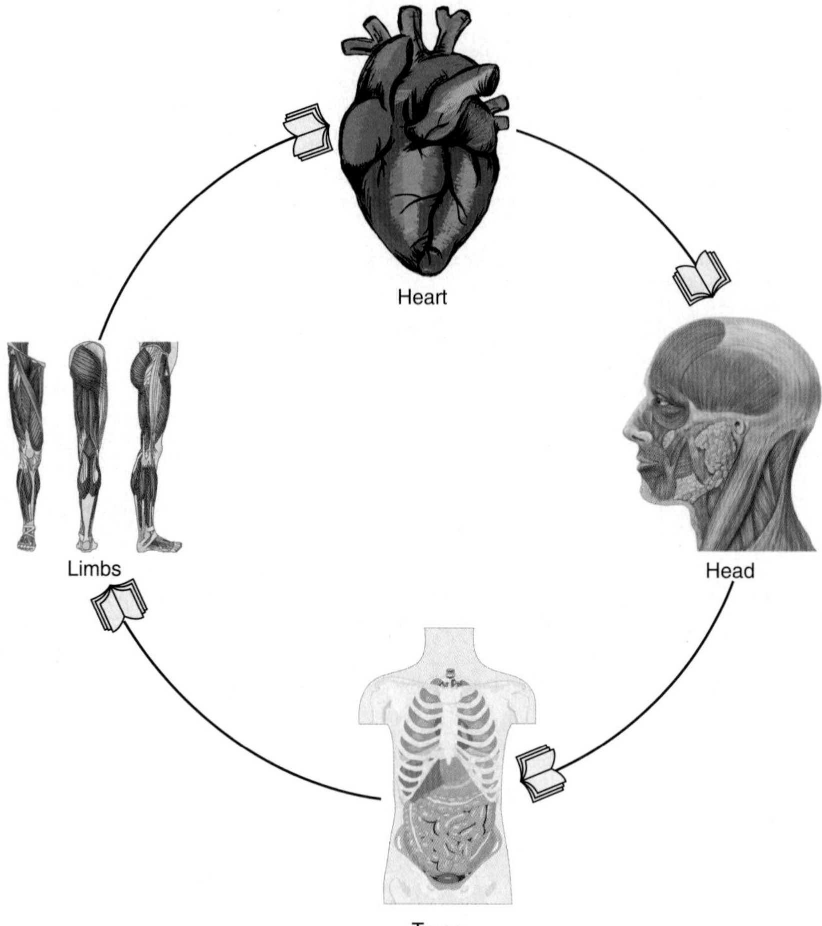

Fig. 8.2 Anatomy of the personal statement.

The torso: This section demonstrates a strong core foundation. You must detail your achievements and involvements, particularly those that make you stand out from the crowd. When you think of the torso, think of extracurricular and voluntary work to spice up your essay. This will give you a different angle, making you stand apart from the rest. For example, if you organised a fun run fundraiser at your school, won a service award for your efforts working with underprivileged children or led a team to reduce energy consumption in your school by a third—these are achievements that remind you how you are unique, with a set of abilities that shows your involvement in your community, as well as your efforts and commitment.

The limbs: This flows smoothly into the next segment—the limbs of the body. These include your hobbies and passions, once again displaying your personality and your life beyond work and academics—a good work–life balance is something that we must achieve to be mentally, physically and emotionally stable. You stand on your legs, just as these hobbies stabilise you and allow you to keep your life in order when things get busy.

Revisiting the heart: This represents the conclusion of your personal statement. This is a short, yet powerful section wrapping everything up, reemphasising the heart (your why) and showing that you are a suitable candidate and future medical student.

In short

The heart

Your passion and reason for doing medicine—the 'why?'

The head

Things you have done in and out of school, e.g. academics, work experience, competitions, etc.—the 'what?'

The torso

Extracurriculars and voluntary experience—the 'wait… you did what? *impressed voice*'

The limbs

Hobbies, passions and personality—demonstrate work–life balance!

> The **start** and **end** of a personal statement form the initial and final thoughts about you in the admission officer's mind, so pay close attention to it!

To explore these components of the personal statement in greater detail, we will delve into each element. In the following sections, you will find excerpts of each element from real personal statements, with both an original copy for you to work on as well as a copy of the same example paragraphs, which have been annotated for you by us. We have also included a few reflection textboxes to act as active reminders and prompts to encourage you to have a go at practising each element of the personal statement at your own pace. Finally, you will find a set of successful personal statement examples that have been left as they were found, without annotations, for you to work on and personally annotate at the very end of the chapter in the appendix.

> Reading these personal statements and annotating them will allow you to identify the differences between a good personal statement and a great personal statement—developing this skill can make the difference between getting into medical school or not. Remember, if you want to satisfy the admission tutors, you need to know what they are looking for and start thinking like them!

THE HEART

The heart of the personal statement is your 'WHY', your passion—the reasoning deep down for your application, your own story behind how you reached this point in your life. This passion I speak of is the dedication that you developed for your subject, which has captivated your heart.

When writing the personal statement and helping others, the majority of students struggle with this part the most. How do you describe a feeling, something that could easily be thought of as a random consequence of several coincidences, as becoming the driving purpose in your life? How do you explain to someone the satisfaction that you get from helping others without sounding the slightest bit clichéd?

The answer is simple—the best way to convey the feeling is to go back to the moment that made you experience it. This is why telling a story is the most effective way to share your thoughts with someone else. It pinpoints a moment so you can better share the emotion and passion that were birthed from that experience. From the very beginning of your essay, you must illustrate this, and what better way to do that than by sharing the story of when you first came to love the subject you have chosen?

Most successful personal statements begin and end with this passion by sharing an experience, telling it as a story of that exact moment of realisation when they knew this was their passion. When going through personal statements, if you have a look at the introduction and conclusions, you will come across a convincing story about why they are dedicated to this subject—and if it's done right, it will convince you too.

This provides a good explanation for why someone is willing to put themselves through the rigours of a course such as medicine. Having passion right at the beginning of your personal statement eases the reader in before you demonstrate the effort and activities in which you have participated. Without evoking this introduction, a list of all your activities can seem quite jarring and purposeless.

We were lucky to receive several lovely personal statements from successful medical students. I've extracted the heart element from these essays, which as a matter of fact were all found directly in the introduction and conclusion. I've left these blank so that you can read it and annotate what you like about it and what you may have done differently yourself.

> Be yourself is the best tip I can give for your personal statement. However, the reason this tip won't work right away is because you have yet to discover who you fully are. For this, you have to think really hard—what is it that made you decide that medicine is your dream career? Take some time and have a 'creative date' with yourself. Get rid of all distractions for 30 minutes and simply ask yourself: What is my story?
>
> **Dr Zeshan Qureshi, Paediatric Registrar**

Excerpts of the *Heart* Component: Nonannotated

Have a go at reading and dissecting this component of the personal statement with a couple of coloured pens.

Example #1

'There and then, I was introduced into the medical world, left the limited and individual laboratory background to contact with doctors and patients, and I understood the importance of the relationship between scientific work and its practical use.'

Example #2

'Yui Kamiji, as well as other wheelchair tennis players suffering from spina bifida, is living proof of the human ambition to overcome difficulties in the attempt to succeed. Stories like hers inspired me to put my empathy, relentlessness and personal experience in the service of those affected by disease. I believe that your medical program will be the perfect means to further develop the necessary skills and fulfil my pledge.'

Example #3

'A woman was wheeled into the emergency ward; she wasn't breathing and her heart was still. Suddenly, the whole ward exploded with activity, as doctors and interns ran forward to save her life. Their composure in this incredibly high-stress environment was remarkable, and each doctor pressed forward and calmly administered the treatment the patient needed. I learned here that there is more to medicine than science; saving a life is more than drugs and surgeries.'

Example #4

'Being the 250th surrogate child born through the agency COTS, I can see the impact that medicine has on individuals and families. These considerations have fuelled my desire to become a doctor and to change others' lives, particularly by specialising in obstetrics and assisted reproduction.'

Next, we annotate two of the four examples to give you an idea as to how we read them.

Excerpts of the *Heart* Component: Annotated

Example #1

There and then, I was introduced into the medical world, left the limited and individual laboratory background to contact with doctors and patients, and I understood the importance of the relationship between scientific work and its practical use.

The use of 'there and then' shows a very specific moment when the applicant realises the importance of what they were doing in the lab.

We can see that they found purpose in the science, through the effect it had on doctors' and patients' lives – we all want a doctor who cares about the person, instead of just seeing them as a disease-ridden laboratory test!

Here, the applicant displays that they are aware of the importance of both human AND scientific sides of medicine, both of which are equally important for good medical practice.

Example #2

Yui Kamiji, as well as other wheelchair tennis players suffering from spina bifida, is living proof of the human ambition to overcome difficulties in the attempt to succeed. Stories like hers inspired me to put my empathy, relentlessness, and personal experience in the service of those affected by disease. I believe that your medical program will be the perfect means to further develop the necessary skills and fulfil my pledge.

By introducing a topic of general relevance, this opening example illustrates the extent to which the applicant understands the significance and implications of the practice of medicine on patients' lives.

Here, they highlight how they have the right attitudes to practice, shaping them to be a good doctor, with a focus on not just the disease but also an interest in the patient's wellbeing. This is the type of doctor that we want for our future, and this applicant demonstrates that very well.

The applicant has not only demonstrated how they have an interest, but also how she wants to further build on that passion by taking the necessary steps. This demonstrates a very strong foundation, conveying right at the beginning that this individual's unique attitude makes them a highly suitable candidate.

? Your turn now. Use a separate sheet of paper to write down your why. What's your unique and original personal story? What made you want to practice medicine in the first place? Simply write it down. It doesn't have to be amazing; it's just a draft! It is important, however, not to cut corners. There's no easy way to get into medical school, you have to go through the motions, so why not give it a go? Brainstorm your thoughts here.

THE HEAD

We all have that moment where we experience a spark, something that can grow into a fire of true passion. For this spark to turn fruitful, one must immerse themselves in the pursuit of that passion. This is what the 'head' entails.

In other words, the head of the personal statement is where you act on your emotions to produce a result. This is where you walk the talk. I like to call this section 'the head' because all our emotions must have some kind of rational foundation. They must have some supporting act to illustrate the sustenance and the value of those emotions by being able to follow through with them.

In simple terms, the **head** usually involves two important aspects:

1. Work experience and clinical placements
2. Academic and intellectual experiences

You choose in what order you focus on the above, depending on what fits best with your first section of the personal statement. For example, if you mention in the heart of your personal statement that you are motivated to explore what medicine entails as a career through work experience, it may be a good place to start with work experience first then.

What can you do to prove your commitment to a lifelong profession? This is where the dreaded work experience comes in. If a student were to attend work experience organised for them just to come out of it with no new learnings or observations, vs a student who after trying numerous times is unable to get experience but commits themselves to volunteering and reading medical literature—who would you think is the more motivated of the two?

Seeing the previous example, I want to take this opportunity to say that it is absolutely fine if you don't get any clinical experience before you join university! This is especially relevant to those unable to get work experience due to COVID-19; for now it is completely okay to reflect on online work experiences. However, universities may be expecting more in-person opportunities (not necessarily clinical) within the next year or two. Most importantly, universities are looking for committed students who make the most of their situation. It is not the resources you are provided with that matter, but the way you utilise a resource and learn from it that admissions officers are looking for. After all, your ability to make the most of all situations will demonstrate the depth of your drive, making you a strong contender. In medical school, all resources will be provided to you. If you are a student who makes the most of what is in *your* hands, you will do well no matter what the availability of the resources, as it is your ability to assess and take the opportunity to learn that matters. This being said, keep knocking on every single door until an opportunity for work experience appears. If I haven't driven this point home enough, we want your attitude to be right, as that is what you're in control of.

In the head of the personal statement, it is good to illustrate the actions that you have taken—your input resulting from your passion will reinforce your desire to study the subject, and you want to convey this desire to the admission officers. Remember, as this is the head, you must show that your focus lies in the medical sciences and healthcare.

In case you're wondering what these actions are, it could be something as simple as picking up a book about oncology, or a weekly shadowing experience at a care home for the elderly. When discussing these commitments, merely describing the experiences is not as valuable as your reflections on them. This is because, as we experience different situations, we may not be able to remember all the details—what is important and valuable is that we are able to pick out the main lessons that we learnt as individuals and see their value in other aspects of our lives and to a career in medicine. Ultimately, communication skills, confidence, listening, etc. are all equally as valuable to a career in medicine as they are to a career in teaching—so, why and how are these skills going to help you to be a better medical student and doctor?

For example, if I were to talk about my work experience in a psychiatric clinic, my observation of a translator being called to support a patient in communicating with the doctor highlighted the importance of breaking down barriers to provide effective communication. This evidenced the value of flexibility and teamwork as the patient, doctor and translator worked together to understand one another and provide an appropriate treatment plan. This allows me to see the value of my background in coaching swimming to people with learning disabilities as I had to be flexible and creative with the methods of communication, e.g. nonverbal/body language, in order to be understood.

If in this way you can pick out the important things in an experience, you can learn by understanding how to apply it to your own life.

I think it's about time that you try your hand at looking through a couple of examples and annotating them, following which I will add my own annotations.

Excerpts of the *Head* Component: Nonannotated

Have a go at reading and dissecting this component of the personal statement with a couple of coloured pens.

Example #1

'Wishing to understand one doctor's daily experience, I did volunteering and doctor shadowing at our local university hospital. This experience definitely strengthened my decision to become a doctor, as it confirmed my belief that helping people overcome diseases is indispensable from being involved in research.'

Example #2

'I chose to take a gap year to enhance my medical knowledge. I am working as a healthcare assistant at BMI Droitwich Spa Hospital where I assist in the provision of quality planned care for patients undergoing an endoscopy procedure. In this role, I have the opportunity to implement my scientific proficiency whilst demonstrating competence, perseverance and teamwork skills in the process. I also come across many emotionally charged situations that call for a calm and composed response.'

Example #3

'Once I decided on studying medicine, I organised work experience for myself by phoning different clinics and hospitals in my hometown, Johor Bahru, and eventually I managed to shadow a few doctors. It was there that I observed the importance of teamwork, where the doctors and nurses worked efficiently and tirelessly to help the patient.'

Example #4

'As a keen feminist, my reading led me to investigate neurosexism, in "Delusions of Gender" by C. Fine and "Living Dolls" by N. Walter. Gender differences supposedly seen in the Corpus Callosum by R Holloway in 1982 became a fascination of mine and the focus of my EPQ, as I delved into the controversy posed by Bishop and Wahlsten surrounding this research. I chose to research the neurological differences in the brain at birth between the genders.'

Excerpts of the *Head* Component: Annotated

Example #2

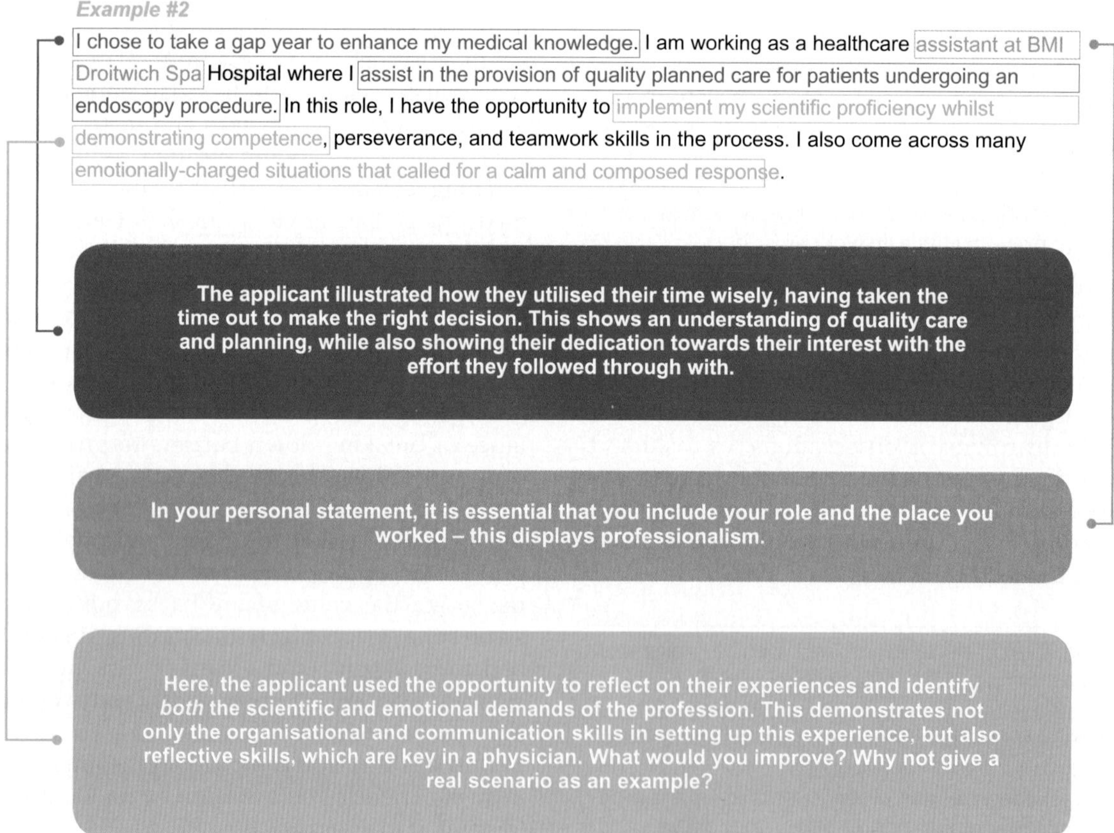

Example #2
I chose to take a gap year to enhance my medical knowledge. I am working as a healthcare assistant at BMI Droitwich Spa Hospital where I assist in the provision of quality planned care for patients undergoing an endoscopy procedure. In this role, I have the opportunity to implement my scientific proficiency whilst demonstrating competence, perseverance, and teamwork skills in the process. I also come across many emotionally-charged situations that called for a calm and composed response.
The applicant illustrated how they utilised their time wisely, having taken the time out to make the right decision. This shows an understanding of quality care and planning, while also showing their dedication towards their interest with the effort they followed through with.
In your personal statement, it is essential that you include your role and the place you worked – this displays professionalism.
Here, the applicant used the opportunity to reflect on their experiences and identify both the scientific and emotional demands of the profession. This demonstrates not only the organisational and communication skills in setting up this experience, but also reflective skills, which are key in a physician. What would you improve? Why not give a real scenario as an example?

Example #4

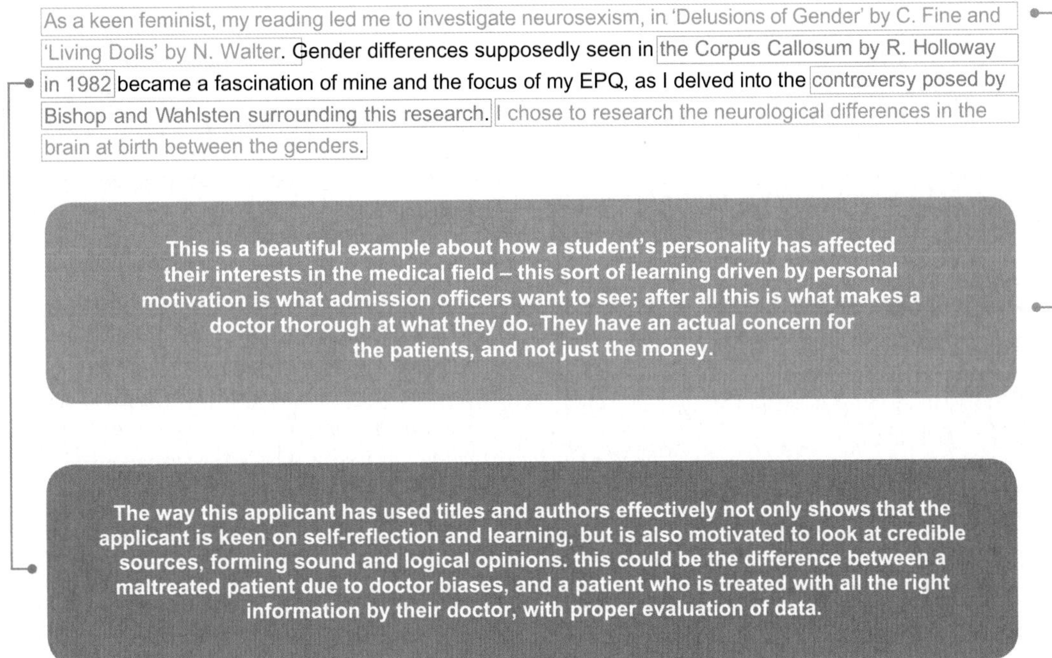

As a keen feminist, my reading led me to investigate neurosexism, in 'Delusions of Gender' by C. Fine and 'Living Dolls' by N. Walter. Gender differences supposedly seen in the Corpus Callosum by R. Holloway in 1982 became a fascination of mine and the focus of my EPQ, as I delved into the controversy posed by Bishop and Wahlsten surrounding this research. I chose to research the neurological differences in the brain at birth between the genders.

This is a beautiful example about how a student's personality has affected their interests in the medical field – this sort of learning driven by personal motivation is what admission officers want to see; after all this is what makes a doctor thorough at what they do. They have an actual concern for the patients, and not just the money.

The way this applicant has used titles and authors effectively not only shows that the applicant is keen on self-reflection and learning, but is also motivated to look at credible sources, forming sound and logical opinions. this could be the difference between a maltreated patient due to doctor biases, and a patient who is treated with all the right information by their doctor, with proper evaluation of data.

? Your turn now. Use a separate sheet of paper to write down your most significant academic achievements as well as work experience placements and encounters. Brainstorm your thoughts here.

THE TORSO

Everyone has something that gives them substance, the so-called 'meat' of the body. This is what they can bring to the table, the things that are ***unique*** to them and the achievements and involvements that describe their ***individual*** personality, which has developed through several extracurricular projects and voluntary jobs. In essence, the torso shows what you as an individual can bring to the field of medicine in terms of personal interests outside academic or shadowing experiences.

But how do you choose what to include? As an individual, I have always been defined both by myself and others, as I am someone who enjoys the act of doing. I saw this as an opportunity, whereby I immersed myself in volunteering for organisations that were close to my passions—this defines me more as a person than anything else that I do. If you are struggling to find what makes you unique, ask a close relative, a friend, a teacher or a tutor. Ask them to describe what sets you apart from others in three words, and see if you agree with them. These descriptive words always align with the majority of the activities in which you take part, and allow you to highlight other traits that make you unique. For instance, working on an organising committee in your school would not only show your interest in contributing to a noble cause, but it would also illustrate your hard-working attitude, your organisation skills and your leadership and communication abilities.

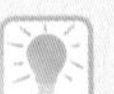

In simple terms, the **Torso** usually involves two important aspects:

1. Voluntary work
2. Other extracurricular activities

Once again, choose wisely in what order you focus on the above depending on what fits best with your previous section about the personal statement. For example, if you talked about developing your teamwork skills as part of your clinical placement in the hospital, it would be a good way to start with 'I have further developed my teamwork skills during a 2-day festival where I worked as a first-aider for St John's Ambulance Charity'.

Need some prompting regarding the various skills that you may have already developed through some of your projects? No problem. Here's a helpful list (Table 8.3). Why not have a think about which ones you've already started building on during your voluntary work and extracurricular activities? Remember, these are key words that stand out to admission tutors. These are, of course, just a couple of the most common examples. This list is endless.

In addition to what makes you unique, you must add into the torso the activities in which you've participated that illustrate the level of effort you've

Table 8.3 **Transferrable Skills List**

TRANSFERRABLE SKILLS
Being punctual
Articulate
Communication
Confidence
Cooperating
Creativity
Critical thinking
Developing rapport
Diplomatic
Able to evaluate
Expressing ideas
Facilitating/coordinating groups
Identifying problems
Imaging alternatives
Interacting effectively with different groups
Listening
Empathetic
Logical
Managing time and stress
Networking
Organising projects
Outgoing
Patience
Paying attention to detail
Perceiving nonverbal messages
Perseverance
Persuasive
Planning ahead
Problem solving
Professionalism
Providing support for others
Resourcefulness

invested in a cause. For instance, if you are an individual who enjoys lab work, creating and organising a chemistry club at your school not only shows your dedication towards subjects that interest you, but also your involvement in bettering your school environment for other students. Describing such efforts make you into a more rounded '3D' person for the admission officers to see.

A common mistake (okay, THE MOST common) many students make is just listing the activities in which they've taken part. For instance, instead of just mentioning that you've run many fundraisers over the weekends and are a part of two organising committees at your school, you must take both of those events and describe how they developed certain skills in you. You must show how you reflected on and learnt from each of these events, developing you into a new person, otherwise it will just sound like a shopping list!

Excerpts of the *Torso* Component: Nonannotated

Example #1

'Mentoring year sevens enhanced my leadership skills as I aided them in their transition from primary to secondary school, helping them with maths, English and enrichments. I formed a bond with younger children and assist them in developing their confidence. This further improved my communication skills, as did my volunteering at a charity shop where I worked alongside the general public.'

Example #2

'I love working as a team member to ensure the safety of others as a voluntary part-time lifeguard. When I react to dangerous situations, I remain calm and act quickly, because I have confidence in both my training and myself. I believe I would act the same way as a doctor. Playing hockey has taught me the importance of playing to each member's strengths to make a successful team. This was mirrored especially in spinal surgery, where I saw a competent team with strong leadership excel in situations where a mistake could have had devastating consequences.'

Example #3

'Last year I had the opportunity to volunteer as a junior counsellor in a month-long international camp run by CISV (Children International Summer Villages) in the Philippines and serve as a young leader in my scout group. Being a role model for younger children, some of whom have disabilities, I further developed commitment and empathy.'

Example #4

'Whilst volunteering at a hospital for neuro-disability over the past year, I not only gained a greater understanding of disorders such as Huntington's disease, but I also learnt the importance of listening to and empathising with the patients. By thinking innovatively, I helped them express themselves through music and art. Similarly, I volunteered at the Whitgift Special Needs Activity Project where I cared for a young person with Mowat-Wilson syndrome. Unable to use conventional methods to interact with him, I improvised through body language and thus learnt to communicate through basic Makaton. Both of these experiences allowed me to develop some of the skills that I witnessed the doctors exhibit and have taught me that communication is key.'

Excerpts of the *Torso* Component: Annotated

Example #2

'I love working as a team member to ensure the safety of others while volunteering as a part-time life-guard. When I react to dangerous situations, I remain calm and act quickly, because I have confidence in both my training and myself. I believe I would act the same way as a doctor. Playing hockey has taught me the Importance of playing to each member's strengths to make a successful team. This was mirrored especially in spinal surgery where I saw a competent team with strong leadership excel in situations where a mistake could have had devastating consequences.'

This excerpt demonstrates rather eloquently the transferrable skills that we can obtain from a variety of different voluntary activities. Here, the applicant's volunteering experience as a lifeguard moulds her skills allowing her to function more effectively in high-pressure situations. She not only highlights this skill, but also skilfully ties it into how it will help her with her medical pursuits.

By drawing a parallel between her extra-curricular involvement in a hockey team and the surgical team she has witnessed, this applicant once again shows how the activities that add depth to her personality also add value towards building her medical career.

Example #4

'Whilst volunteering at a hospital for neuro-disability over the past year, I not only gained a greater understanding of disorders such as Huntington's disease, but I also learnt the importance of listening to and empathising with the patients. By thinking innovatively, I helped them express themselves through music and art. Similarly, I volunteered at the whit gift Special Needs Activity Project where I cared for a young person with Mowat-Wilson syndrome. Unable to use conventional methods to interact with him, I improvised through body language and thus learnt to communicate through basic Makaton. Both of these experiences allowed me to develop some of the skills that I witnessed the doctors exhibit and have taught me that communication is key.'

Make note of the connectors such as 'whilst' and 'similarly' – these can be used to your advantage, allowing for an ease of flow as you move from one thought to another in your PS.

Here, the student shows how one voluntary experience has improved several skillsets and knowledge bases. Most effective and unique, though, is their demonstration of their innovative streak that allows them to think on their feet. Being innovative is a skill that is highly valuable in a field where things are constantly changing, and it is different from the generic list of 'hardworking' and 'effective time management'. they also seamlessly summarised how these experiences honed their communication skills, allowing for one more tick on the checklist!

Your turn now. Use a separate sheet of paper to reflect about the most significant volunteer and extracurricular activities in which you have taken part. What skills have you developed along the way? How did you improve as a person and how will this contribute to you becoming a good medical student and doctor? Brainstorm your thoughts here.

THE LIMBS

Following the torso, this is the penultimate section of your personal statement. This is a completely optional section, but the purpose behind it is to portray you as a complete person. By this I mean to say that the limbs are about conveying your **hobbies**—these are the things that you do to relax and destress. By the way, coping with stress/demonstrating work–life balance is a BIG thing and earns extra marks from admission tutors.

You most likely are wondering why you should waste characters on this. I suggest it because medicine is a very demanding course. There will be moments when you will want to turn to your hobbies—be they running, pottery or taekwondo. By involving yourself in hobbies, you are not only demonstrating your interest and talent in a wide variety of activities, but you are also showing the admission officers that you are capable of handling stressful situations by channelling your energies in appropriate and productive manners.

Once again, just as you did in the torso, you must reflect on your hobbies and not just list them. This will show that you reflect not only on your academic practices, but are also conscious of your daily actions and their consequences on your mental health and wellbeing. As my mother always says, to look after others, one must look after themself. These hobbies show you are invested in yourself, and that is the best sign of a capable medical student—one who is able to look after themselves so as to sustain the rigours of the course that lies ahead of them.

Medicine is all about listening to people, communicating with people, helping them get through difficult times and allowing them to enjoy the good times. If that's something you really enjoy, then medicine is going to be the thing for you, and that's going to shine through your personal statement. Don't be afraid to open up. People want to know what makes you different from other applicants. Yes, everyone loves science and wants to help others, but why are you special?

Dr Carwyn Watkins, Foundation Doctor

Excerpts of the *Limbs* Component: Nonannotated

Example #1

'The importance of language became clear as I saw doctors speaking to patients in their mother tongues. Being fluent in most Indian languages, English and Spanish accentuated my interpersonal skills. Eleven years of Indian classical music has disciplined me to use my time efficiently, doubling as an escape from busy days filled with commitments.'

Example #2

'To relax, I play tennis, sing choir and bake, as the chance to be creative helps me unwind. Having a 1st kup in Taekwondo after 6 years of hard work and dedication, I have learned to keep calm while reacting quickly under pressure. From juggling my school responsibilities with my extracurricular activities, I have also improved my time management skills.'

Example #3

'Studying abroad in the UK for the past 2 years challenged me to thrive on the uncertainty of being away from home, developing my independence, discipline and responsibility. This experience, along with attending an international school, has shaped me into the adaptable person that I am today, at ease with immersing myself with diverse people and cultures. Besides choir, completing the Gold Duke of Edinburgh expedition taught me the importance of interdependence and communication on a team, vital skills for medicine.'

Example #4

'Being a Judoka has required discipline and determination, as training sessions and competitive fights are very strenuous, whilst being a football captain has enhanced my ability to organise and communicate effectively. Gaining the level two sports leadership award, together with my First Aid at Work Qualification, has also improved my ability to make difficult decisions and work confidently as part of a team.'

Excerpts of the *Limbs* Component: Annotated

Example #3

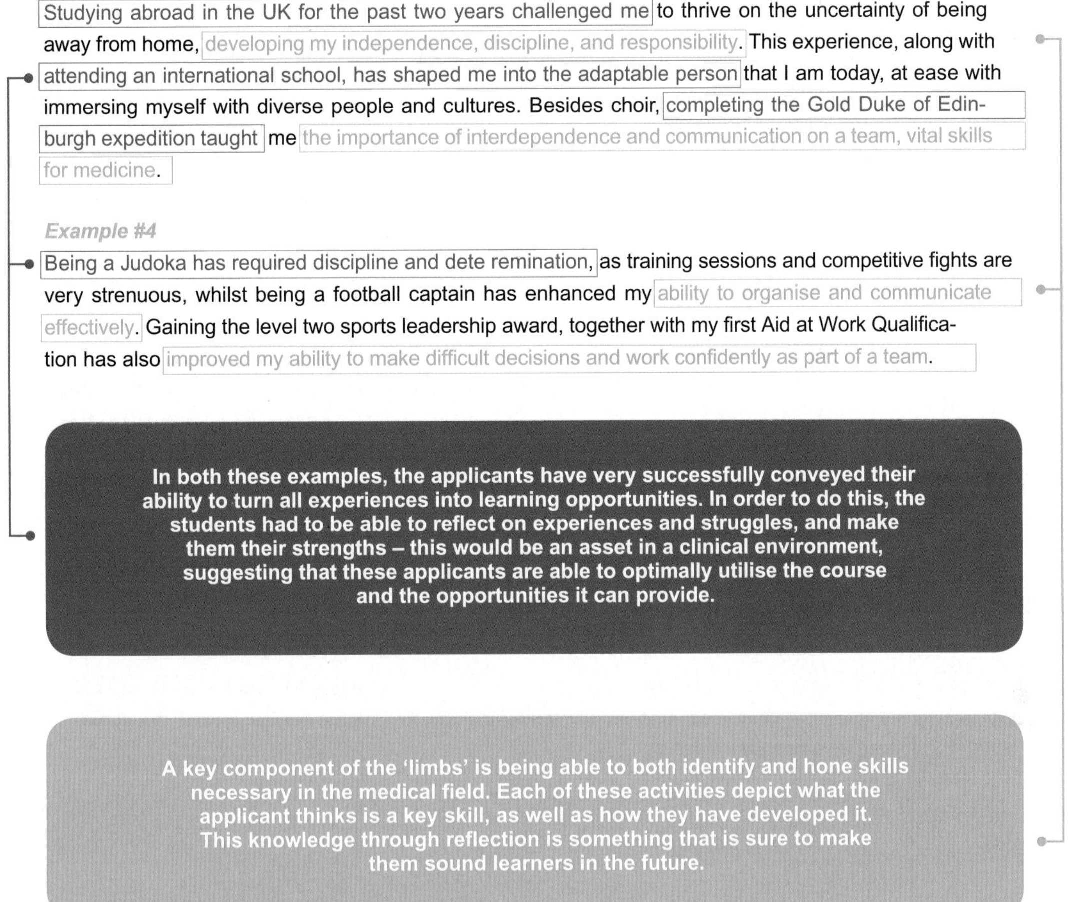
Studying abroad in the UK for the past two years challenged me to thrive on the uncertainty of being away from home, developing my independence, discipline, and responsibility. This experience, along with attending an international school, has shaped me into the adaptable person that I am today, at ease with immersing myself with diverse people and cultures. Besides choir, completing the Gold Duke of Edinburgh expedition taught me the importance of interdependence and communication on a team, vital skills for medicine.
Example #4
Being a Judoka has required discipline and dete remination, as training sessions and competitive fights are very strenuous, whilst being a football captain has enhanced my ability to organise and communicate effectively. Gaining the level two sports leadership award, together with my first Aid at Work Qualification has also improved my ability to make difficult decisions and work confidently as part of a team.
In both these examples, the applicants have very successfully conveyed their ability to turn all experiences into learning opportunities. In order to do this, the students had to be able to reflect on experiences and struggles, and make them their strengths – this would be an asset in a clinical environment, suggesting that these applicants are able to optimally utilise the course and the opportunities it can provide.
A key component of the 'limbs' is being able to both identify and hone skills necessary in the medical field. Each of these activities depict what the applicant thinks is a key skill, as well as how they have developed it. This knowledge through reflection is something that is sure to make them sound learners in the future.

Your turn now. Use a separate sheet of paper to write down your hobbies and other stress-coping strategies. What transferrable skills have you gained from taking part in these activities? Brainstorm your thoughts here.

REVISITING THE HEART

As you would have noticed on your journey through this book and your own personal statement, there is an extensive amount of reflection, both on yourself and your skills. When you reach the end, you might find that you struggle to bring closure to the personal statement. This results in a rather jarring conclusion abruptly trailing off the page. This section of the personal statement can be short but powerful. Here you are giving the course a personal meaning, a meaning no one else can create other than you.

Once we finish mentioning our attributes, personality, skills, achievements and the whole shebang, we need to end on a genuine note. This is one of the most crucial steps, but it is most often neglected by students, leaving the admissions officers wondering, 'Why did you tell me all of this about yourself?'

The conclusion of the personal statement should do justice to your vision of the future and your idea of studying medicine. This is where we loop back to where we started. It should relay back to the initial passion that you conveyed at the start of the personal statement, and demonstrate more dedication than a simple infatuation now that you have backed up your interests with examples.

If you're wondering what I am on about, just answer this question in a sentence or two: Why have you spent an entire 2 to 4 months writing this essay describing all your activities? Because of that vision you have, because of the curiosity medicine has provoked in you, because of your idea of finding fulfilment and purpose through a vocational career such as this? Find an answer for yourself, keep it simple and it will inspire.

All in all, the last couple of sentences impart an important lasting impression—this can sometimes be the deciding factor, as it is key in communicating your conviction to study medicine.

By now, we all know how this works. So it's time to get cracking on another few examples of great and varied personal statement excerpts before you can read what we have to say about them.

> First and final impressions matter most—be it in a personal statement or an interview, people tend to be biased towards the first and final encounter. For this reason, pay special attention to how your personal statement begins and ends.

Excerpts of the *Concluding Heart* Component: Nonannotated

Example #1

'For me to be a doctor is to be an individual who continuously studies to discover new things, carries out research and uses the outcome for people and lives among people assuming social responsibilities. My own purpose as a future doctor is to heal those in need by finding new solutions in combating diseases.'

Example #2

'Not achieving the grades required for medicine the first time round was a devastating setback, but having reconciled with myself, I embraced the task of retaking biology, and my determination has not diminished. By working as a healthcare assistant, I hope to further my development and equip for the future.'

Example #3

'I know that doctors are faced with new hurdles every day, but from my experience I conclude that a sound medical grounding and strength in clinical expertise are the cornerstones of informed practice. This challenge and satisfaction of being a doctor is what inspires me to pursue a medical career, a decision I have carefully and strategically thought through.'

Example #4

'Becoming a doctor requires allegiance and investment of time, and as a science student it is the progressive nature of medicine that draws me to it. The immense satisfaction from this vocation is what I long for, and I know that I have the inquiring mind, dedication and empathy to be a good doctor.'

Excerpts of the *Concluding Heart* Component: Annotated

Example #2

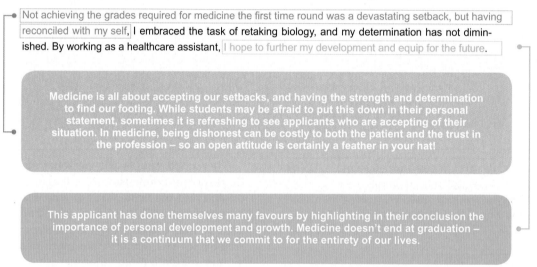

Not achieving the grades required for medicine the first time round was a devastating setback, but having reconciled with my self, I embraced the task of retaking biology, and my determination has not diminished. By working as a healthcare assistant, I hope to further my development and equip for the future.

Medicine is all about accepting our setbacks, and having the strength and determination to find our footing. While students may be afraid to put this down in their personal statement, sometimes it is refreshing to see applicants who are accepting of their situation. In medicine, being dishonest can be costly to both the patient and the trust in the profession – so an open attitude is certainly a feather in your hat!

This applicant has done themselves many favours by highlighting in their conclusion the importance of personal development and growth. Medicine doesn't end at graduation – it is a continuum that we commit to for the entirety of our lives.

Example #4

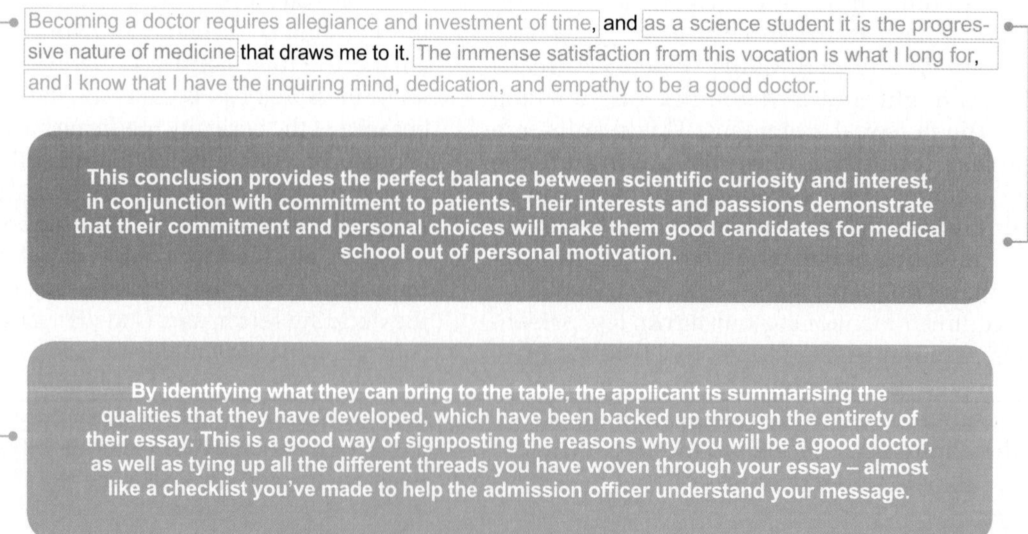

Becoming a doctor requires allegiance and investment of time, and as a science student it is the progressive nature of medicine that draws me to it. The immense satisfaction from this vocation is what I long for, and I know that I have the inquiring mind, dedication, and empathy to be a good doctor.
This conclusion provides the perfect balance between scientific curiosity and interest, in conjunction with commitment to patients. Their interests and passions demonstrate that their commitment and personal choices will make them good candidates for medical school out of personal motivation.
By identifying what they can bring to the table, the applicant is summarising the qualities that they have developed, which have been backed up through the entirety of their essay. This is a good way of signposting the reasons why you will be a good doctor, as well as tying up all the different threads you have woven through your essay – almost like a checklist you've made to help the admission officer understand your message.

Your turn now. Use a separate sheet of paper to remind us why you're interested in medicine and what makes you a suitable candidate, medical student and future doctor. Brainstorm your thoughts here.

REVIEWING AND REFINING YOUR PERSONAL STATEMENT

Just before you think you are done—we are not quite at the end of this journey. I hope you haven't decided to shut your books and submit your personal statements just yet! The review is by far what will help you submit your best personal statement—so you MUST continuously review your essay. In this section of the book, I would like to share with you some tips to make it easier to find the so-called 'red flags' in your personal statement that can put off the admissions office.

Most of the review is just using common sense—so even if you read through it casually, like reading through a newspaper article, you should be able to spot anything odd and change anything that jumps out at you. If you find that you're unable to do so after reading your own personal statement several times over, get someone else to read it. I would highly recommend you do so—after spending so much time on it, the personal statement becomes like your own child and you tend to protect it fiercely. By asking someone else to read it, you may find that in addition to providing you with a new perspective, they might also be able to critique parts of the personal statement that you are emotionally attached to (yeah, it happens to all of us!). Keep in mind that people will have different opinions on the good and bad parts of your personal statement, so be prepared for contradictions as it is a very subjective matter. The most important thing is to have a range of advice and views to help you to understand how the admissions tutors may or may not interpret something—this will help you to adapt the personal statement accordingly. However, ensure that you are happy with what you are submitting because as amazing as advice is, it is still important that you remain genuine throughout.

Check for repetitive vocabulary, and errors in grammar and spelling. Ensure there aren't any acronyms, and that all organisations' names are spelt out clearly and in capitals. Avoid mentioning specific patient names—it is a good time to start getting used to the idea of patient confidentiality. If you are naming books and articles, ensure you mention the author(s) names. Importantly, ensure that the word limit is not breached. In personal statements, there is a *character* limit of 4000, including spaces and punctuation. Make sure you don't go over this limit, as the system will not allow you to enter more characters. The number of lines is equally important as if the personal statement goes beyond 47 lines, UCAS will not accept it. Therefore, you may need to cut down by a few words in order to fit the line count (make sure you check this before the day you plan to submit!).

Asking another person to read it also helps cut out superfluous sentences and makes your personal statement more concise. I remember in my personal statement, I had a very wordy introduction that I loved, but after having my family read it and hearing everyone's opinion, I very begrudgingly removed it. It saved me a good 70 characters though, and I no longer had to struggle with the personal statement being over the limit, just by letting my family and friends guide me through a different perspective.

Read it over and over again, underline it, read it out loud, get someone else to read it, read it out to your parents or siblings, email it to your tutors. The more you review it, the better it will flow and the stronger your personal statement will be. Just reading it every day for a week will take your personal statement a long way! If there is one thing you take away from this book, it should be to go through your essay to do it full justice.

Something we must always keep in mind when writing the personal statement is that we should refrain from listing. Everything that we put down to fill those 4000 characters must remain engaging to the officer and should add value, because the last thing you want is for them to be put off before giving your whole personal statement a chance!

Avoid small grammatical mistakes that can be off-putting by proofreading and spell checking the essay before submission. A good way to do this is to read it out loud to yourself, or by asking a friend or family member to read it. Remember, the key here is to sell yourself, and the best way you can help yourself is by making your personal statement as engaging as possible throughout.

These small changes can make your personal statement seem a lot more slick and professional.

As the old adage goes, practice makes perfect!

THE UCAS REFERENCE: YOUR RECOMMENDATION LETTER

A recommendation letter?! As if the personal statement wasn't stressful enough. While your personal statement makes up the majority of your application, there are other seemingly menial tasks that are of prime importance in giving you that edge in the application process.

Although not as important as your personal statement, a compulsory step of the UCAS application process is to provide a reference. Essentially, the reference is written by someone who's had the opportunity to know you well enough over the years (most likely a teacher or academic tutor), and its purpose is to present to the reader an account of your suitability and motivation to study medicine in the future.

Important to note is that family, friends, relatives and obviously yourself are not allowed to write this reference letter. A common mistake is to think that it is better to get a reference from a doctor rather than a teacher. Just because you've shadowed someone for 1, 2 or even 9 months, it doesn't mean they got to know you. The person who knows you best is the person who observes your behaviour and interacts with you on a daily and weekly basis (i.e. your biology/science teacher/form tutor).

> Your reference is a chance to add in further details that you missed out in your personal statement, which is why you should provide a copy of your final draft along with a 'brag sheet' that contains everything you have done to whoever is writing your reference. I would advise colour coding your brag sheet with different colours for: included in the personal statement, not included (would like to include), not included (not as crucial), not included (will use in interview).
>
> **Dr Zeshan Qureshi, Paediatric Registrar**

Having a great reference that may share some enthusiasm among admission tutors is key. This is why you need to do your best to get a great reference, and not just any reference!

Some final tips:

- Find out early who it is that may write your reference (sometimes schools assign teachers to certain students—if you have someone specific in mind, don't be afraid to reach out and ask them to write your reference. The earlier you ask, the more likely they will be willing to help you out).
- Be proactive and enthusiastic about showing your knowledge during classes (not only where your referee is present, as most teachers talk between themselves and know who the brilliant students are anyway!).
- Schedule a meeting with your referee so you can express your desire and enthusiasm to study medicine at university.
- During the meeting, use your 'Getting into medical school portfolio' to make your teacher's work easier. Using evidence from your portfolio, demonstrate the various volunteer activities that you've been part of, as well as the work experience that you have had so far.
- Give your referee a copy of your personal statement. You may also want to develop your personal statement with them, allowing them to see its growth.

> If there are any activities or mentionable items that you had to exclude from the personal statement, the reference is a great place where you can get your tutor (or reference provider) to add these in!
>
> **Dr Zeshan Qureshi, Paediatric Registrar**

In conclusion, it is very important to build a good rapport and relationship with your referee. You want them to write a recommendation letter that is PERSONAL to you. If they don't get to know what you've been involved in, if you don't show them your portfolio and what you've been up to, how on earth are they supposed to feel motivated to help you get into medical school?

> Our school has a system where each student is assigned a tutor who looks after them over the years. This tutor is also in charge of providing references. Once I found out who they were, I met them to discuss my desire to pursue medicine. They appreciated my enthusiasm. This made me study harder as well as try to be more proactive during lessons. Before the summer term, I met my tutor again and took them through my portfolio of achievements. Not only did I build a great friendship with a tutor that I am still in touch with, but I also received an amazing reference.
>
> **Martin, Medical School Applicant**

The truth is teachers often have a reference letter template that they use for every student. They use the same template for everyone, but the more proactive a student is, the more they get to know a student, the more changes they make to that template and the more personal it becomes. If you tell them who you really are, they will tailor that template to your specific needs and admission tutors will be impressed by it.

EXAMPLE PERSONAL STATEMENTS

As promised, here you have five successful examples followed by six university-specific examples that you can analyse and critique by going through the checklist provided in the beginning of this chapter. We usually recommend not looking at these until you have an idea of what you want to include in your personal statement, mainly because they may simply bias you in one direction or another. As mentioned previously, there is no right or wrong answer. You just need to find the style that suits you best. Happy writing and good luck!

EXAMPLE #1

My interest in medicine originated from watching how my Grandmother who suffered with Alzheimer's disease was treated. I saw the impact the disease had both on the patient and my family. The role of her doctor was key in early diagnosis and treatment, delaying the progress of the disease and giving her valuable time with us.

For 2 years I have volunteered on a dementia ward feeding patients and undertaking ward duties. I have learnt the importance of seeing beyond the medical condition and caring for the emotional needs of the patient. Each week I sit with patients, listen to them and reassure them when they become confused. I have learnt the value of giving time and making every patient feel important. Volunteering at a hospice has shown me that they provide more than just palliative care. I observed the staff giving support to families as well as patients, and was able to emulate their compassionate approach when talking to relatives.

I have also volunteered for the last 4 years with a charity for teenagers with learning disabilities. The initial challenge was learning to communicate using a nonverbal method. The importance of good communication skills became apparent when shadowing an orthopaedic consultant treating a patient with special needs. He treated her with dignity and respect explaining the procedure simply, using her teddy as the go-between. I was impressed with his ability to adapt easily to the needs of the patient. My interest in autism has grown and I am undertaking an EPQ on Autism. I enjoy extending my knowledge and am looking forward to the life-long learning involved in the ever-changing medical field.

To affirm my decision, I have shadowed doctors in different specialisms. While observing a hip replacement, I was impressed by the level of teamwork between the surgeon, scrub nurses and anaesthetist who were all working together for the good of the patient. During an assessment in a clinic, I witnessed a play specialist and a nurse working together to prepare a distressed child for surgery. This made me realise the importance of multidisciplinary teams in all parts of medicine. At a GP surgery I was surprised at the variety of medical conditions handled and the knowledge required. The doctors I observed exhibited professionalism and a commitment to quality care with all patients despite time constraints.

Since July I have demonstrated my ability to work independently as well as alongside colleagues in my job as a Care Assistant. I deal with a wide variety of clients of varying backgrounds each with a story to tell. This has opened my eyes to the idea of patient-centred care, the role of community healthcare and the importance of encouraging healthy lifestyles.

Outside my studies I am a member of the Peer Support team at school and was part of a group running a mental health awareness week as well as discussion groups. I am a highly accomplished oboist, clarinettist and pianist. I am a member of a Philharmonic Youth Orchestra, the school Chamber Orchestra, Big Band and Choir. As Music Captain, I was chosen to run a weekly group at the Junior School which has developed my leadership skills. In the House Music competition I led a group of 40 pupils of varying musical abilities to produce four pieces of music. It was demanding but very enjoyable and gave us all a sense of achievement. I am a keen sportswoman and have represented my school in hockey, netball, swimming and cross-country. Pursuing my interest in sport and music allows me to relax and with careful time management work more effectively on my studies.

During my school career I have thoroughly enjoyed the intellectual challenge of solving scientific questions. A career as a doctor combines my interest in science with my desire to improve the health and wellbeing of each and every patient. I realise medicine is a demanding career and believe I have the enthusiasm, determination and commitment to pursue this course.

EXAMPLE #2

Watching the doctors rush around an obstetrics ward in rural Uganda to observing cardiothoracic surgeons operating in England are two of my most memorable experiences in medicine. They allowed me to appreciate one of the fundamental roles of a doctor: providing the best medical care available to every individual throughout every stage of their treatment. The level of professionalism and empathy I saw confirmed my already deep interest in medicine and I explored this by organising clinical experiences, voluntary work and taking up further reading in medical literature.

Over the past 2 years, I have organised four work experiences including in a general practice to further understand the patient–doctor relationship and in a cardiothoracic ward to observe clinical skills, such as the intricate communication skills required to be a doctor. In the general practice, the sensitivity with which the doctor conducted consultations made patients feel respected, cared for and allowed me to understand their struggles. Alongside this, the doctor used a range of social determinants and the biopsychosocial model to look at patients holistically, ensuring that appropriate treatment was given. Similar themes of trust and understanding were highlighted when I met an anxious 64-year-old patient due to undergo bypass surgery who was reassured by the surgical team. Talking to similar patients made me realise the importance of a doctor's role as a professional in building public trust in the medical profession. This level of trust and communication allows for the active involvement of patients in shared decision making, leading to a more holistic form of health management.

I attended a Social Prescribing conference held at the Royal Society of Medicine which emphasised the pivotal role personalised care plays in lowering dependence on pharmaceutical medicine, a major facet in the NHS's long-term plan. I learnt about the importance of preventative medicine and furthered this interest by taking part in providing personalised care at a charity centre. I also became interested in clinical research and was prompted to read the Neurological Disorders report by the WHO, on which I wrote a literature review. I focused on reducing incidence and mortality rates from stroke in developing countries, discussing potential solutions. The abstract was published on an international medical website and I presented my findings to an audience. This experience helped me to develop an understanding of the crucial role clinical research plays in providing evidence to develop drugs and treatments to improve patient outcomes.

My desire to fulfil my moral responsibility in driving meaningful changes in the lives of others led me to volunteer on a weekly basis at a stroke rehabilitation unit for 1 year. My role there as a student volunteer allowed me to provide companionship in the form of conversation by talking to patients suffering from varying symptoms of stroke. Although difficult to communicate at times, especially with aphasic patients, it was an extremely rewarding experience, and talking to them helped me develop nonverbal and verbal communication skills. A 50-year-old stroke patient with Wernicke's aphasia I met told me about his condition and his struggles with regaining his speech. While seeking to maintain the level of empathy I saw doctors previously demonstrate, I listened and tried to connect with him. These weekly visits taught me to recognise the importance of respect when approaching vulnerable patients and the need for compassion in the medical profession.

A persistent theme throughout my time at the stroke unit was empathy. Providing companionship during one of life's difficult moments, I realised, is what fulfils my moral desire and one which affirmed my decision to become a doctor. I have no doubt that this career, despite it being a lifelong endeavour, will provide me with the greatest possible emotional and intellectual fulfilment.

EXAMPLE #3

'Medicine is a science of uncertainty and an art of probability'—Osler. The study of something as unpredictable yet precise as the human body stimulates my intellectual curiosity and I wish to explore diseases associated with it more deeply. The privilege of learning every day, while combining scientific knowledge and clinical skills to address an issue such as a bleed in the brain, makes me want to pursue a career in medicine.

Since August 2013 I have volunteered every week at a care home, providing assistance with lunch service and talking to the residents about their lives. This experience has been incredibly valuable, as it has highlighted for me the need to treat people with patience both emotionally and physically, and that there can be a more challenging aspect of medicine. Seeing patients' conditions declining over visits and empathising with them as they go through end-of-life care has shown me that being a physician can be emotionally draining, and has underlined that resilience and grit are needed to succeed in such a tough and demanding profession.

Last December I travelled to India to volunteer at an eye hospital and orphanage by helping with tasks such as cooking and cleaning. Through hosting a Bollywood night, charity dinner, numerous cake sales and more, I raised £2600 for four operations and essential classroom equipment. Planning for these events and keeping up with my workload from school tested my organisational and decision-making skills and proved I have the drive to work to the same capacity as the doctors, even when coping with paperwork as well as patient care.

While in India I also managed to shadow the hospital director, a privilege that gave me insight into a doctor's responsibilities and how the multi-disciplinary team is managed. During an outreach camp with the hospital staff, I met a lady who had cataracts in both eyes and facial palsy. We spoke in the local language and as I followed her treatment throughout the next week at the hospital she explained the problems she had in her daily life. Seeing the joy on her face as the dressings came off was one of the most eye-opening experiences, and aside from helping me develop my communication skills, it introduced me to a clinical environment where I observed the defective lens being removed and an intraocular lens being inserted in its place. While I was shown the trust, gratitude and respect in a patient–doctor relationship, I was also able to understand how the healthcare systems differ in countries. This experience prompted me to conduct further research, and I presented my findings on methods of operation and different types of cataracts at the school's medical society.

As of February I worked part-time as a cashier in a theme park, where within a month of employment I was promoted to team leader based on my customer service and selling skills. At the end of the year I got an award for being the company's top seller. Since 2011 I have been an avid member of the school's Combined Cadet Force, attending annual camps and weekly training, both involving treks and tasks requiring a great amount of perseverance. As a senior member I hold the rank of sergeant and therefore have many responsibilities, such as maintaining the welfare and discipline of the younger cadets, while also ensuring they follow my orders. Apart from improving my social skills, the CCF and my job have given me the chance to lead and be part of a team, and have shown me what it is like to work under pressure.

I realise being a doctor is not just a job; it is a lifestyle combining knowledge, skill and commitment. I feel I have developed these qualities through my work experience and am determined to channel my academic ability in science and growing interest for the human body into a vocation as fulfilling as medicine.

EXAMPLE #4

I am interested in understanding the body on a molecular level. Organic chemistry has captured my imagination as it represents the fundamentals of all life. I want to study medicine because exergonic reactions fuel my cells, ligand substitutions keep oxygen moving towards my tissues and condensation reactions build my body. As a result I appreciate the delicacy of the human form and endeavour to treat its vulnerabilities.

When reading 'Mapping the Mind' by Carter, I was struck by the description of agnosia in dementia patients, portraying the harrowingly isolated place many patients must find themselves. This led me to continue my research into dementia, and as a result helped me understand the need to build up relationships with patients I cared for at a nursing home when volunteering in 2014/15. My interest in Lewy body dementia informed how I was able to help patients in distress. After reading McKeith's paper 'Dementia with Lewy bodies', about the neurological characteristics of the abnormally phosphorylated neurofilament proteins seen in the paralimbic cortex, I realised the probable connection between the emotions of the limbic system and the disease. A mental health nurse informed me that rather than denying the reality, it is better to enter into their reality. This was useful for advice when aiding a resident suffering from delusions of abandoned children and so relieved her clear suffering, which brought home to me just how important empathy is when alleviating distress.

I am also interested in the neurological differences seen in Asperger's syndrome and autism, something that encouraged me to read 'The Reason I Jump' by N. Higashida. This informed my approach when helping children at a respite summer camp (2013 & 2015). Overcoming the challenge of poor communication, I saw justification for the research demonstrating high-functioning autistic children show little activity when imitating emotional expressions in the frontal area critical for emotional processing. This experience aided my support of SEN pupils in my role as a volunteer teaching aid. As a keen feminist, my reading also led me to investigate neurosexism, in 'Delusions of Gender' by C. Fine and 'Living Dolls' by N. Walter. Gender differences supposedly seen in the 'Corpus Callosum' by R. Holloway in 1982 became a fascination of mine and the focus of my EPQ, as I delved into the controversy posed by Bishop and Wahlsten surrounding this research. I chose to research the neurological differences in the brain at birth between the genders. 'The Extended Phenotype' by Dawkins helped me hone in on genetic differences between genders, yet opened my eyes to a new way of seeing the ostensible myth of genetic determinism, and this became a further puzzle to me as I read the work of Simon Baron-Cohen to grapple with the conundrum of gender differences.

My 4-week placement on Broadwater Ward, Worthing Hospital, allowed me to explore not only the anatomical intricacy of the human body through analysing bloods, taking X-rays and joining ward rounds, but I also appreciate the compassion, patience and importance of every role in a clinical environment, from the housekeeping team to the consultants, furthering my wish to be a part of that team. I became fascinated with blood as I helped a doctor analyse the blood of an oncology patient suffering from potential septicaemia. When identifying electrolytes in the sample, I got to see how these affected the body.

While learning from a speech and language therapist during my work experience at Worthing Hospital, I realised the physical complexity of a process as simple as swallowing. This opened my mind to the plethora of procedures our bodies must complete every day. My journey to understand the human body, disease and treatments has just begun, and studying medicine at university would provide me with the opportunity to continue this journey.

EXAMPLE #5

A man's choices are influenced by his environment. Witnessing a child's physical and emotional state improve while helping dentists in India was the defining moment when I decided I want to practice medicine. Having an 8-year-old girl I helped treat say, 'I can eat ice cream now and it doesn't hurt' evoked in me satisfaction and the desire to improve the quality of people's lives by removing their pain and suffering. Although the Cartesian theory has defined western medicine as only physical by describing man with distinct mental and physical elements, I believe health entails psychological and social wellbeing too. Candace Pert's book 'Molecules of Emotion' informed me of the science behind emotions, explaining the biochemistry behind opiate receptors and reiterating the importance of emotional welfare in health. My passion for medicine was furthered at weekly art service. Slow but clear improvements in the concentration and motor skills of mentally challenged students made me aware of neurology and art therapy. It highlighted the importance of patience, which I began incorporating in daily interactions. My fascination with the brain's function influenced my service choices, such as with the Institute of Mental Health, showing me the slow onset of mental illness. I noticed how small talk between doctors and patients instantly boosted the latter's spirits, as they felt important and cared for; this taught me the importance of communication regardless of the backgrounds from which patients hail. I believe that healing people is a doctor's priority at any given time. The Médecins Sans Frontières Movement inspired me to equip myself with necessary knowledge through a first aid course to give people minimal but immediate care whenever needed. At my school's medical society, I presented topics like my grandfather's Alzheimer's and autism's prevalence, encouraging reflection on my knowledge both as an initiator and team player. This led me to write my extended essay on the antioxidative effect of phenols on neural degeneration, highlighting the wonders of the convergence between chemical mechanisms and biological structures. Bynum's 'History of Medicine', which illustrates healthcare's development over time, deeply intrigued me; shadowing doctors in Punjab Kesari Charitable Hospital in Mumbai, India, reinforced this with medical procedures from various historical periods. I enjoyed shadowing neurologists and paediatricians. Learning about paediatric febrile convulsions furthered my interest in paediatrics neurology. The importance of language became clear as I saw doctors speaking to patients in their mother tongues. Being fluent in most Indian languages, English and Spanish accentuated my interpersonal skills and proved to be an asset at the Parkway Hospital Singapore, with its broad international patient base. Service alongside clinical experience showed me a doctor's biggest responsibility is a patient's trust. After a bad dental experience where my teeth and trust were both damaged, I realised the key attributes essential in a doctor are integrity, responsibility and ethical judgement, skills I honed while heading global charities (GCs) in my school. My leadership resulted in my winning four service awards. Eleven years of Indian classical music has disciplined me to use my time efficiently, doubling as an escape from busy days filled with commitments. My holistic education applied these skills as the yearbook journalism team's secretary and designer of a magazine for AWARE, a local women's rights institution, drawing on my interest in photography and training in visual arts. I want to pursue medicine, as my passion for science and compassion for people make me suitable for a service-oriented profession. I believe medicine is entering a new phase where empathy and practical science will converge, providing a holistic approach to healing, and it is my dream to be a part of that.

UNIVERSITY-SPECIFIC EXAMPLES

Traditional—University of Cambridge, Undergraduate

My inquisitive mind, fuelled by the influence of my scientist cousins, always provoked new questions about the functioning of atoms to form this bewilderingly complex yet alluringly practical human body. Having experienced bereavements during my childhood opened a new window for my understanding of what medicine entails: a profession where you strive asymptotically towards the best possible patient care, but also take significant responsibilities, knowing that you can lose. Through deep determination and a desire to serve humanity, I have come to view medicine as a lifelong learning experience that embodies a harmony of affability, commitment, science and ethics, all of which enhanced my urge to pave a journey to studying medicine.

My academic interests have been consolidated by my science A levels and the reading I have done around them. While the brain has always intrigued me, its coverage at Biology A Level prompted me to read The Human Brain: A Guided Tour. From Maclean's interpretation of the brain as a hierarchy to a paler substantia nigra due to Parkinson's disease, what I learned from this book and the realisation of what more I could learn captivated me. Chemistry expanded my research abilities through projects and maths improved my analytical and critical abilities in solving problems.

I have worked at a rehabilitation centre for old people, where I helped with physiotherapy and with patients' morale via reading books and talking with them. Observing the doctors there, I was enlightened by their careful employment of empathy and communication. Working at social services and tutoring a vulnerable child voluntarily for 2 years improved my patience. In addition to academic assistance, we played mind games that boosted her cognitive skills and improved her concentration in the long-run. Working with both children and the elderly, I picked up the essential gemstones in engaging with people, listening to them and experienced the pure gratification of putting a smile on a person's face.

In order to widen my understanding of doctor–patient relationships, I did a 2-week internship at a cardiologist's clinic in Nicosia in 2017 summer. Not only did the altruistic manner with which the doctor approached each of his patients impress me, but also observing cardiovascular conditions, such as aneurysms and arrhythmias through ECGs taught me technical skills. I also did a team-based 2-week internship at ICFO Laboratory in Barcelona. Besides accustoming me to systematic teamwork, especially in a practical, activities like using 3D microscopy to explore the finest structures of a cell and doing cell cultures improved my manual dexterity.

My other activities include my participation in the London International Youth Science Forum this year, where I attended lectures on neuroscience and biomedical physics and was selected to give a speech about my project on designing a vaporising device for a novel method of delivering insect repellents. This opportunity benefited my self-expression as well as advancing my communication skills with people of a very diverse range of backgrounds. In addition, completing the bronze level of Duke of Edinburgh as the leader of a group of six taught me to cope with stress and work under pressure. Cyprus Friendship Programme created a bi-communal environment, where I learnt the essence of unity. Working as a section leader in the school magazine further instigated a sense of teamwork and leadership, as I had to ensure that the writers met the deadlines. Playing the piano and folk dancing all inspired confidence in me, while scuba diving and cooking along with exercising fulfil me.

I am highly aware of the demanding aspect of pursuing a career in medicine. Yet, volunteering, medical shadowing and knowledge gained through extensive research all propel me in my journey towards medicine. Therefore, I am prepared to face these challenges and serve humanity as a medical doctor.

Traditional—Cambridge University, Undergraduate

My affinity for science alongside my interest surrounding medical developments has shaped my desire to study medicine. I am enthralled by the intellectual stimulation and progression provided by a career in medicine, as well as the exposure to new experiences when interacting with patients daily. Upon taking every arising opportunity to increase my awareness of the field, my ardour and desire to make a difference to the lives of others are stronger than ever. My decision to practice medicine was consolidated after a wide range of work experience placements over time.

One example is a recent 8-week virtual placement across two London hospitals, where I had the chance to interact with doctors and allied healthcare professionals working during COVID-19. This experience highlighted the value of multidisciplinary teamwork and a holistic approach towards patient care, and gave me the opportunity to witness key changes and challenges occurring across the healthcare system amidst a pandemic. I also got to observe suturing in practice: an advancement on the technique I learnt when attending the Young Doctor Programme. I was able to gain an insight into the principles of surgery and had the opportunity to further my knowledge of anatomy and physiology. This piqued my interest in cardiology, so I participated in a regional quality improvement project on the heart. As part of this, I helped ameliorate an original patient education video to develop understanding of the science around a heart attack, encouraging public engagement in healthcare. The significance of community care became apparent to me during a 6-week placement with Arts4Dementia—an organisation aiming to assist early-stage dementia sufferers through artistic stimulation. By attending weekly online classes and supporting patients, I learnt about the process leading to dementia and the effect it has on victims and their families, both physically and psychologically. Moreover, the power of arts in medicine and its impact on patient wellbeing influenced me to explore the Biopsychosocial Model of Health and Disease. This ultimately led me to Professor Michael Marmot's fascinating research on social determinants of health, illustrated in his book, The Health Gap. My communication skills were strengthened after volunteering at a care home. By building a rapport with patients, I noticed that even a simple gesture can have a profound impact, especially on those who are lonely and suffering the most. This enlightened me to the emotional aspect of this vocation, making me certain that I want to work in a profession where the welfare of individuals is of utmost importance.

After speaking to several doctors, I realised the significance of a work–life balance, something I have built up over the years. Running the medical society at my school helped me acquire leadership experience and confidence in public speaking by holding ethical debates about dilemmas which one may face when working within the NHS. My role entailed various responsibilities: inviting guest speakers, organising sessions and generally aiding my peers. In addition, I am a keen basketball player, I am learning to play the piano and I attend cadets. Currently, I am completing an EPQ where I research stem cells and the controversy surrounding them in depth—this aids my literary, analytical and presentation skills. The Cambridge HE+ programme allowed me to study neurodegeneration in detail, strengthening my ability to conduct and collate effective research while working with new people, thus enhancing my interpersonal skills.

Based on all of my experiences, I firmly believe this is the career that will give me a sense of fulfilment while providing lifelong learning opportunities. I display the required aptitude and enthusiasm to not only achieve but excel in this academically demanding field. I appreciate that there will be challenges, but I am eager to embrace everything my future in medicine will encompass.

Integrated—University of Leeds, Undergraduate

Visiting my Dad in hospital after an accident revealed to me the role of a doctor as a scientist and carer. As he lacked autonomy, his multidisciplinary team were subject to decisions such as whether or not to ventilate. The risk of choosing against was offset by less time in intensive care and recovery. This illuminated how a career as a medic, though subject to personal sacrifice, brings gratification that overrides burden. Few careers embrace elements of human biology, philanthropic conscience and the uncertainties of scientific progress than medicine, which is truly a vocation.

Able to grasp complex theories, I enjoy being challenged. I relish the rigour of A-level Chemistry so entered the Chemistry Olympiad, which developed my application of concepts to find solutions, a skill vital to a doctor. Reading 'This is Going to Hurt' by Adam Kay highlighted the vitality of decision-making when he was faced with delivering a baby to a couple reluctant to have a male obstetrician. This resonated as, growing up in the UAE, I understand and respect different cultures and beliefs.

My burgeoning interest in research and healthcare practices began with my involvement in a project on medical advancements at the British Embassy Abu Dhabi. Inspired, I attended a webinar on heart attacks and wrote a report on psychological trauma and support shortcomings which was endorsed by the British Heart Foundation and led to changing protocols of patient care. Webinar interactions provided insight into how social determinants of health impact access to support, an issue I am keen to resolve.

From research to routine, I shadowed an obstetrician and observed advancements in women's healthcare during a C-section. Fascinated by the intensity of the procedure (due to thick muscle from adhesions of scar tissue), I explored NHS guidelines and learnt optional C-sections are discouraged in the UK. This taught me how patients benefit from medics' varying practice and ability to put personal opinions aside. Through placements with a psychiatrist and a psychologist I explored differing approaches to mental health regarding the complementary nature of social-emotional influences to the biochemical model. This, along with a Bioethics Society debate on homeopathic remedies and my own yoga practice for work–life balance, inspired my EPQ on the extent to which young adults are more inclined to seek out alternative forms of stress management than pharmaceutical medicines. To support this research, I extended my interest from A-level Biology on how drugs affect neurotransmitters to a neuroscience MOOC, which taught me the importance of critical thinking to medics. While science suggests drugs cure patients through altering action potentials in postsynaptic neurons, a journal article by Bushnell G.A. et al., 'Treating Pediatric Anxiety', suggests long-term efficacy of these medications has not been sufficiently studied, raising concern over potential harm. This is a challenge I've been inspired to pursue, prompting me to write a TEDx talk on the less positive side of the pharmaceutical industry. This experience honed my analytical skills, relevant to diagnosing and treating patients appropriately.

In lockdown, I created an Online Medical Society to bring together two schools and pupils from Yr11–13. I engaged in virtual work experience, shared knowledge and created workshops with frontline doctors. This gave me a chance to witness the necessity of resilience in dealing with increased pressures on the healthcare system. I possess this quality, having balanced academics with Gold IA, my Deputy Head Girl role and volunteering since Yr11 with the UAE Special Olympics swimming team, an opportunity that taught me patience is the key to effective communication.

Pandemic-imposed changes have shown that flexibility and endurance are as important as knowledge—attributes that will support me in a medical career that, while unpredictable will be transformative.

Integrated—Anglia Ruskin University, Graduate Example

Blood. Bone. Blue drapes. It was here, standing between surgeons carving out tumours from the patient's exposed brain, that I saw the heart of medicine: a humanitarian application of science and the united mettle of doctors and nurses unrelenting in their desire to help. My week-long experience in the functional neurosurgical clinic and operating theatre consolidated a long-standing ambition to dedicate myself towards a career in medicine.

From the multidisciplinary team meetings and various specialists involved in perioperative care, I saw first-hand how coordinated effort is essential for patient safety. My own teamwork and collaborative skills improved as the regional charity coordinator for a national Muslim youth organisation. Two years of delegating tasks, in order to organise fundraising events with external collaborating charities, taught me the value of harnessing each individual's strength in my team in order to maximise efficiency and output. Consequently, I was able to outperform expectations, maintain standards of professionalism and develop trust with partnering charities. Along with fiscal responsibility, giving presentations on our charitable efforts to local MPs strengthened my composure, time management and public speaking. I saw the importance of this in virtual placements when junior doctors were triaging patients.

But health extends beyond bodily function. Volunteering in a national social prescribing workshop for people with early-stage dementia demonstrated the value of holistic biopsychosocial care. Patient interaction outside of a clinical setting grounded my understanding of the personal effects of illness and how disease can diffuse across relationships, impacting families too. It was in moments of vulnerability that I saw how connection, validation and empathy are the cornerstones of good clinical practice.

In recognition of my voluntary experience, alongside my work as a global coordinator for the National Academy of Social Prescribing, I was awarded a student fellowship from the College of Medicine. This experience affords me several opportunities to speak at national conferences, advocating the need to educate prospective medical students in order to enact real change in future medical practice.

Academically, my undergraduate studies limited disease to biological impairments only. Pursuing global health postgraduate was therefore essential to expand my current knowledge and provide a comprehensive view to the determinants of health. Both degrees have advanced my understanding in the sciences and invested skills in data handling and critical literature appraisal—essential to evaluate evidence in continued professional development. In particular, my undergraduate dissertation project, which looked at the accuracy of a noninvasive diagnostic tool for hearing loss, provided me with the opportunity to write a systematic review.

Beyond studying, I have published opinions in a national report on social prescribing and the British Neuroscience Association. My communication and research skills have strengthened further as co-host of a monthly live radio show, offering a balance to my studies.

Medicine is not without its physical and emotional challenges. However, with its academic rigours and opportunity to induce positive change in people's lives, my desire to pursue this vocation has become resolute. I believe my experiences have primed me with the resilience, discipline and a sincere curiosity needed to succeed in this field.

Problem-based Learning—University of Manchester, Undergraduate

Despite the NHS constitution stating universal access free at the point of entry, healthcare remains unequal in the UK and worldwide. After the death of my brother from malaria due to the healthcare disparity in Gambia, I was driven towards a career in medicine. From experience, notably through reading 'This is Going to Hurt', I learnt that medicine requires a challenging but fulfilling collaboration between academic rigour and good interpersonal skills to ensure excellent care for patients.

In the radiology department at St. Mary's Hospital, I attended multidisciplinary (MDT) meetings and was struck by their complexity and variety. A doctor explained his alteration of a patient's treatment plan, citing her ethical right to autonomy and depicted the variations of health literacy in patients. Another doctor explained his difficulty due to a language barrier and the importance of communication between patients. I was impressed by the honesty in front of their team, showing the realities of medicine. COVID-19 forced more virtual observations, through Observe GP and Brighton and Sussex, where I learnt about the structure of the NHS and the intricacies of primary and secondary care. In other online hospital experiences, I learnt the basis of history-taking and examination skills and the relieving effect of helping a patient with acute and chronic illnesses.

I regularly read the BMJ, where an article focusing on institutional racism in the NHS led me to read 'The Immortal Life of Henrietta Lacks' to research exploitation in science. I was struck by the immortality of HeLa cells and the injustice afflicted on her family due to lack of informed consent. I am a part of the Imperial Pathways to Medicine programme, which allows me to deepen my knowledge and attend conferences such as the Medical Innovations Summit, where I learnt about discoveries such as CRISPR. The complex advancements that are the basis of medicine inspired me to write an essay on monoclonal antibodies. As a Youth Health Champion, I gave presentations on both public and global health, using my public speaking skills to raise awareness about physical and mental wellbeing. I attend Biology Extension, exploring scientific topics such as epidemiology, and the study of this inspired me to read 'The Coming Plague', which illustrated the interdependence of the scientific and socioeconomic spheres. I researched an EPQ regarding the ethical responsibility around Antisocial Personality Disorder as an adjunct to my interest in mental health and medical ethics, developing my time management skills further. I also completed the online course Medical Neuroscience by Duke University. Most notably, I learnt about the Long-Term Potentiation and Long-Term Depression linked to learning and memory and was impressed by the velocity with which such neurological processes occur.

As a community leader and role model, I am a trustee of the Young Advisor's board and raise awareness on issues affecting young people by speaking on CAMHS scrutiny boards and liaising with firms working on neurodiversity. This outlined the importance of community-based medicine. As a founding member of the Team London Youth Advisory board, I use communication and teamwork skills to solve disparities faced by those in the UK, similar to the critical thinking used by doctors to reach a diagnosis. Using my leadership and compassion as Head Girl, I organised a charity event for domestic violence where I tackled emotionally difficult cases requiring empathy and resilience, resulting in my achievement of the Mayor of London's Young Volunteer of the Year award. To balance my commitments, I enjoy martial arts, which helps me destress.

I believe, despite the hardships, medicine is a pioneer in improving the biopsychosocial outcomes for those in our communities. Due to my enthusiasm, love for intellectual stimulation and empathy, I would be a passionate doctor and advocate for the premises which underpin the NHS.

Problem-based Learning—University of Birmingham, Postgraduate

In our society, where death conversations with patients remain highly stigmatised, engaging in open end-of-life discussions is a challenge for doctors. Hence, it was liberating to see the palliative care team maintaining the autonomy of my terminally ill aunt by giving her the choice of dying at home. This moulded my understanding of what medicine entails: an embodiment of the importance of human life and values, coupled with ethics, affability and science, all of which prompted me to consider medicine as a career.

Our limited knowledge of the brain, which, if fully understood, can revolutionise healthcare, incited my desire to study neuroscience, building a strong scientific foundation, which I aim to apply as a clinical doctor. I undertook an 8-week research project, where I explored the potential apoptotic mechanism of motor neuron degeneration in ALS mouse models. Through developing my scientific literacy, the project underlined the ever-evolving nature of medicine and the importance of scepticism in research, inspiring me to read Goldacre's Bad Pharma. Revealing how the pharmaceutical industry misleads doctors through publishing flawed results, I learnt the universal importance of having an evidence-based approach to patient care.

Working within a multidisciplinary team at a COVID-19 vaccination clinic, I helped with the efficient delivery of vaccines by listening to and consoling patients regarding their fear of injections. These conversations shed light on the collective psychological distress in our population amid the pandemic, highlighting the doctor's duty to both physical and emotional wellbeing. This motivated me to complete a 5-week psychiatric placement, where taking patient history enriched my grasp of how social determinants can impact mental health. Thus, I experienced how vital having a biopsychosocial approach, together with empathy and compassion towards patients, is for building rapport and holistic care. I adopted this attitude when volunteering at a rehabilitation centre, where I raised a girl with anorexia's morale simply by conversing with and reassuring her. This benefited my resilience and confidence when managing difficult scenarios under pressure.

My 5-week paediatrics placement introduced me to safeguarding policies and unveiled the ethical dilemmas in healthcare, as I observed a 15-year-old girl wanting to have an abortion without her parents' knowledge. Even though her decision was against the doctor's advice of involving her parents, I learnt that, as a doctor, you still have a duty of confidentiality to a competent child. I also shadowed an ER doctor at a major trauma centre, where I exercised my critical thinking by taking patient histories as part of a structured consultation. Observing the sense of camaraderie among the ED team, despite of the pressure they face from the underfunded and overburdened NHS, was poignant.

To maintain a work–life balance, I do scuba diving and astrophotography. Elected as the Allied Courses President, I organise job fairs, bringing women in healthcare to speak on leadership. My commitment to wider society through cooking at food banks and translating healthcare questions from English to Turkish was recognised with volunteering awards. Overall, embracing roles outside academia furthered my work ethic, time management and organisational skills, which will facilitate my medical degree.

As a Cyprus native, I believe that my cross-cultural empathy and determination will complement my urge to rise to this lifelong endeavour as an NHS doctor—a privilege which I will treasure with alacrity.

SUMMARY, TEST YOURSELF AND REFLECTION

Writing your personal statement clearly isn't an easy task. Most applicants struggle with not knowing where to start. We all tend to procrastinate when a big task lies ahead of us. This chapter has provided you with the starting point. If you've taken part in brainstorming and completing the reflection boxes scattered throughout this chapter, you'll be surprised to find out that your first draft of the personal statement is ready. Don't believe us? Just put together all your reflections in one place. Of course, it's nowhere near completion and it will require 10 or more drafts, but now you have the rough backbone of your personal statement.

Please Remember

- The secret lies in self-reflection and introspection.
- Elaborate and explain what you have learnt, don't provide lists.
- First and last impressions matter most—there's nothing worse than a boring beginning and an abrupt ending.
- Don't worry about the word count when you create your first draft.
- Be prepared to edit as many drafts as required to build the perfect personal statement.
- Be yourself and no one else, this will set yourself apart from the crowd.

As previously discussed, your personal statement is the sum of all your academic, extracurricular and professional encounters. We recommend having a look at your 'Getting into medical school portfolio' and writing down your biggest gaps. What's missing from your personal statement? Is it work experience? Is it volunteer work? Do you need to work harder on your grades? A box for reflection and ideas has been provided here so you can jot down any thoughts you may have.

Test Yourself

- Using the personal statements provided in this chapter, go through each of them using the checklist provided.
- Can you spot the different elements of the personal statement as outlined in this chapter?

Reflection and Notes

RESOURCES

Over a hundred personal statements from The Student Room https://www.thestudentroom.co.uk/university/personal-statements/medicine/medicine-personal-statements.

Oxford tips. https://www.medsci.ox.ac.uk/study/medicine/pre-clinical/applying/ps. Accessed 23 December 2023.

Tips from The Guardian. https://www.theguardian.com/education/2013/oct/01/personal-statement-for-medicine.

UCAS personal statement guide. https://www.ucas.com/undergraduate/applying-university/how-write-ucas-undergraduate-personal-statement.

Universities and Colleges Admissions Service (UCAS). https://www.ucas.com/.

Acing the Medical School Interview

9

Matthew Lau, Bogdan Chiva Giurca and Kiyara Fernando

Chapter Outline

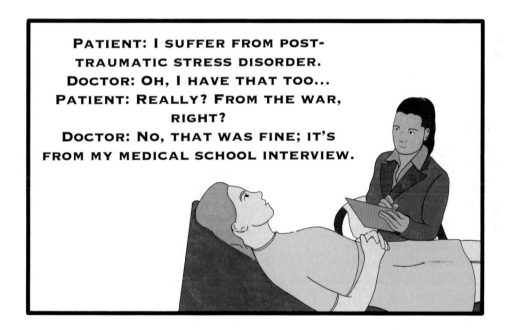

PATIENT: I SUFFER FROM POST-TRAUMATIC STRESS DISORDER.
DOCTOR: OH, I HAVE THAT TOO...
PATIENT: REALLY? FROM THE WAR, RIGHT?
DOCTOR: NO, THAT WAS FINE; IT'S FROM MY MEDICAL SCHOOL INTERVIEW.

INTERVIEW FORMATS

If you've already got an interview, congratulations! You've overcome several obstacles to get here, and it's now your chance to prove to the interviewers that you're worthy of a place at their medical school. This is your chance to shine and show how much you'd love to join their institution. If you're currently waiting for an interview, this chapter will help you prepare in advance.

Interviewing for medical school is a trying time for most students. As you can imagine, combinations of hundreds, if not thousands, of questions could come up in an interview situation. In this chapter, we focus on core themes and principles that can be applied to answer any question that may arise during your medical school interview.

When it comes to tips and examples, we have anonymised real-life scenarios encountered by successful medical students and applicants like you over the years. A selection of tricks for mastering your interview is added towards the end of this chapter, as well as a nonexhaustive list of further questions that you should work through and test yourself in your own time.

As you will see, some aspects are repeated throughout this chapter. This is not the authors repeating themselves again and again. This is to get you used to a few buzzwords that we consider crucial for the medical school interview.

Let's start with the basics and look at the two main types of medical school interviews:

TRADITIONAL INTERVIEWS (FIG. 9.1)

- Panel-style interview
- Held by approximately two to three people
- Perhaps a faculty member as chair
- A student or a junior doctor
- Another doctor or health professional
- This could include a lay member of the public or a patient
- 20 to 40 minutes
- Includes Oxbridge interviews and Group interviews (covered later on in the chapter)

MMI: MULTIPLE MINI-INTERVIEWS (FIG. 9.2)

- Increasingly popular among medical schools
- Consists of several short assessments, each around 10 minutes
- You may be asked a question, asked to solve a problem or take part in role-playing with an actor
- MMI interviews take between 1 and 2 hours, approximately
- Most universities have around eight MMI 'stations'.

WHAT DO INTERVIEWERS LOOK FOR IN A POTENTIAL MEDICAL STUDENT?

- Motivation, insight and passion for studying medicine
- Knowledge of the course, the medical school and the curriculum
- Understanding of the career and its realities—the positives, the negatives, the career options and the role of a medical student
- Transferrable skills and personal aptitudes—teamwork, communication, leadership, empathy, etc.
- Commitment to the course—persistence and determination
- Work experience relevant to medicine—placements, volunteering and extracurriculars
- Insight into the National Health Service (NHS)—structure, core values, as well as past, present and future issues that the NHS may face
- The importance of the work–life balance—coping with stress
- Ethics and medico-legal scenarios
- Professionalism

The most common interview themes are summarised in Fig. 9.3. Most questions encountered usually fall under one of these themes.

As you can see, many of these topics were explored in our previous chapters. The rest are based on your

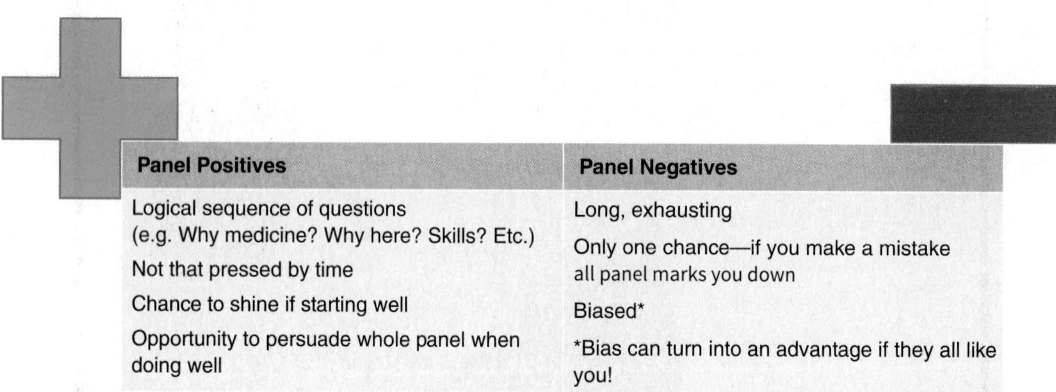

Panel Positives	Panel Negatives
Logical sequence of questions (e.g. Why medicine? Why here? Skills? Etc.)	Long, exhausting
Not that pressed by time	Only one chance—if you make a mistake all panel marks you down
Chance to shine if starting well	Biased*
Opportunity to persuade whole panel when doing well	*Bias can turn into an advantage if they all like you!

Fig. 9.1 Traditional interview.

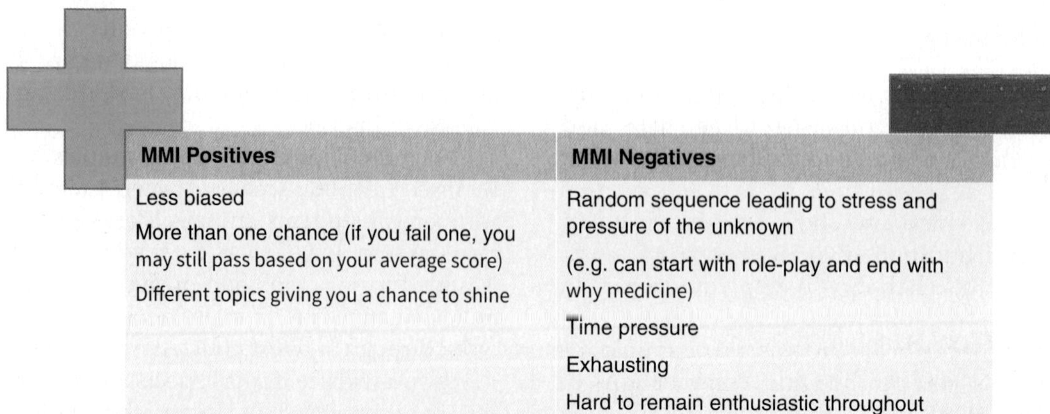

MMI Positives	MMI Negatives
Less biased	Random sequence leading to stress and pressure of the unknown
More than one chance (if you fail one, you may still pass based on your average score)	(e.g. can start with role-play and end with why medicine)
Different topics giving you a chance to shine	Time pressure
	Exhausting
	Hard to remain enthusiastic throughout

Fig. 9.2 MMI interview.

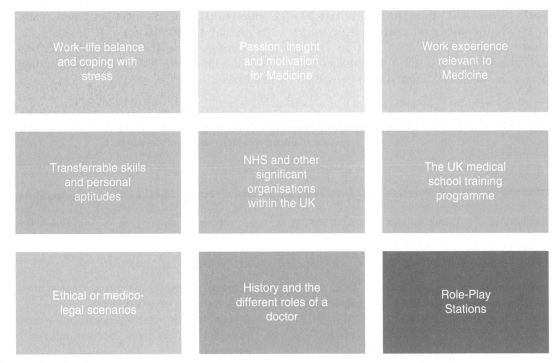

Fig. 9.3 Common interview themes.

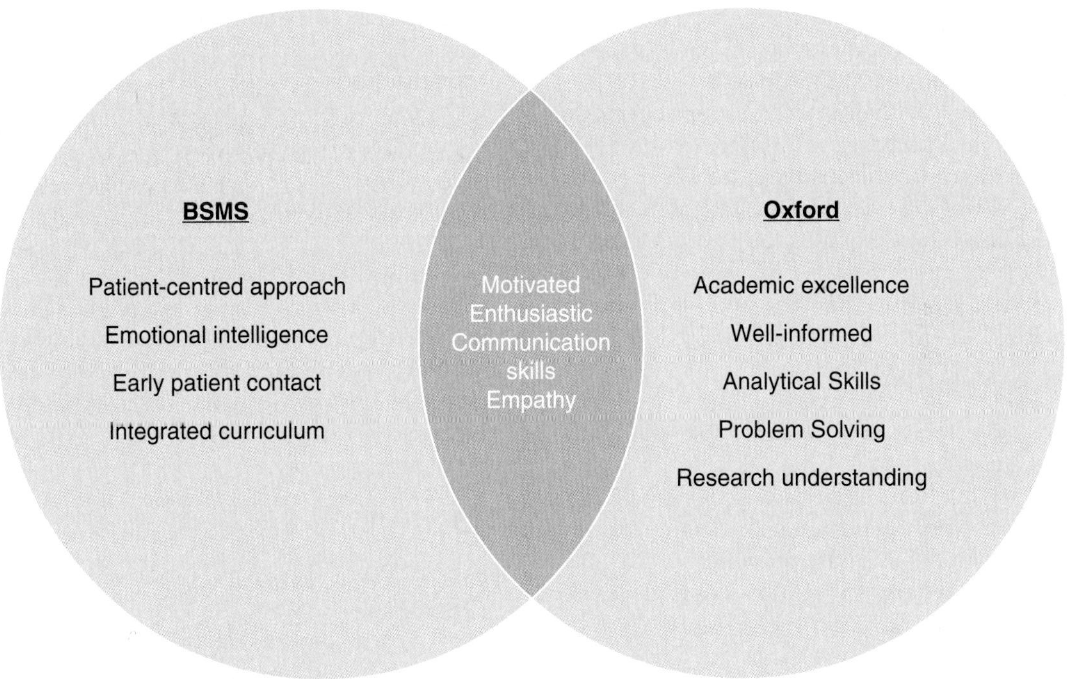

Fig. 9.4 Comparison of two medical schools.

personal experiences and are covered through work experience, volunteering and your personal curiosity.

HOW DO INTERVIEWERS MARK EACH CANDIDATE?

This is a very arbitrary question, although it is essential to understand that different medical schools have different core values. If you spend enough time exploring their websites and reading their admission criteria and 'About Us' sections, you will soon realise what they may ask and what they offer top marks for. Let's take two random medical school courses as an example: Brighton and Sussex Medical School (BSMS) and Oxford Medical School. If you look on their websites, you can spot differences immediately (Fig. 9.4).

Although there are several overlapping items, you can clearly see that each medical school has different core values and, therefore, different aspects that you should focus on more during your interview.

Most medical schools use a grading system (usually 1–10) for each question. Different questions with different themes will focus on different attributes that admission tutors look for.

If, for example, the question is, 'What do you think about euthanasia?' the following marking scheme could be used:

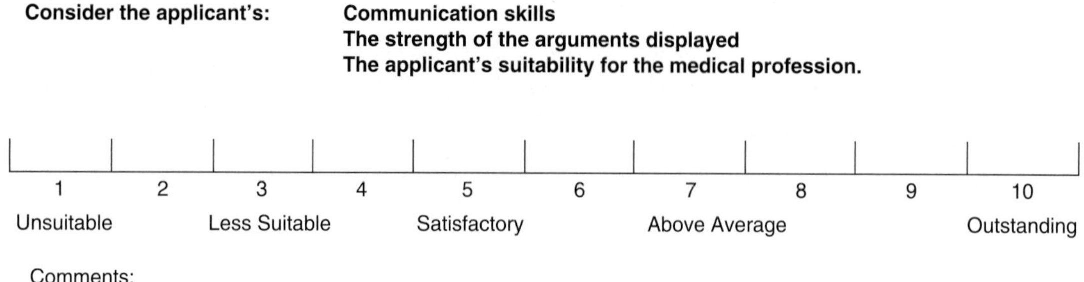

As you can imagine, if the question were 'Why medicine?' admission tutors would look for motivation, insight and passion for studying medicine.

HOW TO STRUCTURE YOUR ANSWER

If there is only one thing you take away from this chapter, it should be the importance of structure when answering a question. Over the years, brilliant applicants with excellent academic achievements have given unstructured answers. They become disorganised and eventually lose their train of thought because they forget their next point.

We all have different styles and preferences. For this reason, we've developed a series of techniques you can use based on your personality. Some are easier to understand, while others require a bit more practice.

Let's start with the one that can save your life in ANY scenario.

THE 'ESSAY TECHNIQUE'

Imagine you have to write an essay. What did your schoolteacher always say? The successful recipe includes an introduction, body and conclusion (Fig. 9.5). Interview answers can be in the exact same format as an essay. They must have the following:

a) **An introduction** where you acknowledge the question, introduce and describe the topic of interest, make a point and state your view
b) **A body** representing your answer's 'meat' (or hummus if you're vegetarian!)
c) **A conclusion** that successfully wraps up your answer and returns to summarise the initial argument

Remember: Introduction, body and conclusion. This is the easiest way to answer a question. Let's see a few examples in action.

'What makes a good doctor?'

Introduction

Several personal skills make a good doctor, including empathy, knowledge, communication and many more. However, the ones that resonate with me most are teamwork, listening skills and leadership.

Observe how you have 'showed off' to the interviewer with how many personal skills you can name, and then focused on a couple that resonate with your personality or previous work experience placements. You are set with a structure in mind—you know where you're heading now!

Body

First teamwork, because medicine requires a multidisciplinary approach where doctors work with colleagues from several departments. They may have different

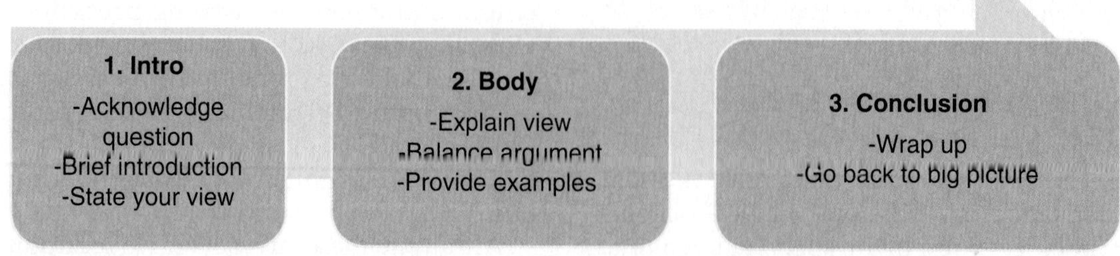

Fig. 9.5 The 'essay technique'.

approaches, but the aim is the same: to ensure top-quality patient care. I was grateful for the chance to observe this during a multidisciplinary meeting as part of my 6-week placement at a local hospital. Several healthcare professionals were in one room, each holding a different piece required to solve the puzzle. Nurses, surgeons, oncologists, radiologists and pathologists shared their knowledge in an organised way to achieve the best outcome for the patient.

Second, listening skills are essential during medical consultations, not only because patients provide valuable information about their condition but also because, as human beings, we need someone to listen to our concerns. During my general practice placement, I saw a 67-year-old woman, afraid she might have cancer. The GP listened attentively without interrupting until the patient finished her story. In the end, he explored her ideas, concerns and expectations. She felt reassured, and with a bright smile, she thanked the doctor for simply listening to her.

Finally, leadership brings structure to a team, which is crucial in medicine. I chose this skill because I recently led a team of four volunteers during a fundraising event for Cancer Research UK. By delegating roles accordingly and setting realistic targets for the team, we organised a marathon and raised £1500 for cancer research.

Observe how each example uses a structure (first, second, third). Each of the three examples also has a precise, logical sequence because it starts with a **POINT**, continues with the **EVIDENCE** for the point you have just made and ends with an **EXPLANATION**. Some of you may remember this as the 'PEE Technique' for each paragraph, taught during primary school.

Conclusion

In conclusion, although several attributes make up a good doctor, and all may be equally important, I chose teamwork, listening skills and leadership because I demonstrated these skills and many others during my recent work experience placements. I plan to improve these skills as a medical student at your institution and put them to good use as a doctor one day.

Observe how you return to the initial picture and explain why you made this particular selection. Observe also how you're 'showing off' by saying that you already have some of the qualities of a good doctor. Finally, you mention the future and use a bit of psychology to indirectly let them know that you hope they choose you (keep this in mind, as this is a trick we'll discuss towards the end of this chapter).

The earlier structure can be adapted and applied to any question.

'What is the most significant discovery in the history of medicine?'

Introduction

There have been many ground-breaking medical discoveries over the years, including insulin, the first successful anaesthetic agent, penicillin and so on. Although all have played an essential role in advancing medicine, I would like to focus on one example that resonates with me the most.

Same model as before. Then move on to the body and conclusion in a similar fashion. Let's try another one, slightly different but with the same principles that can easily be applied.

'Give an example of a time when you were part of a team, and something went wrong'

Introduction

There have been several times when I was a team player, both as part of my work experience and the various volunteering activities I have been involved in over the years, including organising fundraising events for Cancer Research UK. However, the one example that always comes to mind is an important lesson I learned during Year 12 as part of my biology group project.

Although this is a slightly different question asking you for a specific example, the same principle as before can be applied. In the body of your answer, ensure you provide a good description of what happened, how you solved the problem in the end and especially what you learned from this experience.

For extra points, in your conclusion, you can mention how your scenario could be applied to a clinical situation. For example, suppose the theme of your example was 'the importance of delegating tasks'. In that case, you can easily say this is also the case in a busy surgical theatre where the anaesthetist has a clear role of observing the patient while the surgeon carries on the procedure, supported with equipment and various manoeuvres by the theatre assistants.

Remember: Introduction, body and conclusion.

GIBBS' CYCLE: BECOMING A BETTER STORYTELLER

You may have already seen the Gibbs' Cycle in our work experience chapter as a valuable model for reflection (Fig. 9.6). Not surprisingly, this well-known cycle used by medical students and doctors worldwide provides a brilliant way to answer questions that may require examples or personal experiences.

Now, you may have already realised that you don't have to say the beginning of each paragraph out loud (e.g. 'description: what happened', 'feelings'). Just use it as a structure in your head to guide you. As you can see, it is pretty hard to remember each section, and you may require a bit of practice to get used to it. Interviewers will, however, be very impressed by this,

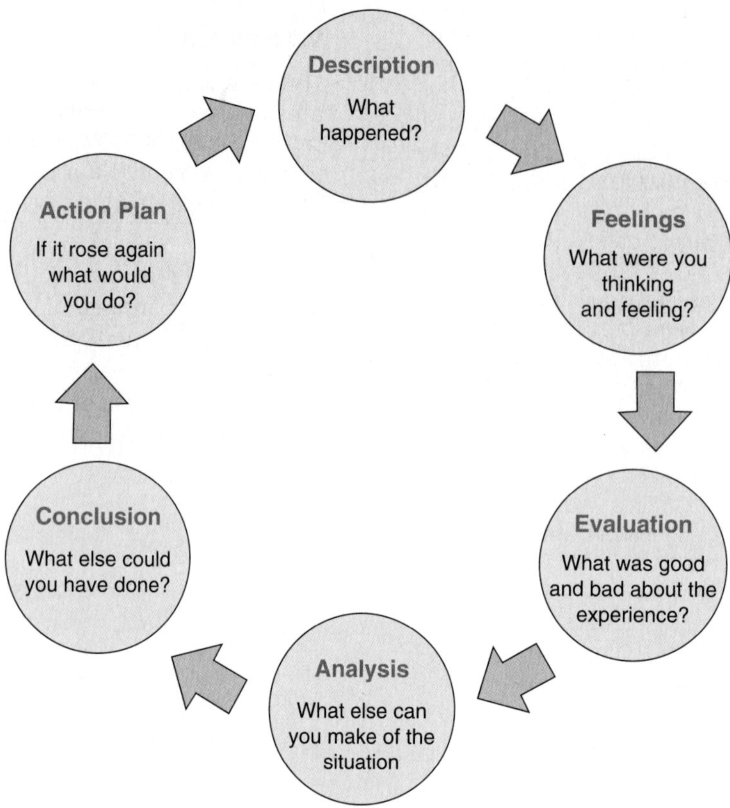

Fig. 9.6 Gibbs' reflective cycle.

I promise. They are often shocked to see applicants have heard of this model and are delighted to see you using it.

> I was asked to describe a time when I showed empathy during my work experience. Step by step, I followed Gibbs' reflective cycle. The interviewer smiled and asked me about the importance of reflection. She seemed delighted to hear that I thought it was an integral part of learning and that I look forward to using it as a medical student and doctor.
>
> **Medical School Applicant**

THE STAR TECHNIQUE

Initially developed as a model for high-performance coaching, the STAR technique has been developed more recently to help interview applicants from all domains answer so-called 'behavioural interviewing' (Fig. 9.7). Essentially, these questions assess the applicant's past experiences to judge their response to similar situations in a future position. This technique can also be used for other general questions and provides a simple structure to follow to avoid getting tangled during your medical school interview.

Situation or Task

Address the situation or task you faced to provide the interviewer with some context. You can use this opportunity to tell the interviewer what the challenge was. For example: When asked to describe an instance where you showed leadership skills, discuss when this happened, why you needed to take control of the situation and so on.

Action

This part of your answer is what interviewers will be keen to hear the most. Use this as an opportunity to highlight your skills and character. You need to explain **how** you dealt with the situation or the task. When doing so, remember:

- Be personal: Talk about **what** YOU did in the situation, not how other people fared. The question is aimed at finding out more about you as a candidate.
- Steer clear of technical jargon unless it is essential to your story.
- Explain **what** you did, **how** you did it and **why** you did it.

Why you did it is crucial. This section judges whether you make well-thought-out and reasoned decisions when faced with tricky situations. The interviewer wants to know about your judgment and whether you can make rational decisions, which is a vital part of being a doctor. When asked to describe a time when you took control of a situation, you may want to pick an instance when you and your team members were in a stressful situation. For example, when part of a sports team, there may have been a requirement for a new strategy and someone to boost the morale of the group, and you decided to take this upon yourself.

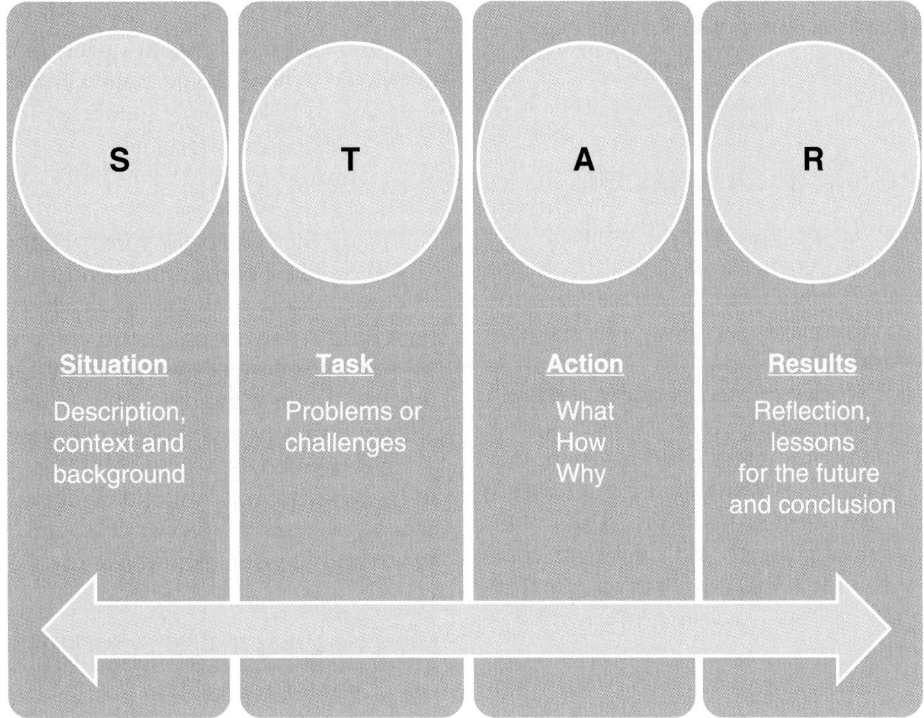

Fig. 9.7 STAR technique.

Result

Explain what happened eventually and how the situation ended. This is an excellent opportunity to reflect on what you accomplished and learned from the situation that could be applied in the future.

> Some people just get this kind of stuff. Not me. I hated talking about why I wanted to do medicine and felt awkward when asked to talk about my feelings or, even worse, about my strengths and weaknesses. Different things work for different people, but for me, it was simply getting friends to ask me stuff like this. I found this challenging, but I started getting better after a bit of practice. I still find it awkward, but maybe that's my personality.
>
> **Medical School Applicant**

'I HATE BOASTING ABOUT MYSELF': HOW TO SELL YOURSELF WITHOUT BOASTING

Trust me; we've all been there. Boasting about yourself can feel arrogant and unnatural. Most prospective medical students we spoke to identify this as a key issue they faced during interview preparation. To combat this, you can avoid bold statements such as, 'I am a great communicator', 'I am a good team player' and so on.

These blunt statements are indeed arrogant. You make a point but don't back it up with any evidence or explanation. There are three key ways to avoid statements like this, so you can build complete answers that portray you as a well-rounded individual.

1. Express your strengths by mentioning that other people have appreciated your skill.
   For example: 'A junior doctor complimented my commitment to gaining as much knowledge as possible during my work experience. This is because I attended numerous workshops held by the hospital'.
2. Justify your skills by discussing their effect on a situation and giving examples.
   For example, 'I have good organisational skills, which helped me organise my school's charity walk, and we raised **£5000 for Alzheimer's UK**'. The example helps to dilute the bold statement.
3. Stay practical and talk about your experiences instead of putting yourself on a pedestal.
   For example: 'Captaining my school basketball team gave me a great deal of experience being a leader; however, I understand the importance of teamwork too, because it is with complete teamwork that we won games'. This statement is much more powerful than simply stating, 'I am an outstanding team player and leader'.

> What do charismatic leaders have in common? Why do people love them, even though they 'show off'? The key here is using expressions and words that make you appear grateful for all the experiences that you've had so far. Examples include, 'I have had the pleasure of winning…', 'I feel honoured to be at this interview…', 'I was fortunate enough to be part of a winning team…' and so on.

Use positive statements and be grateful for every experience which you have been part of. You'll appear more charismatic than you can imagine!

GENERAL PREPARATION FOR AN INTERVIEW

- Mock interviews: Learn about your interview's structure (traditional panel, MMIs, group task or Oxbridge) and ask friends, family or teachers to simulate this environment for you. Remember, practice makes perfect!
- Reflect on all your work experience, wider reading and achievements by reading your personal statement. Think of points of interest in your statement where interviewers could potentially ask questions.
- Record yourself answering questions. This will help you with your confidence and may help you cut down on your 'umm's and 'errr's in an answer. However, be wary of this, as you don't want to sound too rehearsed.

If you hate hearing your own voice, write down answers, but instead of writing them in full, only put down bullet points with your main ideas.

- Question banks help you get a feel for the type of questions you might face in an interview.

Practice your answers. It is not enough to 'think' it out—you must practice saying it out loud. That way, you do not stumble even when asked something simple like 'Tell me about yourself'. But do not over-practice and do not memorise your answers; people can spot that very quickly. Make a list of talking points and let it flow.

Jia Cheng, Medical Student, Manchester Medical School

- Research the medical school, teaching style, societies and strong suits, as you will most likely be asked *why* you chose the university you're interviewing for.
- Refer to the 'What Do Interviewers Look for in a Potential Medical Student?' section. We suggest you take each bullet point individually and think of examples (around two or three) through which you could show your capability. This can be done by reflecting on experiences during volunteering or shadowing. It can also be achieved by drawing from reading you did to prepare for the interview, be it magazines such as *Student BMJ*, *New Scientist*, news articles or books. The 'perfect' answer to address each theme should show the interviewer that you are insightful and well read and can critically think about issues and experiences.

HOW TO BATTLE THROUGH AN MMI

The first and most crucial step is finding out as much as possible about the interview process.

- Speak to medical students at the university that offered you an interview.
- Go through the medical school's website.
- Read student blogs.
- Ensure that you clearly understand the instructions provided by your interviewers via email.

Questions from all themes (as described in this chapter) could come up, so ensure you prepare answers for as many scenarios as possible. By 'prepare', we mean writing down examples and organising thoughts as simple bullet points. You don't want your answer to seem rehearsed, but on the other hand, you don't want to be sweating for 3 minutes looking for that one time when you were the leader of a team. Save yourself the sweat and have an example ready.

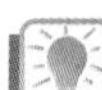

Know Your Personal Statement Inside Out

Often forgotten, the personal statement is a key element that may be brought up during your medical school interview. It is your homework to go through every single remark in your personal statement and ask yourself, 'What did I write here that could lead to a potential question from my interviewers?' If, for example, you mentioned you're interested in surgery, you may want to have a prepared answer for that. On the other hand, if you mentioned a particular disease, ensure you have a general understanding of it, as they may ask you about it. Finally, if you've mentioned reading any books, ensure you can clearly summarise what you learnt from them, as this is also a common question based on personal statements.

WHAT IS AND HOW TO PREPARE FOR A GROUP INTERVIEW

Group interviews are recent addition made by some medical schools.

- Groups of three to six applicants asked to work as a team
  - Take part in a team-building exercise (e.g. build a bridge from paper)
  - Discuss and debate controversial topics (e.g. euthanasia)
  - Take part in any other activity (e.g. problem-based learning [PBL] simulation)
- Short (usually 5–10 minutes)
- Can be set up as one of the stations of an MMI or as a separate exercise upon completion of a panel interview

Be prepared to take part in an icebreaker activity. Many group interviews may ask each person to briefly introduce themselves and mention one interesting fact about themselves. Have one ready just in case.

Do:

- Be friendly and charismatic, and win the respect of the others in the room.
- Support the group—interviewers appreciate when you give a hand to someone rather than being competitive.
- Be confident, but stay humble—there is a very fine line.
- Smile with positive energy that shines bright and lights the room so nobody can resist it!

Don't:

- Talk over people or interrupt
- Be too shy
- Be competitive
- Belittle others, it won't make you look good at all—quite the opposite, in fact

Activities might involve:

- Splitting into two groups and working on a task (e.g. build a tower out of A4 sheets of paper)
  - Ensure you delegate roles by asking everyone what they are good at
  - Depending on your personality, if you feel courageous, act as a leader from the start (but don't be bossy!)
  - If nobody is willing to take responsibility, stand up and take a leadership position, even if this is out of your comfort zone
  - Work together towards the same goal
  - Resolve any conflicts that may arise
  - Communication is key
- Individual follow-up questions upon completion of group activities, such as:
  - What went well/less well?
  - What skills did you personally bring to the team?
  - Reflect on the success or failure of the previous task.

WHAT IS AND HOW TO PREPARE FOR AN OXBRIDGE INTERVIEW

The thought of an Oxford or Cambridge (collectively known as Oxbridge) interview generates much fear and anxiety. Although structurally like a traditional interview, Oxbridge interviews are known for their tendency to ask abstract questions that may throw a student off-guard. Bearing this in mind, it is worth acknowledging that being considered to study medicine at one of these fine institutions is an outstanding achievement. We hope this chapter will help you combat your fear and take advantage of the abstract style of questioning.

- Structurally similar to traditional interviews and focused primarily on problem solving
- Highly academic in nature
- Typically, abstract questions that focus on your reasoning process as opposed to answering 'correctly'
- Usually, two or three 15- to 20-minute-long interviews (varies from one college to another)
- Each interview may have a different focus (e.g. maths, chemistry), then a discussion of questions such as 'Why medicine?'
- Each college takes a different approach—check thoroughly for any information available on their website

The key aspect of an Oxbridge interview is assessing HOW a student thinks. It's about using your knowledge to reach new conclusions. The interviewers place a great deal of emphasis on how you reason out an answer as opposed to arriving at the 'correct' conclusion. Here is an example of a typical question you might experience at an Oxford medical school interview. Remember that the questions tend to be abstract and test how you think; therefore, they are harder to prepare for.

When can you determine when a person is truly 'dead'?

- Biological perspective: Perhaps when a person stops breathing? Or their heart stops beating? Or they are brain dead?
- Philosophical perspective: Does death mean we cease to exist? What about life after death?
- Legal perspective: Territory dependent, e.g. variation between the USA and the UK

The main aim is to:

- Outline your thoughts out loud
- Work out your arguments logically, giving reasons for them
- Consider ideas and arguments other than your own—this demonstrates that you can look at the question from different perspectives
- Expect questions from your interviewer

More than most medical schools, Oxbridge interviews focus on your scientific aptitude. The level of basic scientific knowledge expected to answer these questions is within the A-Level syllabus for chemistry, biology and physics. The tricky part is using this knowledge to answer questions. Additional information by reading around your subjects will improve your answers and, therefore, your chances of impressing the interviewers.

My Oxford interview had two components:

1. Suitability for medicine
   - Ethical concerns (dilemmas/contradictions)
   - News and hot topics in medicine
   - E.g. cloning, postcode prescribing, etc.
2. Academic potential
   - Based on your AS/A-level course
   - Asking you something that would allow you to use current knowledge to reach a new answer
   - Taking things that you know and seeing if you can take them further
   - Understanding WHY things happen

For the most part, the interview is scientific, and they may give you graphs to interpret, open-ended questions like why we have two ears or ask you to design a bladder. They may get you to do basic calculations with information you can obtain from a graph. If you don't know how to do it, please don't panic; they'll teach you. Just be patient.

There might be a question involving about 30 minutes of prereading before you enter the room. You will then be asked questions about what you've just read. For example, it could be an experiment. During the interview, they might ask how you could improve this experiment. Another question could be to provide alternative hypotheses and how you would test for your proposed hypotheses.

Mostly, you can't prepare for it because what they ask you depends on the college. Still, an excellent scientific background will certainly help, as well as loads of practice looking at different sides of a debate (never ever debate solely on one side).

Remember that with both scientific and ethical questions, they want to hear how you think and what you're thinking, not what you really believe. My best tip is to spend a few seconds thinking before you open your mouth, but when you open your mouth, say everything you're thinking and don't be afraid to ask them to repeat a question. Furthermore, you should ask them questions as well. For example, if they give you an ethical dilemma, ask them about the circumstances behind the patient's cases. Does the patient have mental capacity? Is the patient going to get better?

Medical Student

My Cambridge interview had a mixture of questions:

1. Questions they have prepared beforehand
   - They ask everyone the same things
   - Science and academic questions
   - Ethical dilemmas and debates
   - Graphs, objects, anatomy models (e.g. 'What's this bone?'), pictures
2. Questions based on you personally
   - Subjects you are taking at A-Level (e.g. chemistry, maths)
   - Stuff from your personal statement (e.g. a disease, work experience, etc.)
     - 'Tell me about your malaria project that you mentioned in your personal statement'.
   - May ask for extensions depending on how you answer
     - 'What is malaria, and how does it spread?'

They look at how well you keep a clear head if they ask weird or broad questions, so I'd start with a simple, straightforward answer and then expand. This helps for two reasons: First, you don't confuse yourself. Second, it sounds structured!

With the science questions, it's okay if you don't know the answer because everyone learns different stuff from A-Levels/IB, etc., but talk them through your thinking. For example, you can say something along the lines of 'I haven't come across this before, but from what I have learnt, I know that the structure is "X", so one possible solution could be "Y"'. They just want to see how you think and link what you know to their challenges.

I know it seems ironic because it's formal and professional, but keep it conversational, be yourself so you're comfortable, and try to have a good time because it's quite an incredible experience. It's meant to be a discussion rather than an interrogation!

Medical Student

For my Cambridge interview, I walked into a room with a series of bones on the table. I was passed the bones and asked what I knew about them, then asked to explain what movements I thought might happen at each joint. All my friends who did well said that the interviewers are less concerned about actual knowledge and more about applying what you know and problem solving. Obviously, prior knowledge is still good.

Medical Student

I got a bit of a grilling from a set of clinicians in my Cambridge interview. In one of them, they asked me a lot about the heart, and we worked through a problem using Poiseuille's law about blood flow through a vessel, so that was just basic maths. It's amazing how complicated some basic maths concepts can be when you are under pressure! That interview was sitting at a table, working things out on paper, but the other interview with clinicians was sitting on a couch. That didn't mean it was more laid back though!

Those clinicians picked out something from my personal statement (neurosurgery) to ask me about. They asked me about how you might want to control blood pressure during neurosurgery and how these drugs might work with regards to the diameter of a blood vessel. They tried to convince me to go back on a correct statement I had said, i.e. they wanted to catch me out, but I stood my ground, so be careful of stuff like that!

I think my main tip is to take your time; it's better not to make silly mistakes by answering questions too quickly!

Medical Student

PRACTICE QUESTIONS BASED ON OUR COMMON INTERVIEW THEMES

They say, 'Lovers of words have no place where honest work MUST be done'. Let's attempt to answer a selection of the most commonly encountered questions in a panel interview reported by our previous medical school applicants.

Before we start, I want to ask you something: How bad do you want to ace this interview? How bad do you want to succeed? Do you really want it, or do you just 'kind of' want it?

If you want to excel, you must start practising. Before looking at the answer, try writing your own answer. Simply apply the theory and techniques discussed so far.

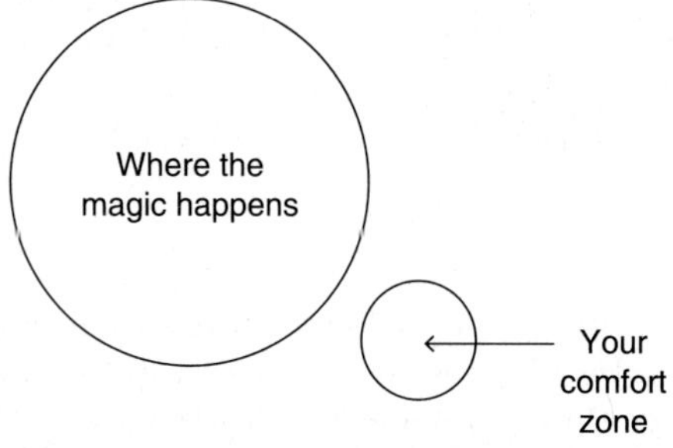

If you 'kind of' want to succeed, you're more than welcome to simply look at the answers without writing your own and without exercising your brain, but remember that as you're doing this, at the same time, someone is working harder than you. Someone is willing to put in the extra work, and if you're not careful, that someone might get a place at medical school instead. Yes, it will be frustrating. Yes, it will be tempting to skip straight to the answer, and you will feel uncomfortable, but that feeling proves that you are growing. Magic always happens when you're out of your comfort zone; always keep this in mind when you're tempted to take the easy path.

***Please note**: These questions can also be asked at an MMI interview during a random station.

PASSION, INSIGHT AND MOTIVATION FOR MEDICINE

Medicine is a challenging career, requiring both commitment and sacrifice. The training pathway is long and arduous, with 5 years at medical school, 2 years of foundation training and around 8 years of further training depending on your chosen speciality, not to mention that this is a career of lifelong learning. The job itself is both physically and emotionally demanding, with long working hours and the possibility of finding yourself in difficult situations. Furthermore, it costs approximately £220,000 to train a doctor!

Medical school admissions teams therefore need to know that you're getting into this profession for the right reasons, know exactly what you're getting yourself into and that you possess the motivation and drive needed to succeed at medical school and beyond. The last thing they want is for you to drop out during the degree, or worse, complete the degree and realise that medicine is something you no longer want to do.

Q1. Why do you want to do medicine?

 Write your draft answer to Q1 on a separate note.

This is perhaps the most important question you will ever encounter. It's essential not only for the application process but also for you as a person. Do you remember our Introduction? If you did write anything down as an answer to this question, compare your answer to see whether there's any difference between the two.

This question can be very daunting. There are several reasons why someone may want to be a doctor, but it is crucial to sit down and identify the real reason YOU want to be a medic. Reasons could include (but are not limited to):

- A strong interest in the sciences
- Wanting to help other people
- Wanting to combine the requirement for intellect and communication into a profession
- Wanting to work in a challenging environment
- Enjoying the dynamic nature of medicine
- Engaging in continuous learning
- Enjoying working with people
- Personal experience

All these reasons are more than valid but ensure that your own motives are clear. Do not simply list the reasons listed here. You may be motivated by some of these points; however, if you develop your answers and give them a personal touch, you are bound to be more memorable. If, for example, you enjoy the scientific element in medicine, you could describe what you enjoy about science. Is it pattern recognition when looking at chemistry assignments? This could help with diagnosing patients in the future. Could it be that it is both intellectual and practical? Dig deeper with your answers to show the interviewers that your answers are well thought out.

'Showing off' Your Work Experience

Remember all those months of work experience placements and volunteering projects? Now's the time to put them to good use. Students will have different work experience levels, whether in a GP clinic or observing a surgeon's work in theatre. What matters is not how fancy and exotic your work experience was but what you gained from it. You could discuss some interesting cases and discuss traits like empathy and good communication skills that the doctors possessed, which helped them deal with different situations. It is essential to go into detail and present how these experiences moulded your career choice.

'I've Always Been Interested in Studying Medicine'

Certain students claim to have been interested in medicine from a very young age. This is very possible if you nursed an elderly relative, experienced illness at a young age or worked with disadvantaged people early on in life...the options are endless! Several individuals could be in the same boat, so personalising your answers is essential. If, for example, you cared for your grandmother when you were younger, which motivated you to explore medicine as a career option, tell the interviewer more about this. Why did it inspire you? What did healthcare professionals do that interested you in medicine? What makes you think that just observing this situation at a young age makes it a suitable career option for you? It would be more beneficial for you to explain what you gained from this experience and why you would be ideal as a medic.

Using Your Personal Story

 If using a personal example involving any disease that you/your family have encountered in the past as a motivation, you must do it right.

Here's our top tip:

It's not about the disease or the suffering it caused; it is about the experience and the extra things you observed.

Stay away from being too personal. Think about it this way: What would I do if I were an engineer and my grandma got ill? Well, what would anyone do? I'd do my best to help her, but does that mean I'd be tempted to switch careers purely because of this? I wouldn't become a doctor in attempt to save my grandmother's life.

EVERYONE wants to help their family and relatives, but that's not what lights up your desire to study medicine; it's simply human evolution and a classic example of the limbic system in action. What fuels your passion is, in fact, the experience itself, being exposed to a particular disease early in life; observing the evolution, progression or regression of a disease; observing the impact of the illness on family relationships; observing the effects of the disease on an individual and so on.

Some optimists may even call it an opportunity to transform the negative burden of the disease into a learning experience. They are grateful for being exposed to such events early in life because this has motivated them to attempt to change the lives of others going through the same disease once they have qualified as doctors.

An extra point is the opportunity to interact with doctors from an early age. Yes, you can talk about all the negatives, but let's be honest, people don't listen to you when you complain. They love hearing about how you turned difficult times into positive learning experiences.

> I grew up with severe allergic asthma and often ended up in the hospital in the middle of the night with life-threatening episodes. It may sound strange, but even if I could, I would not change anything, and I am grateful to be where I am today. That is because I grew up surrounded by doctors and healthcare professionals who indirectly became my mentors and role models. I started dreaming and hoping that one day I could be as knowledgeable as them and remain an approachable and funny doctor who brings joy to children with asthma. It's not the disease that fuelled my passion; it is the encounters I had as a consequence of the disease.
>
> **Medical Student**

My Parents are Doctors

Some students are lucky to have other medics in their families. Although this can be advantageous when gaining work experience and a realistic understanding of the profession, it will not have much impact at an interview. It is more important for the interviewer to figure out whether you have the necessary qualities to be a doctor as opposed to the fact that you come from a medical family. In fact, they would even appreciate your determination to be the first doctor in the family.

Reasons for mentioning that your parents are doctors

- Realistic understanding of the profession
- Access to work experience
- Exposure to the world of medicine

Reasons against mentioning that your parents are doctors

- This interview is about YOU, not your parents
- May be seen as 'Mommy and Daddy's child'
- May seem that your parents are pushing you towards a career in medicine

It's up to you, but the main point is to avoid phrases such as 'Well, my dad always used to say…' because you may seem immature. You are at the moment in life when you need to portray maturity and stability. If your parents have inspired you, that's a great way to say it, but always appear grateful and avoid any comments that may portray you as arrogant.

Applying After Taking a Gap Year

Several students take gap years before applying to medical school. It is essential to explain what you learnt from your gap year. Perhaps you did some volunteer work that prepared you for medical school? Further insight is provided in our final chapter on this topic.

Applying as a Graduate

If you are applying as a graduate who has previously applied to medical school, you should explain how the past few years have helped you prepare. What experiences have you had, and what skills have you developed in your degree that would be useful for a career as a doctor?

As a graduate who hasn't previously applied to medical school, you could explain why your career options changed over the years and how you developed an interest in medicine from your course. Our final chapter dedicated to graduate applicants also fully explores this topic.

Okay, now that's a lot of stuff to remember. As a **summary**, Fig. 9.8 shows a structure you may want to use for 'Why medicine?' questions.

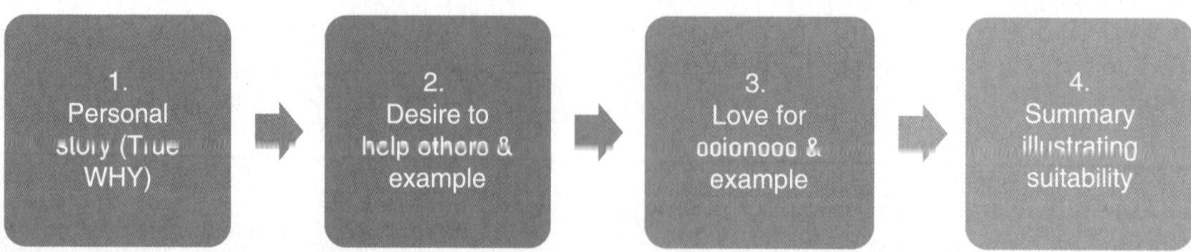

Fig. 9.8 Structuring 'why study medicine' answer.

As you may recall, we collated a couple of 'Why medicine' examples in the introduction chapter of this book. Go back and look again to refresh your memory.

Q2: Where do you see yourself in 5 to 10 years?

? Write your draft answer to Q2 on a separate note.

Most applicants we spoke to tended to give only half the answer that admission tutors look for. They start well, thinking logically, adding up years and thinking about career progression. 'Five or six years medical school plus two years as a foundation, then specialty training in my area of interest…'—perfect so far, but then they stop.

Is that all you'll be doing in 10 years? You see, our brain consists of two hemispheres—left and right. The left is logical, serious, rational and objective. The right is emotional, dreamy and creative. What often happens is that people only answer using their left hemisphere and neglect entirely their dreamer side. What about your family? Ten years is a long time; you may even have children and a happy family. What about your other dreams? What about research, setting up a charity or travelling—taking time to enjoy life?

They want humans, not machines, and even thinking about having a family at your stage makes you appear more mature.

This question should include two aspects (Fig. 9.9):

1. **The realist**: Logical career progression (left hemisphere)
2. **The dreamer**: Family and aims in life (right hemisphere)

Apart from the apparent goal of being a doctor, this question tests your self-awareness. Your answer could revolve around the following two aspects:

Work

- Career path: What stage of training will you be undergoing at the time?
- How have placements, internships, work experience and other courses helped you choose your career path?

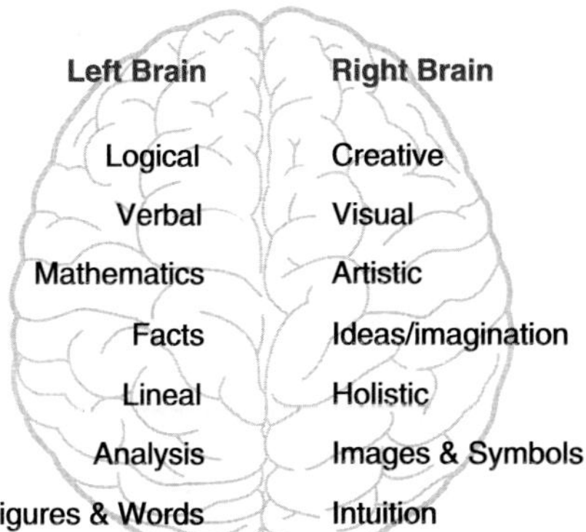

Fig. 9.9 Left and right brain.

- How medical school, conferences and seminars have given you an excellent background to build a career.
- What extra activities have you been involved in during this period (e.g. medical research)?

Play

- How your general life skills may have changed over the years (how you could work on any flaws you may have, e.g. 'I hope the next 5 years at medical school will help me improve my teaching skills. I enjoy teaching and previously taught a fellow student during my GCSEs, but I believe teaching is an avenue I'd like to explore further in the next few years').
- What about any hobbies that you may have developed over the years?
- Where do you hope to have travelled?
- What nonmedical goals do you wish to have achieved in 10 years?
- Finally, don't forget your family and friends!

> Top tip for extra points? Yes, please!
>
> Make your answer as vivid and animated as you can. Use descriptive terms and try to use this opportunity to let them know that you already dream of the moment when you'll receive an offer from them.
>
> For example, one version could be, 'The first image that came to mind when you asked me this question was my graduation ceremony from this medical school 6 to 7 years from now.' Then you can talk about career progression, an area of interest in medicine (or many, since not everyone wants to be a surgeon and most of us need to explore disciplines before committing to one), and conclude with a final remark about your desire to find time for your hobbies and friends, and who knows, perhaps even build a family!

Q3: How would you dissuade someone from going into medicine?

Well, your first instinct might be to say, 'WHY ON EARTH would I even do that after all the painful steps I've been through to apply to medicine?!'

To be honest, you're probably right to think so, but why do you think admission tutors may want to hear an answer to this question? Reflect and attempt to answer this question here.

? Write your draft answer to Q3 on a separate note.

This question can be a tricky one. It tests your understanding of the negatives of medicine. The key is to show an understanding of medicine as a strenuous career while reassuring the interviewer of your commitment to it.

Less positive aspects of medicine:

- Lifelong learning
- Stress
- Staying up to date
- Poor work–life balance
- Challenging encounters (e.g. angry patient)

There are many approaches to this question, but here's a good example given by one of our applicants during one of our mock interviews:

> This is a fascinating question, and I have to say from the beginning that I wouldn't try to dissuade someone from doing medicine in the first place unless I had a solid reason to believe that they may not be able to cope with a future career in medicine (acknowledging the question and keeping an open mind).
>
> However, I am grateful for the chance to learn about the LESS POSITIVE (not negative) aspects of medicine during my numerous discussions with the doctors I shadowed during my work experience placement (showing insight acquired through work experience). The healthcare professionals mentioned stress, lifelong learning and staying up to date as their top reasons. And it is indeed understandable given that doctors never stop learning and are exposed to high-stress situations daily.
>
> This being said, the same doctors I shadowed passionately taught me that they would never change anything in their profession. Lifelong learning keeps their brain active, curious and engaged. Stress has become their friend, and all the rewards that come after a day of work, including the gratitude received from those they help, allow them to love what they do. Although it may sound clichéd, I genuinely believe that if you love what you do, you'll never have to work for the rest of your life.
>
> Finally, I have to be honest. Although many of the less positive aspects of medicine may put others off, I would like to take them as a challenge. After all, they all serve as a positive learning experience. I'd like to use my skills enthusiastically to tackle every single one of these challenges to become a good doctor.
>
> **Medical School Applicant**

Other Example Questions

- Why not apply to nursing?
- You seem to love science, why not apply to a more scientific course (e.g. biomedicine)?
- What do you want to achieve as a doctor?
- What advice would you give to someone considering applying to medical school?

TRANSFERABLE SKILLS AND PERSONAL APTITUDES

This section is an opportunity for you to show off. The key here is to think about the skills you possess, how you have demonstrated them and why they are transferable and necessary for a career in medicine. Essentially, this is to see if you have the key attributes required for the medical profession.

Almost any skill you have can be tailored to fit the skills you may deem essential to be a doctor. Still, this chapter will help you focus on the key attributes sought after in medical school applicants. You may be asked to give evidence, so we strongly recommend that you have an example to show for the commonly tested skills!

Q4: Are you a leader or a follower?

 Write your draft answer to Q4 on a separate note.

The key to this question is establishing that you can be a leader OR a follower depending on the situation. In other words, you're just like a river—you are malleable, fluid and adaptable when encountering an obstacle along your journey.

Start by acknowledging the question and mention that through your projects, work experience and extracurricular activities, you had the opportunity to gain skills for both roles.

It would be helpful to give an example of a time when you were a leader and why it was necessary. For instance, 'During my sixth form, I was the athletics team captain. This experience taught me that strong leadership helps bring out the best in all team members. I helped organise athletic meets between schools and developed strategies that all sports team members would weigh in on instead of enforcing what I felt was right. After all, it is important to have input from all team members'.

Use an additional example to describe a time when you've been part of a team. You could then discuss that you would follow someone's lead as a team player. Following someone's lead helps you observe other people in charge. As a medic, you would not be the most senior member there in many situations. You would often have to follow someone in charge, and it is essential to the interviewer that you understand that sometimes it is just as important to take instruction as it is to give it.

Want to get some extra points? Talk about the concept of 'Shared Leadership'. If you want to refresh your memory about this, go back to Chapter 4.

> I was asked whether I was a follower or a leader. I gave two examples and thought I'd bring in some theory too. I explained what shared leadership is and how big of a crossover there is between teamwork and leadership. I think they really liked my personal example. I mentioned how leadership and teamwork are a must in an orchestra and how I observed this as a young violinist. During a concert, the role of the conductor was important, but it was as important as all our individual parts were!
>
> **Medical School Applicant**

Q5: How do you cope with conflict?

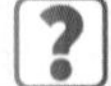 Write your draft answer to Q5 on a separate note.

The situation could be between team members, family members, colleagues in school, etc. Just remember to personalise the issue by giving an example. It doesn't matter what you choose as an example—be it when you fought with your sister because you ate her cookies or that one time when you and your best friend fought, simply use the following principles to help you.

1. **Acknowledge the conflict**—'I realise it's upsetting you, and I'm trying my best to understand why.'
2. **Gather further information**—'Let's talk about it. Could you tell me more about it? I want to get this right.'
3. **Identify the problem and apologise**—'I did not know you felt this way; I am truly sorry about this.'
4. **Ask for ideas and choose the solution together**—'What do you think we should do? Perhaps we could… What are your thoughts?'
5. **Action plan**—'If this were to happen again, what can we do differently?'

If you can't remember any of these steps, I saw a straightforward diagram in a children's book that always reminds me of what you can do to resolve a conflict (Fig. 9.10). In summary, don't be a mouse or a monster. Be yourself.

Q6: Give me an example of a time you showed leadership and something went wrong.

? Write your draft answer to Q6 on a separate note.

Description: When I started the medical society with two of my peers, we were not confident regarding public speaking, open presentations and teaching. Looking back, I must admit that our first session lacked the necessary preparation and engagement techniques that I later learned about. Needless to say, the attendance rate for our next session dropped, and the remaining ones looked disinterested.

Feelings: Despite the initial frustration and disappointment, I didn't feel demotivated and called a team meeting. We came up with suggestions such as more active involvement. I also proposed a structured session with multiple segments, allowing me to delegate tasks to different members, which increased involvement and added variety.

Evaluation/Analysis: This experience was helpful as it helped me develop communication skills and learn how to teach effectively. I also learnt how to overcome the initial setback and use leadership skills to try and improve the situation.

Conclusion (try to wrap it up here): Overall, this was a significant learning experience, and through it, I feel more prepared for the future. Over time, attendance increased, and the next school year saw an extra 11 pupils sign up compared to the previous year.

Action plan (If the same situation came up): If the same problem came up in the future, I feel I would know what to do. I genuinely hope to apply these leadership and communication skills in medical school and in the future.

Look at the structure here and how it elevates the content of the answer. The experience itself isn't the focus here, but rather the lessons learnt and the reflections the student has made. Medical schools love seeing students reflecting and learning from their mistakes, you'll be doing it a lot in your career!

Other Potential Questions

- What is your greatest strength?
- What is your greatest weakness?
- What attributes do you possess that would make you a good doctor?
- Give an example of a time where you demonstrated communication skills.
- Talk about a time where you were in a position of leadership.

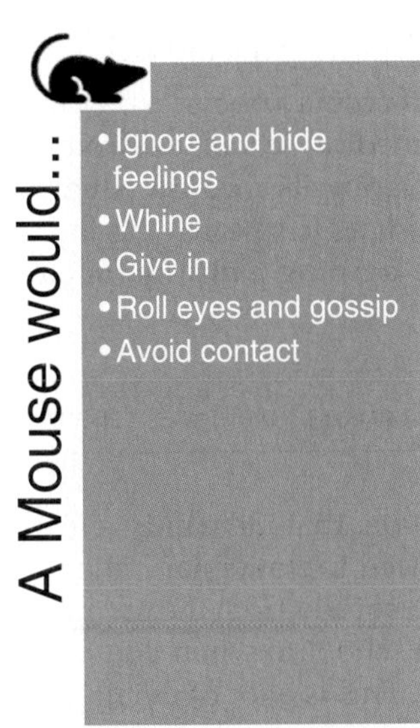

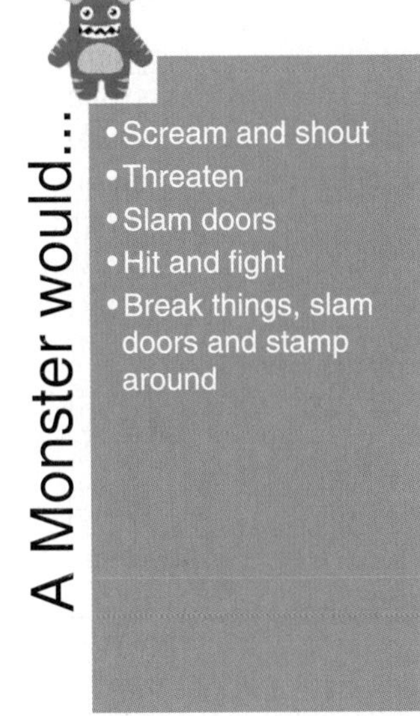

A Mouse would...
• Ignore and hide feelings

• Roll eyes and gossip

A Monster would...
• Scream and shout

• Slam doors
• Hit and fight
• Break things, slam doors and stamp around

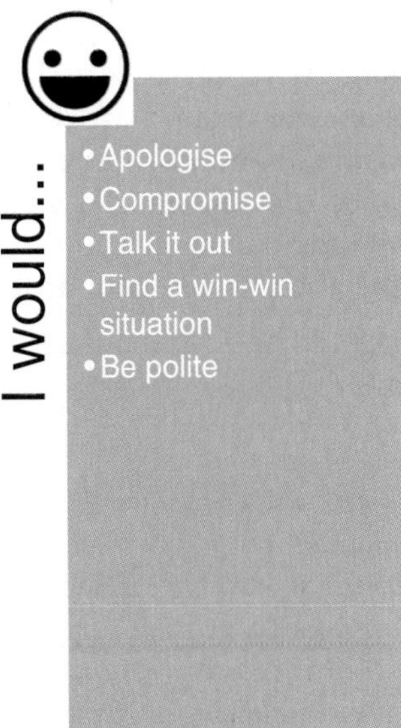
I would...
• Apologise
• Compromise
• Talk it out
• Find a win-win situation
• Be polite

Fig. 9.10 Models of handling conflict.

WORK–LIFE BALANCE AND COPING WITH STRESS

Stress can affect everyone in different ways. If unidentified or poorly managed, this can hinder your performance and negatively affect your wellbeing. However, if harnessed and utilised correctly, some people find that their performance thrives when put under stress.

It is healthy to identify areas of stress in your life. Although eliminating those factors is not always possible, developing methods to deal with them is crucial. Medical school can be a challenging time for students, and the interviewers want to see that you can cope. The last thing they want is someone dropping out halfway through the course!

Q7: How do you deal with stress?

 Write your draft answer to Q7 on a separate note.

There are three main facets you should consider when answering these questions:

Mind: What do you do to relax your mind?—'I like to keep a journal and reflect on how I'm feeling at the end of the day. It helps me to release any built-up emotions'.

Body: How do you take care of your physical fitness?—'I also recognise the importance of activities that keep me physically fit. I believe that a healthy body leads to a healthy mind, so I go on a 5-km run twice a week to take care of myself. It also releases a lot of endorphins which helps with my mood'.

Social circle: Doctors also need social support! Applicants often neglect this theme: 'It's helpful for me to discuss personal issues, and I often go to my friends for support. I'm looking forward to maintaining my current friendships while developing new ones at medical school!'

In your answers, make sure to go over all three aspects! Applicants often talk about individual activities such as listening to music or playing sports without addressing why these actually help them. By basing your answer around aspects of mental health instead of basing it around what you actually do, your response stands out and makes you look capable of handling anything that comes your way.

Q8: Tell me about a time you dealt with stress.

 Write your draft answer to Q8 on a separate note.

'A notable time I felt stressed was last year in the lead-up to my netball trials. I play goal shoot, so a substantial skill I have to master is shooting the ball through the hoop. I ensured I left myself a reasonable amount to practice and prepare for the trials; however, I could feel myself getting anxious in the weeks leading up to the trial. As a result, my sleep was poor, and my energy levels were reduced. This had a detrimental effect on my practice, meaning I kept missing sessions and worked myself up into an even more stressed mindset, negatively impacting my performance. This started to become a downward cycle.

However, I am pleased to say I identified that my lack of sleep and poor performance was likely stress related. Once I identified this, I was able to put into place steps to manage my stress. For example, I would only allow myself to practice an hour a day and would not punish myself for my performance. This helped alleviate the pressure from my practice. I would also allow myself to unwind before going to sleep, vastly improving my sleep quality. By putting these measures into practice, I felt better prepared, rested and calmer by the time the trials came around.'

Notice the structure here! The answer uses the Gibbs' reflective cycle to effectively convey what happened. The first paragraph is the description, feelings and analysis stages, and the second paragraph talks about her conclusion and action plan. Make use of these reflective cycles to effectively convey your message!

Other Questions

- How can stress be beneficial to a doctor?
- What hobbies do you have?
- Why is work–life balance important?

THE UK MEDICAL SCHOOL TRAINING PROGRAMME

Part 1: Career Progression

Medicine is not a career for the faint-hearted, so interviewers will want to find out if you have done your homework and are aware of what lies ahead of you. The goal here is to ensure that you have reasonable expectations of the challenges ahead and the skills required to cope with these pressures in the future. By showing that you have thought about the training pathway and career progression, you will illustrate to the interviewer that you fully understand how you will progress after starting medical school.

To gain insight into the path of medicine in the UK, we recommend that each student have a reasonable knowledge of the steps to become a doctor and eventually reach consultancy. Each medical school will have a totally different way of delivering its medical education, so it is important for candidates to research this thoroughly.

Q9: What is the training pathway for a doctor after graduation?

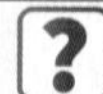 Write your draft answer to Q9 on a separate note.

This is a question that demands a chronological answer. You will need to understand the process from start to finish—specifically from the moment you graduate from medical school to when you complete your speciality training. This is a lot of detail to convey in a short period of time but provided you can outline the general process, this will provide a suitable answer, as the interviewer only wants to see that you understand how the training pathway works and will ask you for further detail only if required. It is important to keep your answer succinct and relatively brief; it is all too easy to get bogged down in detail!

> *'After graduating from medical school, graduates will become provisionally registered with the General Medical Council and join the National Foundation Training Programme. The programme lasts for 2 years, during which they will work as junior doctors to gain experience and exposure to medicine under supervision and whilst completing core competencies.*
>
> *The junior doctors will then gain full GMC registration upon successful completion of foundation year one. In foundation year two, the junior doctors work more independently whilst developing their portfolio and taking on greater responsibilities.*
>
> *After completion of the foundation years, the training diverges into a few pathways: General Practice Specialty Training (GPST), Internal Medicine and Medical Specialty Training or Surgical Specialty Training. These pathways vary in length, with the GPST being the shortest at 3 years. Still, all pathways overlap in a few ways—you will be expected to pass the examinations for membership or fellowship of the appropriate Royal College, and all pathways culminate in a Certificate of Completion of Training (CCT). The CCT allows you to apply for consultant posts, and many doctors voluntarily undertake further training and professional development. Additionally, many pathways require annual revalidation.'*

However, do keep in mind that this answer goes into a lot of detail. Only a general understanding is necessary for this question, but students are still expected to know a few different pathways and the overall progression pathway.

Part 2: Picking an Individual Medical School

This is a MUST prepare question as over half of our applicants have encountered it in both panel and MMI scenarios. If this comes up, I am afraid you can't just tell them that you've only decided to go there because of their lower UCAT and BMAT threshold, even if that may be the case!

Preparation for 'Why this medical school?':

- Thoroughly research their website.
- Visit the medical school during open days.
- Speak to students or friends from there if possible.
- Access online forum groups and join the discussion.

Key points to cover in your answer (Fig. 9.11):

1. Course structure (e.g. early patient contact, dissections)
2. Teaching style (e.g. integrated, PBL, traditional)—what makes it unique?
3. Community feeling, extracurricular and location
4. Extra: Research interests/reputation

We suggest starting with the academic side, rather than going into societies or how fun the city is at the beginning.

Answer using a simple, three-point structure as explained in our 'Introduction, Body and Conclusion' technique described earlier. Here's a rough structure for you to adapt and build upon.

Introduction

Selecting the right medical school certainly wasn't easy, but after I researched and read about X Medical School, I knew this was where I would like to train as a medical student. Several things made me choose this medical school; however, I would like to focus on three aspects that truly resonate with me as a person.

Body

1. The medical school's values of placing patients at the centre of their teaching, providing early patient exposure (continue explaining why).
2. The PBL approach not only makes this course unique but also matches my personality and skills perfectly (continue with evidence of teamwork skills, self-motivated attitude and so on in this case).
3. The sense of belonging and community emphasised by current medical students at your institution (continue with the importance of stress relief, extracurricular activities, etc.).

Conclusion

These three reasons explain my strong desire to join this medical school instead of any other. I hope that one day I will be part of this fast-growing, internationally renowned institution and give something back as a student (providing vision).

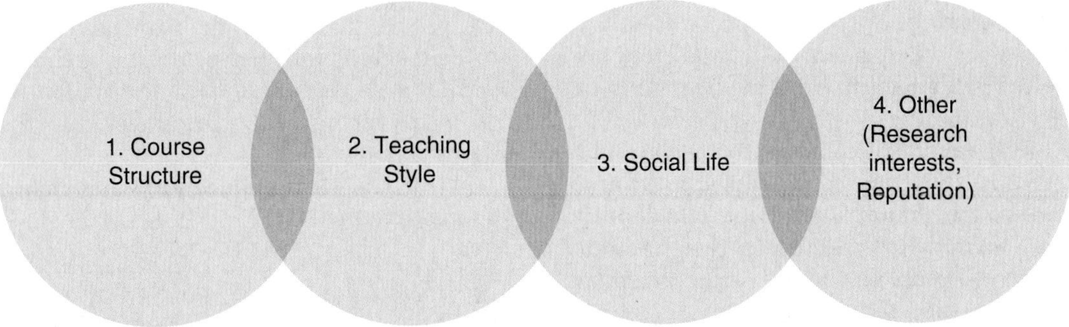

Fig. 9.11 Picking an individual medical school.

The previous structure is relatively general and must be personalised with real examples that can be taken either from the university's website, your conversation with medical students or any friends you may have from there.

Avoid generalising statements that could apply to ANY medical school in the UK. For example, if you talk about their PBL approach, you need to be more specific about how that fits into their whole curriculum and what may make it unique from other medical schools that do PBL too. Another example would be mentioning the reputation of a medical school, especially if it isn't at the top of the league table. The interviewers could challenge you and say, 'Well if you wanted a high reputation, why did you not choose Cambridge or Oxford instead of us?'

Q10: What do you know about PBL compared to traditional teaching methods?

 Write your draft answer to Q10 on a separate note.

This is a knowledge-based question that looks at your understanding of the different teaching methods in medical schools in the UK. It assesses how well you know your own way of learning and if you have considered this when choosing medical schools.

Traditional teaching

For the traditional courses, students begin their training with 2 years of 'preclinical' work involving the study of the basic medical sciences. This is followed by a 'clinical' course of approximately 3 years, during which they work in hospital wards under the supervision of consultants.

Throughout the final 3 years, they also attend lectures on all aspects of medical practice. This is a subject-based course of lectures, where, for example, you would undertake anatomy, physiology, biochemistry, etc., all as separate courses.

This type of teaching tends to have the traditional preclinical/clinical break after the third year, with almost all teaching being lecture based.

Medical schools in the UK that offer this style include Oxford, Cambridge, UCL, Imperial and a few select others.

Problem-based learning

PBL is a very patient-oriented approach, and students can expect to see patients right from the beginning of their course.

Students are given medical cases to resolve and learn from, guided by group work with a tutor and self-directed learning. On top of academic and clinical learning, group work helps students develop communication, teamwork, problem-solving skills, personal responsibility and respect for others.

PBL has an 'open inquiry' approach, where facilitators play a minimal role and do not guide the discussion. There are now very few medical schools in the UK using a pure PBL approach to curriculum delivery. Generally, there is a more blended approach with more facilitator interaction and the provision of lectures and seminars to support the individuals' learning.

Medical schools in the UK that offer this style include Liverpool, Manchester, Glasgow, Queen Mary, Peninsula, Sheffield, Keele, Hull and York, Bart's and East Anglia.

My question was based on the various medical school teaching methods. I gave a thorough description, which seemed to please the interviewers. 'Excellent, well done—so which one's better?' My brain froze, and the only thing I could think of at the time was that PBL is innovative and new, and because this medical school was using it, I thought it had to be better. Not surprisingly, the interviewer concluded the question: 'Oh okay, so then Cambridge has got it totally wrong...'

Medical School Applicant

Avoid choosing one over the other, as there isn't clear evidence to favour one teaching style over another. Come up with examples of positives and negatives for each teaching method and conclude by saying that it does, in the end, depend on the personality of the individual applying. Use your own personal skills and learning style as examples and say why you prefer a particular teaching style over the other (hopefully the one that the institution interviewing you uses) but mention that this may differ from person to person. Just keep an open mind.

Other Potential Questions

- What is your plan after you graduate from medical school?
- What is foundation training?
- Are you planning on doing an iBSc (if noncompulsory) or an MBPhD (if available)?

NHS AND OTHER SIGNIFICANT ORGANISATIONS WITHIN THE UK

This is an important theme that is likely to come up in your interviews. Be sure to know all the major health-related organisations in the UK (including the NHS, CQC, GMC and NICE), their role and any important details (such as the core principles and values of the NHS). It's also a good idea to learn about the current challenges facing healthcare systems in the UK and internationally.

Q11: If you were chancellor, what changes would you make to the NHS?

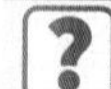 Write your draft answer to Q11 on a separate note.

This question tests your understanding of the problems in the NHS, the national budget and whether you have a realistic approach to the issues.

It is essential to address key issues faced by the NHS today:

An Ageing Population

The NHS was set up to treat people with diseases. Many diseases that would have killed people 65 years ago have been cured, which is brilliant. While it means people are living for longer, they often live with one or more illnesses (complex long-term conditions) such as diabetes, heart and kidney disease. In turn, this needs ongoing treatment and specialist care. Example solution: There is a lack of local services such as district nurses, beds in community hospitals and mental health support due to the ever-rising demand for care from accident and emergency (A&E) units and hospitals running out of beds. All those services are hectic because of the rising number of older people with complex medical needs and therefore have waiting lists.

Lifestyle Factors

Drinking too much alcohol, smoking, a poor diet with not enough fruit and vegetables and not doing enough exercise are all primary reasons for becoming unwell and needing to rely on health services. The increasing prevalence of overweight children encapsulates the upwards trend of this issue. Examples of a solution: awareness programmes, sugar tax, compulsory exercise programmes for children in school and healthier school lunches.

Accident and Emergency Departments

An ageing population, increased illnesses and falls during the winter, cuts to social welfare, long general practice (GP) wait times and NHS 111 sending more people to A&E are all reasons why A&E is experiencing a strain. Examples of a solution: helping patients' access primary, social and preventative care to stop unplanned admissions to A&E and freeing up acute beds for patients who need them.

Mental Health Support

More people are diagnosed every year with mental health issues. Providing support to patients is of utmost importance, and we need accessible psychological services and public health campaigns destigmatising mental health issues and increasing self-awareness of warning signs. There has been an increase in the number of children suffering from anxiety, mood disorders or challenging behaviour, such as anger and aggression. Due to cuts in social care, voluntary sector services and preventative care, the number of cases being referred to services has doubled. Capacity is much less than the demand, so waiting lists are growing exponentially. Example solutions: have children and adult services work hand in hand and increase the budget for mental health services.

It is estimated that without radical changes to how the system works, the rise in demand and costs will mean the NHS will become unsustainable, with tremendous financial pressures and debts. If no changes are made, there may be a £30 billion funding gap for the NHS nationally by 2020.

Staffing Crisis

The NHS has always struggled with retaining staff, despite being the 10th biggest employer in the world! This has recently worsened, and healthcare services across the UK have suffered from increased waiting times, poorer quality of care and increased demand on existing healthcare staff. More and more NHS staff are leaving for better pay and better conditions in the private sector, other industries or even overseas. This is worsening due to the effects of Brexit and the pandemic, which is driving the NHS to the breaking point.

Of course, this issue has been summarised to ease your understanding. It is up to you to learn more and focus on one aspect extensively in preparation for your interview.

Q12: What are the arguments for and against the sale of tobacco?

 Write your draft answer to Q12 on a separate note.

Yet another classic question encountered in both panel and MMI situations.

For

- Tobacco sales generate revenue for the government via taxation. This money is pumped into social services, i.e. the NHS.
- Tobacco farmers in developing countries get their income from the industry, and banning tobacco sales would lead to severe unemployment in such countries.
- People have the right to choose if they want to damage their bodies via smoking.
- Banning tobacco would lead to the development of a black market—one that would not be under government regulation; this would mean that people with tobacco-related illnesses would be less likely to seek medical attention for fear of prosecution.

Against

- Tobacco leads to severe respiratory diseases that are burdening the NHS, such as emphysema and COPD.
- Smoking impacts other people as well as those who are exposed to second-hand smoke. They have not actively made the choice that smokers have. Babies of mothers who smoke have no choice, and the government has to protect innocents such as these.
- Cigarette addiction could perhaps act as a gateway to addiction to other harmful substances.

It is crucial to produce a balanced argument. This applies to any 'for' and 'against' type of question.

Remember, if there's a debate, keep an open mind and don't make any assumptions. Another tip is to avoid using strong words such as 'obviously', 'must', 'definitely', 'always' and so on. Instead, try leaving room for doubt and different opinions by using words such as 'should', 'may', 'perhaps', 'could' or 'might'.

Other Questions to Consider

- What is the role of the GMC in the UK?
- How do you think modern technological developments could impact the challenges the NHS is currently facing?
- What are the founding principles of the NHS?
- Name one core value of the NHS and explain it.
- What are your views on the privatisation of the NHS?

ETHICAL OR MEDICO-LEGAL SCENARIOS

In life, we face ethical dilemmas quite often. But as a doctor, your decision to handle the difficulties will have long-lasting or even life-changing effects on your patients and their relatives.

This is one of the most common sections tested in interviews and assesses your ethical reasoning. For these questions, ensure you know the four main ethical pillars, important concepts such as competence, and relevant historical cases. It's also a good idea to be up to date with any current medical cases worldwide.

The interviewers here are looking for sensible and logical thinking, going down every possible path and seeing the issue from different angles and lenses.

You should, therefore:

- Demonstrate your coherent chain of thoughts
- Balancing the pros and cons, and the interests of all the stakeholders
- Act in the best interest of your patients

You will learn more regulations in medical school and beyond. But if you cannot think and act ethically, knowing all the regulations will not enable you to practise medicine ethically. This is important as one unethical act by a doctor could jeopardise the integrity of medical professionals, affecting doctors' relationships with patients and the general public.

Q13: What would you do if a mother comes into A&E with a child who is profusely bleeding and refuses to administer a blood transfusion?

 Write your draft answer to Q13 on a separate note.

This is a typical example of an ethics question you may face in an interview. If you started thinking back to the ethical principles discussed in our previous chapter, that's fantastic! Here are a few extra things to consider here:

Do not be quick to conclude that this mother is a Jehovah's Witness. It is a known fact that Jehovah's Witnesses do not accept blood donations due to religious beliefs; however, the mother in this situation may fear the procedure itself. It is important to understand why she is against the transfusion—she might not understand the severity of the situation, what a blood transfusion entails, dislike the idea of having someone else's blood in her child, etc. Once you identify the issue, you can decide what approach to take.

If the child is deemed competent per the 'Fraser guidelines' (look into this!), they can make their own decisions. If the child is conscious *and* able to decide, this is considered. Your communication skills will be tested when dealing with the mother whom your decision may anger.

If the child is not considered competent, consent must be obtained from the mother. Suppose the mother is concerned about the practical issues surrounding the procedure. In that case, it is your job to use your listening skills and empathy to reassure her about the cleanliness of the procedure and the risks of not having a blood transfusion. You could involve senior members of staff who could help with this.

If the mother still refuses treatment, either on principle or underlying religious belief, the decision to treat would have to be based on the child's best interests. As the situation is an emergency, you need to be sure that you can be held accountable for your decisions should there be a case made against you in court. If the situation is not an emergency, discussing the case at a multidisciplinary team meeting and/or getting a court order to carry out the treatment would be advisable. In any case, try to speak with senior members or the hospital's legal team when making decisions of this nature.

Make sure you mention the core ethical principles to get full marks. Do go back to our Medical Ethics chapter and refresh your memory about how to tackle an ethical dilemma.

Q14: A 15-year-old girl has been in a car accident and no longer has brain activity (is brain-dead). However, the parents still believe she is alive and will wake up if given enough time to heal. She currently depends on external assistance to survive (mechanical ventilation, artificial nutrition, etc.), and you know that her recovery is extremely unlikely. Given her parents' wishes to keep her 'alive', would you, as the doctor responsible, keep life support on or turn it off?

 Write your draft answer to Q14 on a separate note.

This is a common ethical scenario in interviews and is a challenging exercise to reason through. Remember to use the pillars of medical ethics in all questions to do with ethics to break them down! We've put together a step-by-step guide to reasoning through any case in the following:

Step 1: Start by identifying which pillars are relevant in the case and why they are relevant. Note that only some pillars are applicable in each ethical case! In this case, all four are relevant, but it is very rare; most cases only involve two to three ethical pillars. You could say something similar to:

'This is a challenging case as it involves all the ethical pillars of justice, beneficence, non-maleficence and autonomy.'

Justice: This child is taking up a lot of hospital resources in a stressful time for the NHS (using up a bed on a ward, multiple life support machines and lots of staff), which could be used to treat other patients.

Beneficence: Could letting this child peacefully pass away be better than keeping her alive with machines? In this case, the act of taking away her life may actually be in her best interest.

Nonmaleficence: Ending life support could be seen as directly harming the patient as it will lead to her death. Is this an ethical thing to do?

Autonomy: Her parents arguably have autonomy as their child currently lacks capacity. They want to keep their child on life support, so would it be a violation of autonomy to go against their wishes?

Step 2: Explain that the reason why these cases are complex is that the ethical pillars conflict with each other or that each ethical pillar can be interpreted differently. For example:

'Beneficence and non-maleficence here are conflicting as, on the one hand, you could argue that keeping life support on is cruel and harms the patient. However, turning off life support will kill the patient and prevent her from waking up, which could be interpreted as causing harm.

Furthermore, the pillar of justice could also be debated in this case. Some could argue that everyone has a right to treatment and that even if the chances of recovery are low, everyone is entitled to an opportunity to do so. However, this case takes a lot of resources that could otherwise be used to save others' lives who have a higher chance of recovery. Is it fair to others that the resources are being spent on someone unlikely to survive?'

Step 3: If they ask you what you would do, try to keep your answer as loose as possible. If you give a solid and firm answer that you think is 'correct', you open yourself up to be challenged. A good technique to use is the 'ideal world' technique which goes as follows:

'In an ideal world, I would try to communicate with the parents and answer any of their concerns first. This may be a case of them not understanding what no brain activity means, or they may be in shock, in which case I would involve other team members, such as a palliative specialist or psychologist. I would try to make the parents understand that it may be beneficial for everyone to turn off life support and provide them with additional help on dealing with grief and other mental health support.'

In this answer, you can see how you give the most ideal scenario, which means that if challenged, you can move on to the next point like this:

'However, I realise that we don't live in a perfect world, and there may be a case where the parents refuse to turn off life support. In this case, I would first escalate the issue to my superiors and ask for advice on how to proceed. I may also seek legal advice to assess whether to bring this to court for intervention. It is a challenging case involving a lot of emotion, so I would not attempt to solve this by myself, and I would work with the team to ensure we come up with an adequate solution.'

You can see how you can use this format whenever you're challenged. Keep talking about different situations with different variables, and never firmly say that this is what you would do. Always come across as someone flexible who changes what they would do based on what's presented.

Example Questions

Assume two patients come in needing a liver transplant. One patient is a 56-year-old man with liver cirrhosis due to his drinking habits. The other patient is a 13-year-old girl who has a congenital liver disease. Assume both operations have an equal chance of success.

- Who would you give the liver to and why?
- What factors should and shouldn't be considered in cases like these?
- What are the four pillars of medical ethics, and why are they important?
- How would you approach providing contraception to someone under the age of 16?
- What is consent?
- What is confidentiality?
- What is capacity?
- What is the difference between ethics and law?

HISTORY AND THE DIFFERENT ROLES OF A DOCTOR

Part 1: History

Knowing a bit about the history of medicine is crucial for medical school interviews! We recommend learning at least five key events and why they were significant. We also recommend knowing about current developments and potential future discoveries so remember to keep up to date on your healthcare news.

Q15: Ten years ago, doctors used to wear white coats and now very few do. Why do you think this is the case?

 Write your draft answer to Q15 on a separate note.

Two issues need to be addressed in this situation:

- **Infection control:** White coats were initially designed as protection from infection in a hospital.

However, they were later realised to be carriers of infectious agents as they were rarely cleaned.

- **Doctor–patient relationship:** Medicine has moved from a 'doctor knows best' approach, where doctors were pedestaled, to a more 'patient-centred' approach. White coats acted as an artificial barrier between the medical professional and the layperson. As doctors now aim to get closer to patients and build better doctor–patient relationships, patients must see doctors as people they can trust, not so different from themselves.

Q16: What do you think is the most significant discovery in medical history?

 Write your draft answer to Q16 on a separate note.

'There have been several notable discoveries in the history of medicine, including the discovery of antibiotics, anaesthesia and the structures of the human body.'

Show off that you know multiple notable events! The interviewers will be impressed that you can name so many.

'However, the one that resonates with me most is the development of the vaccine by Edward Jenner. He was the pioneer of the first ever vaccine and was directly responsible for the eradication of smallpox which at that time was a major disease which killed hundreds of millions of people. Vaccines have already saved more than this number and are perhaps the most significant lifesaving discovery in history.'

Then dive into more detail about your selected one. Show off some knowledge and understanding of the topic.

'I particularly like the development of vaccinations as it uses evidence-based medicine. Edward Jenner used observations and results to test a hypothesis and developed a medical treatment using this evidence. I hope to use similar scientific techniques in the future in my research to develop something of my own which is beneficial to the medical field.'

Then in the final bit, relate it to yourself and why you chose the example. Don't be afraid to throw in a few keywords and personal reflections

Other questions

- Who do you think was the most influential individual in the history of medicine?
- What discoveries do you think will be the most important in the future?
  Choose three significant events in the history of medicine and discuss how relevant they are today.
- Which significant figure in the history of medicine do you think made the biggest impact?
- What current pieces of research interest you?

Part 2: Roles of a Doctor

Most of the general public has the impression that all doctors do is practical work, from surgeries to clinics. However, the role of a doctor encompasses more than that and includes teaching, research and managing.

Q17: What are the different roles of a doctor?

 Write your draft answer to Q17 on a separate note.

You should have a basic idea of what doctors do! The following is an answer that details the different roles and what they encompass. Be sure to demonstrate you know what being a doctor entails and that you know about the job!

'Although doctors are often only seen as practitioners, doctors have multiple roles, including research, teaching and managing.

Firstly, as practitioners, doctors are responsible for diagnosing diseases, carrying out consultations, communicating effectively with patients and colleagues, prescribing drugs and much more.

However, they also have a significant role in research and academia. Research plays an essential role in medicine by influencing clinical guidelines and ensuring efficacious clinical decision making. It is essential at each stage of the treatment process, from prevention to cure. I hope to explore this further in an intercalated degree while studying at medical school.

Furthermore, teaching is another core responsibility of a doctor. In hospitals and local practices, there are staff members at different levels of seniority. To ensure the next generation of healthcare practitioners can effectively learn and develop their skills to improve patient outcomes, those with more experience often teach and pass on their knowledge. This is crucial in maintaining quality clinical care and is a major part of the training pathway.

Lastly, doctors also have a role as leaders and managers. Being a good doctor entails working effectively in teams, providing leadership to colleagues and sharing a vision with the organisations and hospitals in which they work.'

Again, keep it brief and don't bore the interviewer with an essay in each role. You should demonstrate an understanding of the different roles but be careful not to go beyond this! If, for example, you focus too much on research, you open yourself up to being asked, 'so why not study biomedicine and go into research?'

Other questions to consider

- Why is research an important part of being a doctor?
- Do you want to teach in the future?
- Why are leadership skills important in medicine?

WORK EXPERIENCE

The majority of medical schools will have a station or a question about work experience as part of their interview. This is a relatively simple station providing you put in a bit of preparation in advance and reflect on your experiences. Remember that medical schools are aware that candidates will have had varying opportunities to obtain clinical shadowing, so while it is helpful if you can gain that, it is arguably more important to obtain hands-on experience where you are developing and demonstrating skills, whether that be in the caring setting or elsewhere. Always check the requirements of individual medical schools, as some require hands-on experience specifically of a caring nature, while others do not.

A common mistake is to think that work experience is a simple box that can only be ticked if you shadow doctors in the hospital environment. Witnessing extensive surgeries and innovative patient care is not helpful if you cannot explain exactly what you gained from it. It is also not about assisting surgeons and trying to appear more knowledgeable than you are. You need to be able to show **TRANSFERRABLE SKILLS**. You need to have the building blocks—the foundation on which you can add through your time at medical school.

Q18: Discuss a work experience you've had and what you learnt from it.

? Write your draft answer to Q18 on a separate note.

This question aims to explore what you feel you have gained from your work experience and/or volunteering. It is not focused on **how much** experience you have gained or how clinical it is. You should be able to reflect on the experiences and why they will make you a good medical student, i.e. in the form of skills developed or insight into a medical career.

'I undertook 2 years of weekly volunteering in a care home as the activities coordinator. This involved helping with organising events such as bingo and sing-a-longs for the residents, as well as spending time with residents on a one-to-one basis, providing them with company and providing some personal care.

From this, I developed my team working skills when organising events with other volunteers and care home staff. Contact with residents with dementia has increased my confidence in communicating with individuals with cognitive issues, triggering me to reflect on my approachability and develop different communication techniques. I have also undertaken a week of work experience on the respiratory ward of a hospital. Here I was able to observe the importance of being able to work as part of a team, particularly emphasised when I attended multidisciplinary team meetings.

For example, an elderly postoperative patient was found to have no care system at home. Communication within the team and input from staff members with different skills (e.g. OT, physio) enabled the discharge coordinator to arrange home care and ensure that they were adequately supported. This also emphasised the importance of holistic care.'

Remember that medical schools are aware that some candidates have more opportunities than others to arrange work experience, especially in a clinical setting. They will not penalise you for not having extensive clinical experience but will expect you to demonstrate that you have developed skills through something extracurricular. This may be a role in the school student leadership team, involvement with sports or volunteering in the community. Anything that gives you transferrable skills can be reflected on and made relevant to a medical career.

Q19: What makes a good doctor?

 Write your draft answer to Q19 on a separate note.

Although this question isn't directly related to work experience, don't be fooled! It is very important to include observations and reflections that you have made on your experiences. You may be able to talk about how you read about the important skills of a doctor, but it is much more powerful to draw from experience. A sample answer could be something similar to the following:

'I believe that several qualities make up a good doctor such as empathy, compassion, communication and many more. However, from my work experiences, the skills I want to focus the most on are communication skills, leadership and teamwork.

Firstly, communication is a skill that is necessary across every aspect and speciality of medicine. I got the chance to shadow a GP whom I saw listen attentively without interrupting the patient and then further explored the patient's potential treatments with them. The patient felt reassured and thanked the doctor with a smile for simply taking the time to listen to her. With recent developments in the NHS long-term plan with themes such as wider integration of shared decision-making, this skill is necessary in today's world.

Secondly, leadership brings structure to the team and is often crucial. I chose this skill as I saw the necessity of decision-making through my work experience in the surgical theatre, where the chief surgeon would effectively delegate tasks and ensure the team worked together efficiently.

Lastly, teamwork is a skill that I've seen and one which I have developed in my own time. Medicine is a subject which involves a multidisciplinary approach, and doctors work with colleagues in different departments. I was fortunate enough to join an MDT meeting where different members, including nurses, oncologists, heart surgeons and radiologists, all worked together to develop the best treatment for a patient. The use of shared leadership in cases like these, where leadership is distributed among all members of a team, ensures coordination and the highest quality care for a patient.

As you can see, several good qualities make up a good doctor, and I have tried to develop these skills in my own time through extracurriculars and other activities.'

Although this isn't the most extended answer, it is very well structured and will keep the listener engaged. Most of the time, the interviewer will cut you off if your answer gets too long, as they have other questions to get through, so you may not be able to finish your answer. Remember to keep it short and succinct; if they do cut you off, it could be a good thing! The interviewers often move on to the next question when they're satisfied that you know what you're talking about.

Follow-up Questions

- What key skills have you observed during your work experience, and how have you developed them?
- Discuss a situation from your work experience or volunteering where something could have been done better. What would you have done differently?
- What communication skills did you observe/develop during your work experiences, and why is it important?

MMIS

Before we jump into various examples, two essential tips have been shared by tens, if not hundreds, of applicants and medical students:

The first secret to acing MMIs is practising as much as possible before your real attempt. We've had quotes in different shapes and forms—some students feeling grateful for putting in the hard work to practice, others feeling sorry for not doing more mock interviews as they found the actual interview very distressing.

> During my first mocks, I could not concentrate and could not get the previous questions out of my mind. What if I said something stupid? What if I failed that station? During one question, I almost started crying. However, the more I practised, the more the process became mechanical, and habitual even, up to the point where I would read a question and be able to concentrate purely on that without considering what I may have messed up previously. My top tip would be: Get as much practice under simulated interview conditions as possible; it will save your life.
>
> **Medical School Applicant**

The second secret is to remember that your performance doesn't carry over to other stations! The interviewers don't know whether you've completely failed the previous one, so you can still get a high mark by performing well on the others.

What could come up in an MMI? The following are classic recurring themes:

- Ethical scenarios. For example, the interviewer will present you with an ethical scenario you must discuss. Please refer to our Medical Ethics chapter on using the core pillars to answer ethical dilemmas.
- Role-play with an actor in different situations. For example: To encourage someone to stop smoking or break bad news to a patient.
- Describe what you see, which involves objects and materials such as a particular bone, a diagram, a picture or any type of art.
- Dealing with data, for example: Calculating the drug dosage for a patient.
- Traditional interview questions that we've covered earlier. For example: Why did you choose medicine? Why should we choose you instead of other applicants?

A key concern for most students is the fast-paced nature of MMIs. Don't worry; you're not alone in this! You have come this far, so it is probable that you already possess the necessary qualities and will one day make a fine doctor. You will develop the knack to answer the MMI stations through practice and learning to formulate well-reasoned answers that draw on your personal experience and ideas in a ten-minute window.

Examples of Common Role-Play MMI Stations

Although most MMI stations will be similar to questions asked during a traditional interview, role-play is often only employed in MMI situations. Here, we've highlighted a few scenarios that often come up, but the themes in all of them are the same! Make sure you listen, don't say anything rash and always be empathetic. Even if you have no idea how to approach a role-play scenario, simply employing those skills will get you a passing mark.

Station 1: Breaking Bad News

Before we start with the questions, it's important to know that over half of our applicants have recently encountered a question revolving around death, bereavement and breaking bad news. This is often labelled as 'Difficult Communication'; believe me, it can cause A LOT of distress, especially when you have a crying actor in front of you.

This is an extensive topic you'll undoubtedly encounter again during medical school. Our aim here is to give you the basic knowledge so you can ace any related question.

There's a lot of theory around, but if there's one thing you should remember, that is the following acronym: **'SPIKES'** (Fig. 9.12).

S: Setting

- A quiet, private, comfortable area where no one can interrupt your conversation

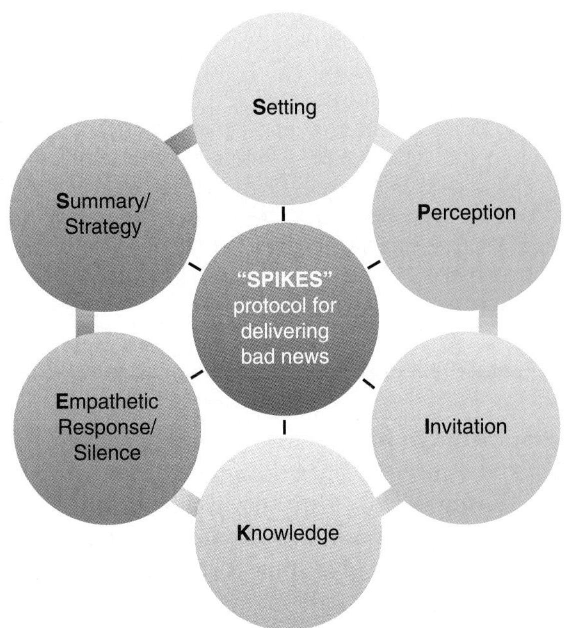

Fig. 9.12 SPIKES technique.

- Tissues and water at hand
- Are there any family members with them that they'd like to have in the room? (This often also acts as a very subtle warning shot too.)

P: Perception

- Understanding what patients already know and what they don't
- For example, 'Could you tell me what's happened so far?'

I: Invitation

- Check if this is a good time to discuss this—in an MMI situation, they will always say yes, but it's essential to ask as there are extra points just for asking
- A friendly, kind and empathetic way could be, 'Mrs Smith, I'm wondering if this is a good time for us to discuss this; what do you think?'

K: Knowledge

- Chunk and check, i.e. deliver information in small chunks, checking that it's been understood afterwards
- Start slow, but don't beat around the bush too much
- Start by using a warning shot such as, 'As you may know, we did a test last week. Unfortunately, the results were not what we hoped.' (WARNING SHOT for the patient)
- STOP, PAUSE, BREATHE
- 'I am afraid the tests show that you have got cancer. I am very sorry.'
- STOP, LONG PAUSE, BREATHE

E: Emotions and Empathy

- Use touch if appropriate—e.g. hold their hand or place your hand kindly on their shoulder (this is situation dependent as some people may find it awkward).
- Reassure that it's normal to feel the way they feel: 'I know this is hard, and it is normal to feel this way/I cannot even imagine what you're going through, but I am doing my best to understand and to support you through this.'
- Give them time; stay silent until they calm down—please don't keep talking at this point; silence is the best thing you can give them.
- Even though it may feel awkward, maintain silence until they are ready to speak again.

> Make use of 'imaginary aids' such as a glass of water or some tissues. 'I've left a box of tissues and a glass of water next to you. Take your time; I'll be here whenever you want to talk'—then be silent and wait for them to approach you. Saying that you're sorry ten times in a row will irritate them, so don't do that, please.

S: Strategy and Summary

- People usually forget everything apart from the fact that they've just been diagnosed with something horrible.
- Ask whether they'd like you to call anyone from their family to have a conversation together.
- Ensure support and that you and your team will do your best to be there for them.

> If all fails, **just be yourself**, act as a normal human being and imagine that the person in front of you is a friend or a relative so that you can easily empathise with them.

Here's a simple, funny, real-life example to help you remember SPIKES better. Let's say you spilt coffee on your flatmate's laptop. That's bad, right? How do you NORMALLY break the bad news to your flatmate?

Setting—Hey man, how are you feeling today? Look, I was wondering whether this might be a good time to have a quick chat about something.

Perception—Do you remember your laptop? The one you kept on the kitchen table? Well, I was wondering whether you've tried turning it on this afternoon…

Invitation—There are many reasons the laptop may not work, but I think I know what happened with it, and I am afraid it's not good news. Would you like to know what happened?

Knowledge—You know I always drink coffee in the kitchen, right? I am afraid I spilt coffee on your laptop this morning (pause, breathe, allow them time to realise what has happened, then continue). I am afraid your laptop has flatlined.

Empathy—I am very sorry; I can only try to understand what you're going through. I've left a glass of water and some tissues here.

Strategy—I just want to reassure you that I'll do my best to help you with whatever I can. We need to do further tests to see whether a 'keyboard transplant' might work. Otherwise, we may have to opt for palliative care and buy a new one for you.

Yes, the previous example is indeed very silly and perhaps something that only a medical student could come up with, but I hope it proves a point that all you need to do is be supportive as you would be with a friend!

So that's the approach, but what do interviewers mean by 'applicants should portray effective and empathetic communication skills'? It involves:

- Active listening
- Eye contact
- Nonverbal (body language)
- Open questions
- Empathy
- Silence
- Touch

> Remember that you can't make bad news good and that 90% of successful clinical communication involves careful active listening.
>
> **Dr James Gilbert, Consultant in Palliative Medicine**

Station 2: Breaking Bad News

An actor plays the role of your elderly neighbour. You have accidentally run over your neighbour's cat while reversing your car. You have 5 minutes to break the bad news to her.

This role-play tests insight, integrity, communication skills and empathy. Try to use the SPIKES method we just discussed; take it slow and put yourself in their shoes!

> I was asked to comfort my friend whose dog had died the day before. I did well initially, trying to cheer him up, although I made the massive mistake of saying, 'I'm happy to help you find a new one'. It was something I said without thinking. No wonder my station ended abruptly when the actor started shouting that his dog was not 'just' an object. I've learnt my lesson—put yourself into the other person's shoes and consider their values!
>
> I guess you all know whether I passed or failed that station.
>
> **Medical School Applicant**

Station 3: Teaching Task

Without using your hands, explain how to tie their shoelaces to the actor.

Tests verbal communication skills, the ability to break down the task into a series of small steps and your ability to check that the actor understands what you are saying.

> This was perhaps my most challenging station. A blindfolded child was in front of a short labyrinth throughout the room. I was asked to give him clear instructions, but the child would do something wrong whenever I gave an instruction. I said 2 metres; the child would go 4 metres. I said left; the child would turn right. He kept doing this until I was one step from having a nervous breakdown. I then remembered what my mentors used to say—it's just a game! The child plays a role; he does it on purpose. As soon as I realised this, I calmed down and started saying things like, 'Well done, you're doing well, let's keep working together, and we'll make it in the end'. The child's behaviour changed instantly. I passed that station.
>
> **Medical School Applicant**

Station 4: Giving Health Advice

This is a more recent addition to interviews, especially during MMIs. Our surveys over the past few years have shown a large number of applicants who have been asked to give some form of health advice to a patient or group of patients.

The most common question we have encountered is advising a patient who wants to quit smoking. The number one reason for failing such stations is students becoming judgmental and not showing empathy. Applicants fail to consider WHY that patient smokes. Here are a few key things to remember:

1. The scenario says they are a heavy smoker but don't jump to conclusions; ask yourself:
   Do you smoke at all? How much do you smoke?
   If they say 60 cigarettes per day (at which point you might think 'wow'), try not to be judgmental.
   Simply ask, 'Do you think that's a lot?' Chances are, they may tell you they think it is.
   How long have they smoked for?
2. WHY do they smoke?
   Is there anything in particular that makes you smoke more during the day?
   E.g. at work, at home, when having a lot of free time, in high-stress situations, etc.
   Does anyone else in your family smoke (e.g. wife)?
3. Show understanding
   'Given your history, I do realise this will be hard for you, but we're here to help.'
   'Is there anything we can do that you think might help?' (e.g. if the wife smokes, what about a joint consultation to discuss this together?)
4. Use signposting
   Smoking cessation clinics
   Leaflets
   NHS Choices/Patient.co.uk websites

Similar to breaking bad news, it all comes down to something anyone would do if they were talking to a friend or relative. Claudia, one of our successful applicants, is the perfect example. You see, Claudia used to hate talking about herself, she had to work very hard at questions like that, but when it came to giving health advice, she was brilliant. Surprised, I'd ask, 'How did you just do that?!' Claudia always said: 'I don't know, I didn't actually have a structure, I just imagined someone who was genuinely struggling with that problem, so I wanted to first know why and then do my best to help'.

> Often unhealthy habits occur due to some sort of social factor. Enquire about their life, job, family and any stress they may be exposed to. If you help them deal with their current situation, they'll be more likely to quit and change the unhealthy habit.

You can imagine how other similar questions can follow the same pattern (e.g. what health advice would you give to someone who drinks a lot/who has an unhealthy diet?).

The most commonly asked question from an applicant's perspective is, 'What if I don't know any of the side effects or medical implications of a particular topic?'

The simple answer to that is: You don't have to. The General Medical Council (GMC) states that you should always 'acknowledge your limitations' and 'work within the boundaries of your knowledge'. For example, if a patient asks you about anything you are clueless about, simply acknowledge their question and say that, unfortunately, this is not something you are confident in discussing but that you are very happy to signpost them to your supervisor, who will gladly answer their questions.

> I was asked to advise a heavy smoker who was about to have surgery. I was challenged several times about the specific side effects that they may be exposed to and how smoking could affect wound healing. I knew some basic principles, but I was afraid I would get marked down for not being able to explain any specifics. I passed the interview in the end—I think it's because I simply said that this knowledge was beyond my role and that I would signpost them to the rest of my team instead.
>
> **Medical School Applicant**

Station 5: Communication and Empathy

A close friend in your first-year medical school class tells you that his mother was recently diagnosed with breast cancer. He feels overwhelmed by his studies and is considering dropping out of medical school to spend more time with his mother. Please console your friend.

This would look at your ability to empathise and counsel a friend. It tests your listening skills and ability to comfort a patient when they experience bad news or are going through tough times.

The more common version of this station is that your colleague (a medical student) and your best friend have asked you to sign him in for a lecture when he is not attending. What would you say in that case? Please think twice before you answer; it's important to realise how difficult a scenario like this could be in real life, where your friendship is on the line.

Other Common MMI Stations

Here are five bonus rounds of topics based on the most encountered questions by our applicants over the past few years. The following topics could appear in any type of interview, be it a traditional one or an MMI.

Bonus Station 1: Alternative Medicine

Acupuncture is an ancient Chinese therapy that has been reported to treat insomnia. It is a heavily debated therapy as it is considered 'alternative medicine', and limited research has been conducted on its benefits. Studies carried out have small sample sizes and large standard errors. As a healthcare policymaker, your job is to weigh the pros and cons of introducing acupuncture into the NHS. Please discuss the issues you would consider during an approval process for acupuncture.

This question addresses your ability to use given information and prior knowledge to reason out an ethical issue. It would look at your practicality and general knowledge, and you would have to provide a balanced argument.

Cast your mind back to the start of the chapter, where we discussed answer structure! This would be a great question to use the 'essay structure' in which you make a point, back it up with evidence and then explain it further.

Bonus Station 2: Organ Prioritisation

You have two patients. One is the mother of three young children, while the second patient is a middle-aged man and a previously known alcoholic. You only have one liver, and both patients will die without a liver transplant. Who would you offer the liver transplant to and why?

This is a prioritisation exercise that also involves medical ethics. The emphasis is on problem solving and rational thinking under pressure.

Read the ethics section earlier in the book to better understand how to answer this. Remember that you should always go down as many avenues as possible and never stick to only one answer. Compare and contrast the ethical pillars clashing in this case, ask for further clarification and argue for both sides!

Bonus Station 3: Give Us a Time When…

This is perhaps the most common category of questions encountered by medical school applicants in both panel and MMI settings. They probably come up in most, if not all, interviews, and they are relatively easy to predict.

This question could apply to absolutely any skill that you can think of. Here are a few examples:

- Give an example of a time when you showed empathy (most common).
- Give an example of a time when you were the leader of a team, and something went wrong.
- Give an example of a time when you showed problem-solving skills.

- Give an example of a time when you showed good communication skills.

Your homework is to jot down the most common skills and develop an example for each. Here's when your 'Getting into medical school portfolio' and the work experience reflective templates described previously in this book come in handy. Look through your work experience placements and assign several skills to as few examples as possible so you have a higher chance of remembering them on your interview day.

For example, empathy, communication and listening skills can always be portrayed by a single example from your work experience where you've had the chance to interact with a patient. Similarly, teamwork, leadership, problem solving and creativity can be grouped and discussed using an example from extracurricular activities.

Don't write down an entire answer for each question; it would look rehearsed. Instead, come up with an example and be prepared to talk about a skill as part of that example. The worst thing that could happen is they ask you to give an example of a time when you've shown empathy, and you have to think for 5 minutes and come up with something that seems rushed and forced.

Bonus Station 4: Hot Topics in Medicine

The topics shown in Fig. 9.13 are keywords that you may like to familiarise yourself with. These are some issues (for example NHS related) that are specific to the UK. In contrast, there are other issues, such as the ethics of abortion, which need to be considered by all potential medical students. These are considered 'hot topics' as they are relevant in today's environment and are likely avenues interviewers could discuss.

Bonus Station 5: History Taking

The chances that this might come up are low, but we've had a few disappointed applicants over the past year who did not know how to approach this scenario. It's always best to be prepared, so here's a simple plan.

First things first—don't forget to introduce yourself (including name and role), seek their consent for this conversation and reassure them everything will be kept confidential (only shared with senior colleagues for the purposes of their care). When it comes to the conversation, the most important thing is to start with an open question and LISTEN: 'What's brought you in?' Follow this up with slightly more specific closed questions based on what they say (e.g. when did it start, where is the pain, does it get better or worse, etc.). Include questions about their well-being in the past, including other diseases or whether this episode has been present before (e.g. has this been present in the past, did anything make it better? What about medication? Did it help? Do they see their doctor often for any reasons?).

Make sure you cover their social and family life to look for any stress causes or diseases that run in the family. Conclude by summarising everything to the patient and ask whether there's anything else they'd like to mention before the end of the consultation.

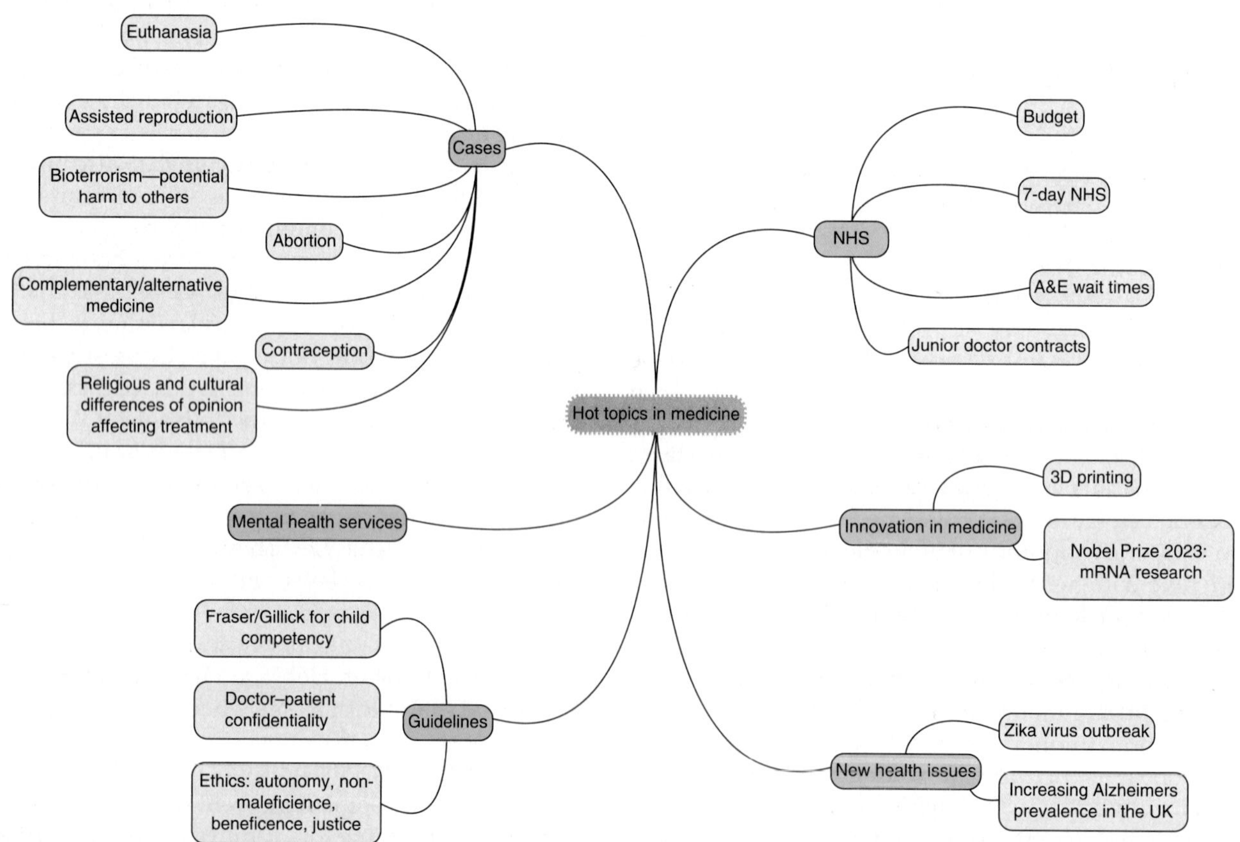

Fig. 9.13 Hot topics in medicine.

Use ICE:
I—Ideas: 'Do you have any ideas what this cough might be?'
C—Concerns: 'What is your biggest concern?'
E—Expectations: 'What would you like to get out of this consultation?'

This can be used in any circumstance, whenever talking to a patient. This is what bridges the gap between the patient and the doctor or, in your case, the medical school applicant. By the end of any consultation or discussion, you need to ensure that you've matched your agenda with theirs. You may assume that someone wants pills for pain when all they needed was a letter to take time off work until they recover.

So, for history taking:

1. Introduce yourself, seek consent and reassure them this remains confidential.
2. Start with an open question and listen.
3. Follow this up with closed questions.
4. Discuss the past.
5. Discuss family and social history.
6. Use ICE (Ideas, Concerns, Expectations).
7. Enquire about general health.
8. Summarise and check for anything you might have missed.

VIRTUAL INTERVIEWS AND THE PANDEMIC

Although the pandemic is over, virtual medical school interviews are here to stay. Medical schools will increasingly offer these to international applicants as well as those who may find it challenging to attend the interview in person. Although some are obvious, we have included an inclusive list of essential tips to make sure that these run as smoothly as possible:

- Make sure your internet connection is smooth! Try and get a wired connection/LAN cable if possible or make sure you're in a place where the WiFi is strong. You can even conduct it at a friend's house, a private library booth or at school if necessary.
- Make sure your camera and microphone are working flawlessly. If you don't know what platform the medical school will use, hop onto a private zoom call, and make sure everything works.
- Dress well! It might be virtual, but first impressions do count. Please remember to wear pants, even if you're tempted not to—save yourself the embarrassment in case you're being asked to stand up.
- Don't move tabs around or open/close your notes during your interview. The interviewers have years of experience; they'll sense if you are distracted or reading straight from a preprepared document. They'll also be able to see if you're swapping between apps on your computer from the flashes on your face, so be very careful.
- Make sure you're in a quiet environment with no distractions or background noise. If you're doing it at home, let your family members know you're having an interview so they can avoid making loud noises during that time.

However, keep in mind that you may still be asked COVID-19-specific questions, so we've included a few examples. The method to answer these questions is the same as the questions in the rest of the chapter; the only difference is the content. Make sure to write down all your relevant personal experiences regarding the pandemic and use the questions below as inspiration in case you've forgotten a few.

COVID-19 Questions and Scenarios

- Should COVID vaccines be made mandatory for the general public? What about mandating them for healthcare workers?
- Lockdowns—good or bad during a pandemic?
- You are a medical student on placement in the hospital. One of your classmates confides in you that they have not had their COVID vaccination. How would you persuade them to get vaccinated? (Role-play or discussion station)
- What is the impact of COVID-19 on the NHS?
- Have there been any positive aspects for healthcare that have emerged out of the COVID pandemic?
- What are the pros and cons of virtual consultations?
- How do you think COVID has affected children/young adults?
- Try to convince your friend not to go out to a party during a national lockdown. (Role-play or discussion station)

These questions are just a few examples of COVID-focused questions you could be asked, and there are plenty more that you may come up with yourself. Some common themes may surround:

- Safeguarding: How do you ensure children are safe online? How do you ensure patient data is securely kept?
- Quality: How do you ensure that the quality of care received in virtual consultations is of high quality? How do you build trust and connect with the patient if it's online?
- Inequality: If we move to a more virtual world, what happens to those who cannot afford internet/devices/don't have the literacy skills to navigate such technology? What positives will there be if we become more virtual?

Again, there are several items to consider, so do have a careful think about them!

BEFORE, DURING AND AFTER YOUR IN-PERSON INTERVIEW

THE RUN-UP TO THE BIG DAY: HOW TO PREPARE FOR THE INTERVIEW

- Practice discussing topics in your A-Levels that may be of interest with teachers and peers. This will prepare you for the interviews like the Oxbridge one,

which is essentially a discussion of thoughts about various scientific ideas.
- Speak to older students who have been through the same process and ask for advice.
- Browse the internet for tips from students who may have been through the same experience. Be wary of sites like *Student Room*; take everything you read with a pinch of salt! Only a few students share their experiences online, and this may not be representative of the entire cohort's interview experience.
- Record yourself answering questions and note any nervous habits you may have. Common ones include repeating the word 'like', cracking knuckles, avoiding eye contact and adjusting hair. These habits are normal but could distract the interviewer from what you're trying to say.
- Do any prereading that the university may have asked you to do. Certain universities may ask you to bring an interesting health news article to discuss. Ensure you choose one that is current and about which you have a great deal of knowledge. As this is a topic you were asked to prepare for, the interviewers will expect you to be confident enough to discuss the article fully.
- Prepare all documents you may need to take to the interview, for example, any forms that require filling, etc.
- Make sure to double-check your invitation to interview so you know what time your interview is, where it is and how you would get there.

WHAT TO WEAR ON THE DAY

The idea behind dressing for a medical school interview is to look the part. It is important to look well groomed and professional. This may be the first time you have had to dress formally, so here are a few guidelines for you:

Women
- A knee-length dress or skirt with a blouse works for women. Alternatively, you could opt for smart trousers with a shirt and/or a blazer.
- Dress conservatively. We suggest perhaps tights with your skirt and tops that cover the chest and upper arms.
- We recommend that if you're wearing makeup, ensure that it is light and natural—you are not getting ready for a night out!
- Jewellery, similar to makeup, should be kept to the bare minimum.
- Comfortable shoes are essential. For MMIs, you need to walk between stations, and the last thing you want would be to fall over. Opt for a shoe with a slight heel or flat pumps.
- Try not to overdo the perfume!

Men
- For men, a smart suit or shirt, tie (optional) and trousers are your safest option.
- Shoes should be cleaned and polished.
- Although it might seem an excellent occasion to bring out something from your wacky tie collection, we would suggest that you keep your tie simple and professional (if you decide to wear one).
- Facial hair should be trimmed and clean.
- Try not to overdo the aftershave!

THE BIG DAY

- Eat a balanced meal the morning before your interview to focus on the task at hand instead of any grumbling noises your stomach might make!
- Caffeine is a stimulant. Some of you may be used to consuming copious amounts of coffee, but some of you are not and might think that it is advisable to neck a *venti* or a *Red Bull* before your interview. Remember that caffeine can also make you jittery… which is not very desirable!
- Arrive well in advance of your interview so that you have time to acclimatise and settle your nerves before you walk in.
- Nerves are normal. Interviews are a stressful time, so remember to take some deep breaths and keep calm before walking into your interview.

? Stress: Good or Bad?

A pounding heart, breathing quickly and sweating are ways stress manifests itself. The most common questions we encounter are, 'Do you ever get stressed?' and 'How can I get rid of stress?' First of all, the fact that you get stressed about your interview means that you care about its outcome and would not want to miss this opportunity.

Second, can you think of another time when you might have had a pounding heart, and your breathing rate got faster and faster? Perhaps when you received the invitation for the interview?

Excitement, joy and courage usually accompany the same physiological responses as stress. In other words, your body is preparing you for the task you need to undertake. Your heart beats faster to pump more blood to your brain, and you breathe rapidly to receive more oxygen. It's up to us whether we consider stress a friend or an enemy. Next time you're anxious, smile and think that this is to give you enough resources and courage to cope with your challenges! You have worked hard, and you deserve to be there.

- Remember, the answer is in the journey and not the destination. If you're finding a question hard, the chances are that most students are in the same position as you. Reason out your answer and show the interviewers that you're able to think critically about a topic.
- Take your time with your answers. Don't pre-empt the question and rush to answer. It is important to show the interviewer that you are thoughtful and not flustered.
- Some universities give you the opportunity to speak with medical students before your interview. This may be an excellent opportunity to ask them any

questions you may have and to practice speaking to someone (i.e. calm your nerves before the interview and get into the interview mindset).

- Don't be distracted by students in the waiting room. They may seem intimidating, but you are all capable and in the exact same position!
- Walk in with confidence…you've worked hard for this!

DURING THE INTERVIEW

- Be confident—you have been invited to the interview for a reason. The university believes you to be competent, and it is your chance to show the interviewers that you are!
- Be friendly—at the end of the day, the interviewers are looking for approachable and competent medics whom they would enjoy teaching.
- You may be confronted with a sensitive situation. For example, you may be asked why you want to be a doctor instead of a nurse. Think carefully about this and ensure you don't offend any panel members while attempting to answer this (there may well be a nurse interviewing you!).
- Listen carefully to the question. Your interviewer will often provide cues or prompts designed to direct you and give you key bits of information.
- ASK if you need clarification rather than trying to answer a question you don't fully understand.
- Don't worry if you go blank. Ask the interviewer to repeat themselves, as this will give you some time to recollect your thoughts and get some structure to your answers.

> Remember, not all interviewers will look at you or agree with you, and they might even question you even though you appear to have reached the correct answer. They might attempt to stump you and intimidate you slightly to see how you respond to pressure and intense questioning. If you have a two-person panel, there may be a situation of good cop, bad cop. Be aware of this!
>
> **Dr Zeshan Qureshi, Paediatric Registrar**

POST INTERVIEW

Be in the top 1% of applicants who ACTUALLY enjoy the interview and don't sigh with relief when you walk out of the room at the end of the interview.

Your work here is done! You've made it through an incredibly trying experience so take a moment to sit back and relax. The next few days or weeks are a waiting game. You've done the best you can, and now it's time to get your mind off it and hope for the best!

Best of luck, and remember, all your hard work will pay off in the end. One day, you will be a medical student. You will reach your dream, and when you do, you'll look back to all the hard work and smile because you'll realise that 'luck' plays only a tiny part.

TOP 12 TRICKS AND HACKS TO BOOST YOUR INTERVIEW PERFORMANCE

1. **It's Just a Game**

The people interviewing you are generally very friendly but may not appear so during your interview. This is because everyone has a role. The actors play a role, and the interviewers play a role, so you must also play a role. Your part is to be the perfect candidate, ready to shine a light on your vast amount of experience and acquired knowledge.

Did someone say something slightly inappropriate that put a lot of pressure on you? Did an actor challenge you in any way? Does the interviewer look scary and serious and doesn't smile at all? Whenever this happens, keep smiling to your inner self, and remember that everything is just a game. They are doing this to see whether you crack under pressure and whether you can cope with challenges. If you do this long enough, even the most serious and scary interviewer will smile in the end.

> During one of my stations, an actor played a patient concerned about OCD. I can't remember what I said, but I must have upset the actor as he started shouting, 'Are you saying I'm crazy?!' I panicked when challenged but soon realised it was all 'just a game'. Instead of defending myself, I smiled kindly and said that I apologise for coming across that way—I was trying to understand how they felt about this situation to do my best to help. The actor calmed down, and I passed my station eventually.
>
> **Medical School Applicant**

2. **How to Avoid Brain Freeze**

This is perhaps one of my top tips for anyone out there. It's simple but not easy. Have a good STRUCTURE, and the rest will follow. Do you remember our 'Introduction, Body and Conclusion' technique earlier in the chapter? Your introduction must include a clear skeleton for your answer.

For example, if you say, 'There are three reasons for which I want to do medicine:

1. My personal story
2. My love for sciences
3. My desire to help others'

It doesn't matter if your brain freezes in the middle of an argument, as you can quickly move on to the next point in a structured way. You now know where you're heading!

Did your mind freeze towards the end of your personal story? No worries, end it there and move on to your love for sciences. Did your mind freeze when you talked about your passion for science? No worries, move on to your desire to help others. Did your brain freeze again? Conclude the question by going back to the overall three reasons, and you'll be fine.

The second reason this is extremely helpful is that the interviewer can easily follow you through. You already set a direction for your answer, and even if they are bored or look out the window at some point, they will still catch up on your next point because you've set a clear structure inside their head.

3. **Planting a 'Seed' in the Interviewer's Head**

Psychological research has shown that our brains are very weird, and there are many ways to persuade someone subconsciously. In your case, this can be achieved by using phrases that will make them more likely to remember and choose you. These include phrases that paint a vivid image of the future of you as a doctor or as a medical student as part of their institution.

Let's take 'What makes up a good doctor?' for example. Towards the end of your answer, you can say something along these lines: 'The skills I have demonstrated throughout my work experience are something that I hope to build upon during my time as a medical student, hopefully as part of your institution, and as a future doctor'. Another example could be 'Why our medical school?'. Here you can say something like this: 'I hope one day, I will be part of this amazing community of medical students and use my skills and knowledge to give something back'.

These are just a few examples that can be adapted to several questions that may come up. Essentially, always think of ways to help them imagine why you are already acting like a medical student they'd wish to have.

4. **Put Yourself in the Interviewer's Shoes**

When preparing for interview questions and during the interview, try to ask yourself, 'Why did they ask me this particular question?' What would you usually say as opposed to what they'd want to hear?

The best example is the 'How do doctors cope with stress?' type of question. Many students drop out of medicine; sadly, some even end up with severe mental health problems. If you're being asked this question, it is because they want to see whether YOU 'have what it takes' to cope with medicine. The question sounds general. For this reason, most applicants only give a general answer about how doctors cope but never use their own personal examples. Of course, you'll start by showing an understanding of the prevalence of stress among doctors, but then you must talk about yourself. After all, this interview demonstrates your suitability for becoming a doctor.

We've already covered it earlier in the chapter, but just as a refresher, there are three aspects to this question. You can imagine it as a tick-box exercise for interviewers and admission tutors:

- **Mind**. What do you do to relax your mind at the end of a tough day? (Reflection, action plans, meditation, etc.)
- **Body**. The Romans got it right: '*Mens sana in corpore sano*', which roughly translates to 'A healthy mind in a healthy body'. What do you do to relax your body? (Sports, hobbies, gym, etc.)
- **Family, friends and colleagues**. An essential element often neglected by applicants, which interviewers assess, is your ability to make new relationships and maintain old ones. Here it would help if you said that you find it helpful to discuss problems with friends and family and often seek support from your peers. You can even end the question by saying that you're looking forward to collaborating with your peers as part of medical school and making new friends (again, this is planting a 'seed' in their head that you are already planning and thinking about the future).

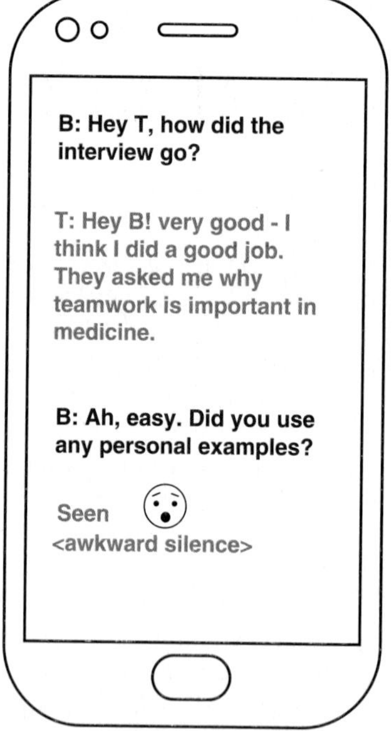

Another example could be 'Why is teamwork important?' You cannot answer that question without using personal examples from your own work experience and extracurricular activities.

Have a look at this awkward conversation between one of the authors of this book and an applicant.

Hopefully, this will help you remember always to think 'WHY' they might ask you something.

5. **Dealing with Challenging Interviewers and How to Avoid Losing Any Marks**

Okay, this is perhaps one of the most common reasons for losing marks during interviews, and we've had hundreds of applicants who have highlighted that they don't know how to react when challenged.

First, you must recognise when you're about to be challenged. Pay attention to how they phrase their questions, together with their voice and body language. Here are some examples:

- 'You mentioned X, but what about…?'
- 'Did you mean…?'
- 'Does that mean that…?'
- Voice—inquisitive, curious, confused
- Body language—closed, curious

Second, once you know something terrible is coming, try to anticipate the question or mistake that you have made. Very often, you'll be able to repair it. There are three possibilities here:

a) You forgot to mention something.
b) You said something debatable and didn't mention the other side of the argument.
c) You said something wrong or didn't know the answer.

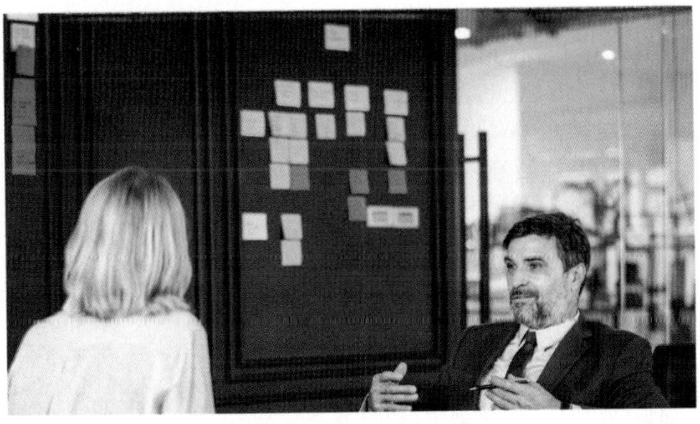

Let's break them down one by one.

a) **You forgot to mention something.**

If this is the case and you realise what you forgot to mention by the time they finish their question (in most questions, you will!), here's a trick to repair it: as soon as you realise, start SMILING and NODDING your head slowly. This will indicate that you know what they're about to ask you. The interviewer may not even finish their question because you've already signalled you're ready to go. Once they stop talking, start with something positive: 'I'm glad you've asked me this…' or 'This is something I was hoping you would ask, as it's an important aspect to be covered…' This way, you say what you forgot, answer the question, and don't lose points as the interviewer will be satisfied that you've matched his agenda.

Obviously, if you have no clue what they were talking about, DO NOT LIE. They will catch you.

b) **You said something debatable.**

This is very similar to the previous situation. The only thing to add is that if you said something controversial or something that might have been misunderstood, you have to apologise for coming across in a certain way. Be professional. The absolute DON'T in this situation is to say, 'That's not what I said; what I meant was…' You said it, so take responsibility, apologise for your action and repair it.

c) **You said something wrong or didn't know the answer.**

In this situation, same as earlier, be professional, apologise politely and try to repair it. If you don't know the answer, you must say that although you do not know the answer, you would be prepared to do your best to answer it if they could provide further information or guide you along the way. If they refuse to give more information, mention that although you haven't come across this subject, this is something you are keen to explore in the future, as it does sound important.

6. **Pause Before You Answer**

Take time to think, and DO NOT RUSH to answer. Count to three in your mind before you answer. If you need more time, no problem; ask for 15 to 30 seconds. You may wonder, do I lose points for this? No. What would you prefer, someone who opens their mouth and stupid things come out, or someone who's considerate and says, 'This is a complex question—would it be okay if I think about it for 15 seconds so I can give you a full and structured answer?' or 'A few seconds would very much help to organise my thoughts if possible?'

Obviously, don't say, 'May I please have 30 seconds to think?' if they ask you, 'Why medicine?' You should know that already (hopefully?!).

7. **Balance Your Arguments**

Often, applicants lose precious marks during the interview because they come across as single-minded. Always do your best to present the other side of the argument in a nonjudgmental manner.

Another tip is to think about the ideal scenario when presented with a situation, then mention that we don't live in an ideal world. If that failed, try 'in a less ideal scenario, I would do x, y and z'. For example, if they ask what you would do if a patient shouts at you, you can use conflict resolution techniques to calm them down in an ideal world. In a less ideal scenario, you'd have to call security if they couldn't be calmed down.

8. **Don't Forget to Signpost**

   Keep in mind any services, leaflets, websites, colleagues, supervisors or any other areas where you might be able to signpost during any scenario that could come up. It is essential to demonstrate awareness that you are not alone, and that medicine is a discipline that involves a multidisciplinary approach. Don't put the problem on your shoulders.

9. **Practice Visualisation**

   If you want to succeed, you need to be confident and believe that you deserve a place at medical school. Look in the mirror, dream and imagine exactly how it will be. Imagine what you'll wear, visualise the steps taken to the venue, imagine how you'll walk in, shake hands, how you'll smile, how they'll ask you what you know and how if they ask you something you don't know, you'll be able to deal with it anyway. Just imagine every single detail and visualise the end when you thank them for having you there and how happy and proud of yourself you will be. You deserve to be there. It's not luck; it's based on all your hard work, so never even think about doubting yourself!

10. **Use Everything You've Got to Succeed (Words, Voice, Body Language)**

    This is simple psychology. Research has shown that the information and actual content (i.e. spoken words) represent only 7% of how you come across to an interviewer. Your voice and tone represent 38%, while the big chunk is made by body language, occupying a massive piece of 55% (Fig. 9.14).

11. **A Few 'Always' Situations**

    Always maintain eye contact with everyone in the room, not just with the person asking the question. Try to acknowledge the presence of every interviewer, even if they keep writing stuff down.

    Second, always shake their hand and introduce yourself to EVERY SINGLE PERSON in the room. Often applicants ask us if this is awkward in situations where the interviewer is not looking or is writing something down. It isn't awkward at all (unless you make it awkward!). Let's say you walk into the room and say hello, but only look down as they write something. Your role is to go to them with confidence, put your hand out and introduce yourself. Many of them will be surprised because probably you're in the 5% of applicants who dare to introduce themselves. They will look up and might even apologise for not seeing your hand earlier, and they will introduce themselves too. They will remember you.

    Another reason to shake hands is the research and science behind the human touch. Why do you think the baby is placed on the mother's chest after birth? You can argue that it's because there's a maternal connection, but what about the times when you're out with your friends, someone makes a funny joke and you pat them on the back and say, 'Haha, so funny!' That's a perfect example of how human touch brings us closer to each other.

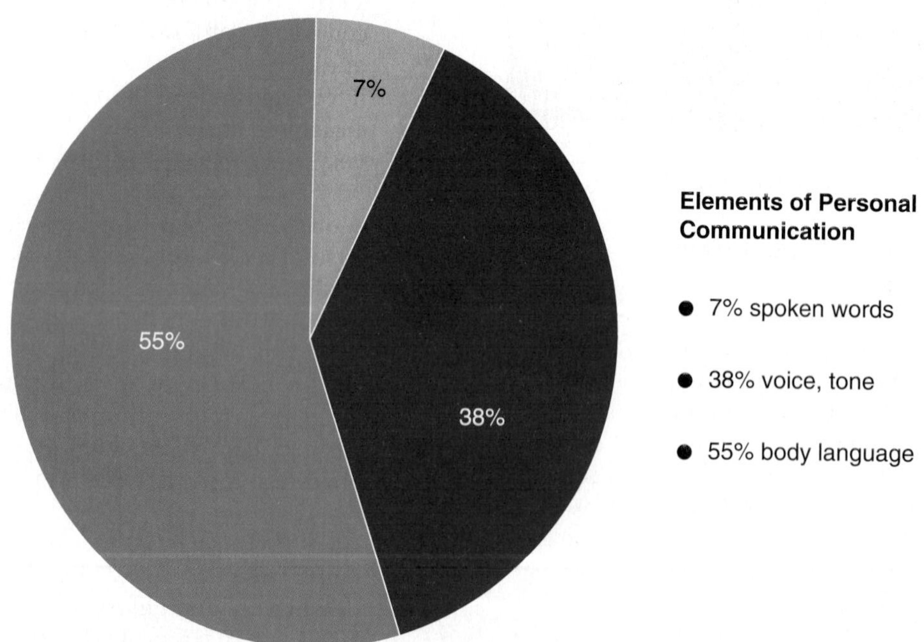

Fig. 9.14 Elements of communication.

12. **First and Final Impressions Matter Most**

This may sound like common sense, but one of the best tips is to be enthusiastic and grateful for being there and having the chance to meet these people.

When you are waiting to be called in, think about the opportunity you have been given. Think how hard you have worked for it, how long you have been waiting to meet these people and how close you are to reaching your goal. Thinking about this will undoubtedly make you smile and make it easier to express your burning passion. When you enter the room, show appreciation, and demonstrate that it is a pleasure to be there. This will give you an advantage over students who see the interview as a daunting task or a necessity instead of an opportunity.

When your interview ends, you want to ensure that you are still enthusiastic and passionate. Many students sigh in the end as if a burden has been lifted off their shoulders. Although the pressure is officially over, try holding it inside for at least a few more minutes! Rather than feeling relieved, stay enthusiastic and show them that you loved being there. Give them the impression that you would do it again because you are confident and love talking about your passion. This may be hard to achieve, but it will give you some extra points.

Bonus Tip: The Real Secret

I want to leave you with a final thought. Everyone will have the same resources and access to tips and information. The question then becomes: **What makes the difference between success and failure?** Although everyone will have the same resources, NOT EVERYONE will be ready to practice and fail for as long as it takes until they master this topic. If you're feeling enthusiastic and can't wait to start doing things, that's amazing; I am delighted to hear it. But, remember: Enthusiasm is easy. Endurance is hard.

Best of luck. One day, we hope to receive an email from you telling us how excited you are because you've received an offer. This is what keeps us going. This is our motivation for writing this book. It's you.

TEST YOURSELF: 130+ MOST COMMON MEDICAL SCHOOL INTERVIEW QUESTIONS

People always say, 'Knowledge is power', right? Well, that's only partly true. Knowledge becomes power, but only if you use it. Are you keen to ace your medical school interviews? Here you will find a selection of the most commonly encountered panel and MMI questions and scenarios. Use them to practice with family, friends, teachers or just yourself in the mirror!

Many of these questions have already been covered in our previous chapters. Still, if you are like millions of students from all over the world, you have probably already started to forget A LOT of the stuff mentioned previously. Use these questions to test yourself and aid memory consolidation. Have a go—I promise you'll be surprised to see how much you know once you apply the techniques uncovered throughout this chapter.

PASSION, INSIGHT AND MOTIVATION FOR MEDICINE

1. Tell us a bit about yourself.
2. Why medicine?
3. Why not nursing?
4. Why not research?
5. Why in the UK? (If international)
6. If you are not successful with your application, what will you do?
7. What aspects of medicine attract you to this career?
8. What do you see as the drawbacks of studying medicine?
9. What intimidates you most about studying medicine?
10. What interests do you have that would make you a suitable candidate to study medicine?
11. What do you hope to achieve from a degree in medicine?
12. Tell us about a recent article/book/publication you read that shows your interest in medicine.
13. What do you think you would like to specialise in?
14. What have you learnt about medicine from peers, doctors and medical students?
15. Tell me about something/someone who had a significant influence on your life.

WORK EXPERIENCE RELEVANT TO MEDICINE

16. Tell us about your work experience.
17. What have you learnt from your work experience?
18. From your work experience, tell me about a challenging situation you had to deal with/observe.
19. What are the most important skills a doctor must possess?
20. How does the skillset of a doctor vary from that of a nurse?
21. What is the importance of work experience?
22. Has anything from your work experience changed your view on medicine?
23. What is your experience of the relationship between doctors and nurses, pharmacists, lab technicians, etc.?
24. What is the role of a doctor, in your understanding?

TRANSFERRABLE SKILLS AND PERSONAL APTITUDES

25. Give an example of a time when you've shown empathy.
26. Why is teamwork essential?
27. Give an example of a time when you were part of a team, and something went wrong. How did you solve it, and what did you learn from it?

28. Give an example of a time when you were a team leader.
29. What makes a good doctor, and do you think you have any of these personal skills?
30. Do you think empathy is a skill that can be learnt?
31. How important is empathy in the medical profession?
32. What is the distinction between empathy and sympathy in medicine?
33. If your friends could describe you in three words, what would they be?
34. Give us an example of when you worked on a team and it was unsuccessful. Explain why you were unsuccessful and what you would do to change this in hindsight.
35. What are the qualities of a good leader?
36. As a doctor, is it more important to be a leader or a follower?
37. You are part of a team, and there is a great deal of conflict between team members. How would you go about remedying this?
38. How would you cope with a team member not pulling their weight in a group project?
39. Is delegation important in medicine? If so, why?
40. How have you coped with independent study?

INSIGHT INTO THE NHS AND OTHER SIGNIFICANT ORGANISATIONS WITHIN THE UK

41. What does the BMA do?
42. What does the GMC do?
43. What are CCGs?
44. What are the Royal Colleges, and what is their role?
45. What do you think the role of public health campaigns is?
46. What would you change about the current NHS, if at all?
47. What do you think the most important development in medicine has been?
48. What do you think the impact of Brexit has been on healthcare?
49. How would you fix the current staffing crisis?
50. What is your opinion on the privatisation of the NHS?
51. How well do you think the NHS provides mental healthcare for patients?
52. What is your opinion on alternative medicine?
53. What is your opinion on the opt-out system for organ donation?
54. How do you think organ donation should be determined due to the scarce availability of donors?
55. Can you think of ways in which A&E wait times could be reduced?
56. What do you think are the consequences of increased primary care pressures on the NHS?
57. What are some funding challenges for the NHS?
58. How do you think the NHS could cope with increasing antibiotic resistance?
59. Should vaccination for children be made compulsory?
60. Is the increasing prevalence of obesity a concern for the NHS?
61. What are the implications of the increased ageing population?
62. What are the stresses for a GP today?
63. How has technology changed healthcare today?
64. What is your opinion on nurses being given more responsibilities in the NHS and doing work that used to be a doctor's job?
65. How can doctors promote health in addition to treating illnesses?
66. How has the role of the doctor changed in the modern healthcare system?
67. What is the influence of the media on the role of the doctor?
68. Why do you think most doctors do not wear white coats in hospitals today?
69. What does 'holistic medicine' mean to you?
70. What do you think the most significant healthcare issue will be in the next 10 years?
71. Should nonessential surgery be available through the NHS?

INSIGHT INTO THE UK MEDICAL SCHOOL TRAINING PROGRAMME

72. What is the duration of training for a UK medical school graduate?
73. What are intercalated degrees?
74. What are the different teaching styles? What are their advantages and disadvantages?
75. Are there any features of the course that attracts you to it?
76. What about extracurricular activities and societies?
77. Do you believe cadaver dissection is essential to medical school teaching?
78. How would you contribute to this medical school?
79. If you were struggling in medical school, how would you handle this?
80. Sixty percent of medical students are women. Why do you think this is the case? What are the consequences of this?

ETHICAL OR MEDICO-LEGAL SCENARIOS

81. What is autonomy? (same question for other ethical principles)
82. What are the four different pillars of medical ethics?
83. What are the different types of consent?
84. Why is consent necessary?
85. What is confidentiality, and why is it important?
86. What is the Hippocratic Oath? Is it relevant in today's world?
87. What is euthanasia? How would you handle a case for euthanasia using the four pillars of ethics?
88. What <u>are</u> the ethics surrounding compulsory vaccination?
89. What <u>are</u> the ethics surrounding abortion?

90. What are the ethics surrounding a patient refusing a lifesaving blood transfusion?
91. What are the ethics surrounding a 13-year-old patient refusing a lifesaving treatment?
92. A patient diagnosed with HIV refuses to tell their partner they are HIV positive. What would you do as their doctor?
93. As a junior doctor, your consultant arrives at work with their breath smelling of alcohol. What is your course of action?
94. At medical school, your peer contacts you, reveals that she is failing her exams and asks to copy your assignment to help her through the year. What do you do?
95. Do you think the NHS should treat smokers?
96. You have one liver available and have to choose between a mother of two and a 17-year-old boy with congenital liver disease. Whom would you choose and why?

HISTORY AND THE DIFFERENT ROLES OF A DOCTOR

97. What are the different duties of a doctor?
98. Why is research necessary?
99. Why is teaching important for doctors?
100. What is the most significant discovery in medicine?
101. What does a doctor do apart from seeing patients?
102. What does shared leadership stand for?

ROLE-PLAY

103. How would you convince someone to quit smoking?
104. How do you deal with angry patients?
105. A patient gives you a £20 note and a 'thank you' card and insists you take it. What do you do?
106. A patient asks you to go for a drink at the end of your hospital shift. What do you tell the patient?
107. A patient comes to you with early-stage respiratory disease and has a history of smoking. Please speak to the patient about cutting down on their smoking habits.
108. The interviewer asks you what ethical pillar of medicine you believe to be the most important and to explain it to a child.
109. A male patient who is 32 years old has just been diagnosed with pancreatic cancer and breaks down in tears in front of you. How would you go about consoling him?
110. A 16-year-old girl enters the clinic wanting to be tested for STIs. She asks you not to tell her parents that she has come in. How would you go about handling this?
111. You are a surgeon who has just performed a procedure on a young male. During the procedure, there was severe nerve damage, and it was found that the male patient would not be able to move his arm again. How would you go about breaking the bad news?

WORK–LIFE BALANCE AND COPING WITH STRESS

112. How do you cope with stress?
113. Why is stress important?
114. What are your hobbies?
115. How do you cope with failure?
116. In your opinion, what do you think is your biggest weakness?
117. If you are struggling with an assignment or with the course, when would you seek help?
118. What is your biggest strength?
119. Whom do you admire and why?
120. What was the last book you read? Would you recommend it? Why?

COVID-19 AND THE PANDEMIC

121. Should COVID-19 vaccines be made compulsory?
122. Should COVID-19 vaccines be made compulsory for healthcare workers?
123. What do you think of the UK government's response to the COVID-19 pandemic?
124. During the initial outbreak of COVID-19, ventilators and intensive care beds were in extremely short supply. During this time, doctors were having to make decisions about who should get a ventilator and who should not. In this scenario, you will be given two patients and asked to choose whom you would give the ventilator to
    Patient 1—54 y/o father of two with asthma
    Patient 2—85 y/o woman with no underlying health conditions
125. You are a medical student on placement in the hospital. One of your classmates confides in you that they have not had their COVID-19 vaccinations. How would you persuade them to get vaccinated? (Role-play or discussion station)
126. What is the impact of COVID-19 on the NHS?
127. Have there been any positives for healthcare that have emerged out of the COVID-19 pandemic?
128. Do you think virtual consultations should be continued in the future of medicine?
129. What are the pros and cons of virtual consultations?
130. How might COVID have affected children?
131. How would you address inequalities if the NHS moved to virtual consultations?
132. How would you ensure that quality of care and healthcare standards were maintained in a virtual environment?
133. If you were the dean of the medical school, how would you deal with the course being oversubscribed?
    a. We also have to inform some people that we are unable to provide a place; how would you do this?
134. You're talking to your friend about a party happening while lockdown measures are active. Try to convince her not to go out.

SUMMARY, TEST YOURSELF AND REFLECTION

This chapter has taken you through what to expect from all the different interview types and how to practice.

If You Want to Succeed, You Need To

- Practice likely interview questions and scenarios.
- Prepare short-answer models and know your personal statement inside out.
- Seek additional experience to fill in any gaps for answering common interview questions.

Test Yourself

- Go through the practice questions with a colleague or friend and provide constructive criticism of each other's answers.

Reflection and Notes

RESOURCES

General Medical Council, 2020, Good medical practice. Available at https://www.gmc-uk.org/-/media/documents/good-medical-practice___english-20200128_pdf-51527435.pdf.

General Medical Council. Learning materials for ethical questions. Available at https://www.gmc-uk.org/ethical-guidance/learning-materials.

General Medical Council, 2018. Outcomes for graduates. Available at https://www.gmc-uk.org/-/media/documents/outcomes-for-graduates-jul-15-1216_pdf-61408029.pdf.

NHS England, 2016. NHS five-year forward view. Available at https://www.england.nhs.uk/wp-content/uploads/2016/05/fyfv-tech-note-090516.pdf.

Oxford interview samples. Available at https://www.ox.ac.uk/admissions/undergraduate/applying-to-oxford/guide/interviews.

SPIKES and breaking bad news. Available at http://theoncologist.alphamedpress.org/content/5/4/302.long.

TED Talks. Hot topics in medicine. Available at https://www.ted.com/talks?topics%5B%5D=medicine.

A Guide for Nontraditional Applicants

10

Aisha Sharif, Polen Bareke, Jamie Christian Charlton, Caroline Gu and Gareth Lau

Chapter Outline

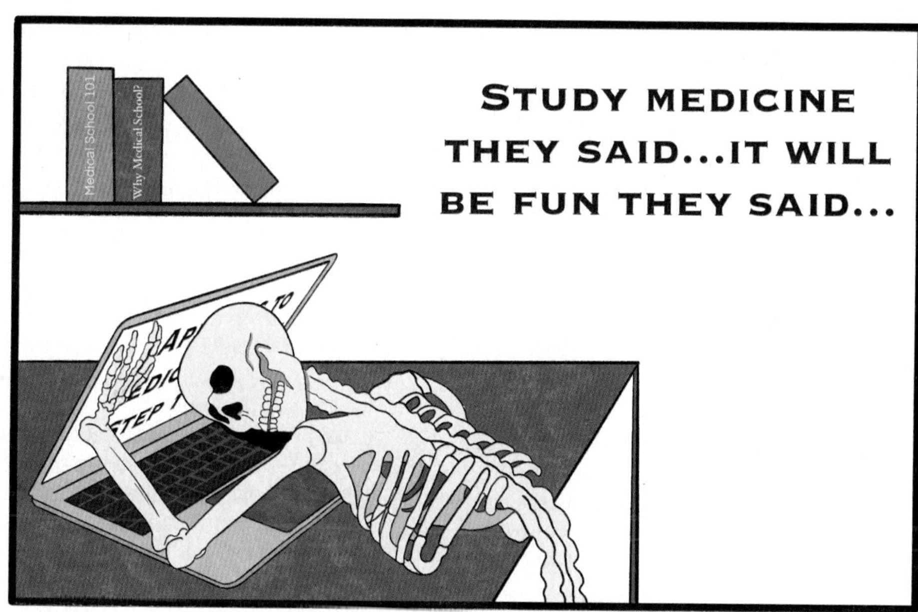

Being different is a good thing. It means you're brave enough to be yourself.

NONTRADITIONAL APPLICANTS

We have dedicated our final chapter to those of you who may have an extra thing or two to think about when applying to medical school. Be it something to add to your personal statement, useful information regarding relevant differences in your medical school interview structure or extra tests that you may have to go through, this chapter has got it covered.

In the first section of this chapter, we cover key information regarding **Graduate Entry to Medical School**. This includes key differences and exams of which you should take careful note. We then move on to discussing special aspects that **International Students** should consider when applying, including quotes from successful international medical students.

We hope you'll never even have to think about this, but the truth is, there are a certain percentage of medical school applicants each year that will be rejected. This doesn't mean that you will never get into medical school and that your journey has ended here. This is why we've named our third section **'Not Ready Yet'**—to prove that all you have to do is be persistent and one day you will end up doing what you love.

Finally, over the years, we have also received a lot of questions about taking a gap year and reapplying. Our last section aims to answer some of the most frequently asked questions about these topics.

GRADUATE ENTRY TO MEDICINE

Most people have the impression that all future medics are taken straight from secondary school with their impressive collection of A stars, commendations, medals and trophies, but what is becoming increasingly recognised is the contribution of non-school-leavers—in other words, graduates. It wasn't until 2000 that the first graduate entry medicine (GEM) courses were offered by medical schools. Since then, the popularity and success of the scheme have seen the enrolment of graduates soar, particularly since it provides a route into medicine for people who made the decision to become a medic later in life, or for people like me who couldn't decide what they wanted to do with their first set of post-nominals.

This chapter isn't designed to contemplate the pros and cons of school-leavers vs graduates (freshers vs oldies)—there will undoubtedly be sports matches and drinking games to that effect later on, but what this chapter aims to do is explain the process and concept of GEM to those who may be considering it. If, like me, you are joining medicine straight after receiving your degree, or several decades after it, then GEM is specifically designed to be your route into the profession. Make no mistake, having a degree already is not an automatic ticket into medical school, but it gives you an alternative way to prove yourself as a worthy potential future physician in a way that school-leavers aren't able to do. Medical schools have come to realise that not every applicant has wanted to be a medic since primary school, and many people try other careers or have families before they consider medicine as something they can envisage doing.

Medical schools also realise that academic qualifications aren't the sole determinant of an amazing doctor; rather, they look at the person as a whole, including their lived experiences and personality. It's all well and good being a Mensa 180 IQ genius, but if you haven't done anything else, then you won't stand out as much as someone who has done other things to better themselves. This is where my bias for GEM surfaces, because school-leavers have a very slim window to prove themselves ahead of their colleagues; they have 2 years during their A-Levels (or International Baccalaureate (IB)) to get their work experience, study, play their sports and gain their distinctions to try and gain an advantage in the interview. That's a lot to accomplish in a limited time, and kudos to those who make it, but graduates already have a degree (so they are already familiar with higher education), they have more life experience and they possess a different perspective, because they have had time to see how medical school, and life as a doctor, would fit into their own lives, and maybe their partner's. Medical school, and the process of applying as a graduate, is going to be a long, difficult and emotional journey, regardless of what stage in your life you go for it. However, you are not in any way disadvantaged by applying to medicine as a graduate. If anything, you have advantages that you bring to the table that you might not even realise.

This section aims to expand on what GEM is, how it works and whether it is for you. I am able to relate my own experience to this chapter, as can many other people who have been through the process, and I believe this insight is useful, as it not only explains how it works, but I can relate my own thoughts and emotions to the process in a way that a detached observer might not be able to do.

I didn't come out of the womb knowing that I wanted to be a doctor more than anything else in the world. It was a career I placed on the back burner during secondary school, and took off the hob and binned when I opened my first set of A-Level results. It was a crushing disappointment—my A-Levels were terrible, I'd failed chemistry and the only doctorate I thought I would ever get was doctor of self-pity. It wasn't as bad as it sounds, my A-Levels went okay in the end, and I was delighted to be accepted to study geography at a Russell Group university. I am very happy with my first degree. I still love geography and I have no regrets, but it wasn't until I did a bit of digging that I discovered that I could actually apply to medicine with a degree already. Better yet, it didn't have to be a medical or biological subject! That was when my ambition to become a doctor got back on track. Even though your A-Levels might be wrong or you already have a degree, you can still have the 'right stuff'.

Jamie, Graduate Entry Medical School Applicant, UK

When I started completing my A-Levels, I had the opportunity to shadow a GP for a week and I absolutely loved what the GP was doing. I decided to do more research to really see if being a doctor was for me. I was doing Biology, Chemistry and Maths at the time, so the stars were really starting to align so I decided to go for it. On results day, my grades weren't enough to get me into my firm choice or my insurance. I was gutted and ended up doing a degree in Chemistry. This isn't the typical degree like doing biomedicine or biochemistry. It did limit my choices because some universities have specific requirements so make sure you check beforehand. However, in the end, I worked hard, graduated and now I'm studying medicine. You don't always have to opt for the more traditional degree, there are plenty of ways to reach your goal of studying medicine—the real question is: Do you have the motivation and discipline to persevere?

Aisha, Graduate Entry Medical School Applicant, UK

Although I knew that I wanted to become a doctor from a young age, I could not get into medicine on my first try as I missed my offer by one grade. However, I got into my insurance choice and studied neuroscience instead, which, at the time, I saw as a 'failure'. Even though people around me kept telling me that doing this degree would benefit me in many aspects of my life, I refused to believe them, as I thought they were only saying this to comfort me and make me feel better about not getting into medicine. The environment I grew up in made me believe that there is only one route into medicine: Straight after finishing school. It is very difficult not to see yourself as a 'failure' if you're brought up in such an environment (at least, it was for me!). However, reflecting on my experiences during my neuroscience degree made me realise that I was not mentally ready to go into medicine on my first try. I am now very grateful that I got into medicine at the age of 21, rather than 18, having done some character development in between these years. If you are reading this as a graduate applicant to medical school, I want you to know that not getting into medicine on your first attempt is not a measure of your intelligence or academic capabilities. There is more to you than scoring high in your exams, and contrary to the belief of some of our teachers and academic advisers, a good doctor is not always the highest-scoring person in the class; instead, it is someone who takes their time to listen to the concerns of the patient, actively showing empathy and compassion to them. Therefore, my advice to you is that if medicine is really the career you want to pursue in the future, do not give up on this dream—stay focused, driven and hard-working, but also—be kind, humble and caring.

Polen, Graduate Entry Medical School Applicant, UK

SO, WHAT IS GRADUATE ENTRY MEDICINE?

Graduate Entry Medicine is actually quite a broad term. On the whole, it is the different set of entry requirements that apply solely to a graduate, in order to be considered for medical school entry fairly alongside other candidates. After a long consultation, the first GEM schemes opened to applications in 2000, and the scheme has only been growing since. At the time of this writing, there are now 14 UK medical schools that take graduates for GEM training. Good news, right? Well, this is where it gets complicated. There is currently no standardised way in which medical schools assess their graduate candidates. Each school has different prerequisites. Some may need a certain combination of A-Levels while others don't even look at them; some may need a certain admissions test while others don't, and they all set their own requirements. Just because you don't meet the requirements of one school doesn't mean that is the case for all of them! Do your research and find out what they want—what is their version of the 'right stuff'. Do you have it?

Broadly speaking, medical schools place a lot of weight on A-Level predicted or achieved grades for school-leavers, whereas in GEM, more emphasis is on your degree. Most processes will look at your degree subject and mark, your extracurricular experiences, admissions test marks, interview performance and personal statement. I hate to break it to you, but just because you're a graduate doesn't mean you don't have to do homework anymore!

Just as there are different methods of entry between schools, there are also different types of GEM courses. I'm not talking about the differences between MBBS, MbChB or MB BChir (they're all the same thing), but how the schools actually teach graduates. Some schools, like Warwick, knock a year off for graduates, who can join a 4-year 'accelerated' course. These courses are more intense and they have shorter holidays, but you get your degree faster. Other schools teach you no differently; you join your cohort as an equal with the school-leavers. It is entirely your decision what you think suits you, but hold that thought until I have broken down GEM a bit more first.

WHAT BACKGROUND DO I NEED? WHAT IS THE 'RIGHT STUFF'?

I'll start this section by dispelling a myth straightaway—you DON'T need to have a science degree or science A-Levels to do GEM. Let that sink in—you can get into medicine having (almost) no formal science qualifications. There is a caveat though; it will limit your options a bit more. Let me explain.

Some medical schools require a specific degree and/or grade for GEM. For example, Liverpool states that candidates must have a 2:1 degree classification in a biomedical/health science subject. Other schools, like Warwick or Exeter, don't mind what subject you studied. Most schools do require a 2:1 or better, although they make dispensations if you do a master's course and you had a 2:2, for instance. If you haven't done a science degree or A-Levels, it will limit your choices a bit more to those schools that don't require it. Why, then, don't all schools require sciences? This all comes down to admissions tests. You may have heard the terms UCAT, BMAT or GAMSAT. If not, don't worry, there's a whole section on those beauties coming up, but they are rather nasty exams that are quite sciencey. They are designed to assess a candidate's abilities in scientific reasoning and logic, sometimes with an essay or two thrown in. The mark you gain in these tests means more to some schools than your previous scientific background, so yes, you can still apply to GEM even if you studied history, art, drama, underwater basket weaving or Justin Bieber, but you can't quite get away with being completely scientifically illiterate unfortunately—you'll just have to do a long exam on science instead.

When it comes to entry requirements, you need to do your research. Each school publishes its own grades and subjects, and you need to align with their minimum requirements. If something isn't entirely clear (as is often the case in applying) phone them and ask. What do you have to lose? If your grades aren't good enough, cross that school off your list and try your next one. There'll probably be a place for you out there somewhere.

Make sure you always check the universities' websites for entry requirements before you apply. Each university is different, and some have specific requirements you ought to find out about prior to applying to maximise your chances and avoid potential hiccups. If you're unsure, you can always ring them and ask; that's what they're there for after all.

As I mentioned previously, there is more to the ideal candidate than their qualifications. Your life and work experience factor into your personal statement and interview. Let me present you with a scenario—you have two candidates and one medical school vacancy. Candidate A has a first class degree in biomedical science. They have no medical work experience, and they were not a member of any university societies. They have been in a paid role for 5 years but have never sought any type of leadership position. Candidate B has a low 2:1 in geography; they have been a first aid society president, advanced first aider in St John Ambulance, member of two medical societies and employed full time since leaving university.

Which candidate would you choose? I'll give you a clue; Candidate B was me. I had a (low) 2:1 but I was still invited to interview. They loved the extracurricular angle, and it gave me loads of examples to bear in the interviews! Academia isn't everything, because being a doctor isn't just an academic role. Doctors also perform the role of counsellor, physician, report writer, speaker, researcher, tea maker and note taker. We've all known people who are absolute geniuses in their field but have the social skills of a brick. Imagine if you have to break the worst possible news to a family—patients don't want a doctor with no empathy, and medical schools don't either. Lived experiences build one's character. The longer you've been around, and the more you learn and participate in things, the more strings you have to your bow. See the section on work experience where I elaborate more, but the right stuff is also about your personality and your experience. As a graduate, you have done things that school-leavers haven't, and that gives you a unique edge.

> You don't necessarily have to have a scientific background to get into medical school but be aware, qualifications aren't the only thing they look for. Future doctors need to be good 'all-rounders', people who have acceptable academic backgrounds but also put a lot of time into extracurricular pursuits and work experience.
>
> **Jamie, Graduate Entry Medical School Applicant, UK**

> As a graduate, you have more time to look for work experiences and volunteering opportunities. Use that extra time wisely. Manage your time effectively so your studies don't fall behind either. Always remember, it's not what you did but what you learnt from it; reflection is key. Medicine admissions don't expect you to have scrubbed in on a rare surgery—quite the opposite—what they expect is enthusiasm, commitment and passion whether that is through volunteering in a care home or on a hospital ward.
>
> **Aisha, Graduate Entry Medical School Applicant, UK**

WHICH MEDICAL SCHOOLS OFFER GRADUATE COURSE IN MEDICINE (4-YEAR)?

Which schools accept graduates? The best ones, of course! On a serious note, there are currently 14 schools that accept graduates directly. The schools and their programmes can be found quickly on Google, but the ones currently offering GEM are:

- Birmingham
- Cambridge
- Cardiff
- Imperial
- King's College London
- Liverpool
- Newcastle
- Nottingham
- Oxford
- Barts and the London (Queen Mary's University of London)
- Southampton
- St George's University London
- Swansea
- Warwick

These schools offer the accelerated GEM course (Universities and Colleges Admissions Service (UCAS) code A101), but you can apply to almost any school with a degree; you'll just have to enter as an undergraduate. Hopefully, more schools will be added in the future, but a consideration of GEM is that you may need to relocate if you get accepted in a school somewhere other than where you live.

HOW DO I APPLY AS A GRADUATE?

When I was told I'd have to go through UCAS and write my personal statement again, I nearly shrivelled up in a corner and cried. As much as we dread it, unfortunately, you still have to apply for GEM in the same way as an undergraduate degree. You apply through UCAS, submit your personal statement and admissions test results, sit your interview and then (if the stars align) get an offer. Let's go through the process sequentially:

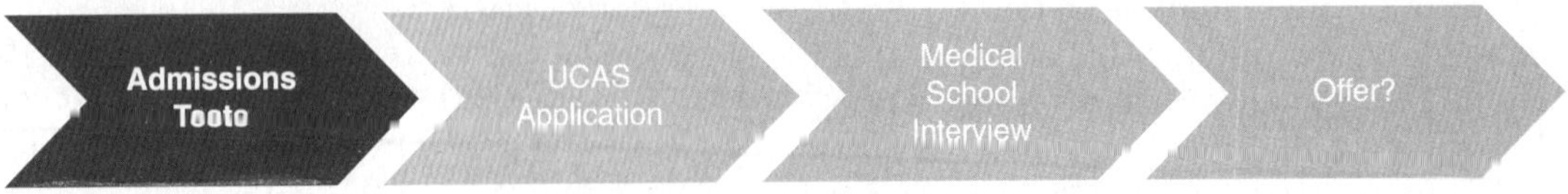

Admissions Tests → UCAS Application → Medical School Interview → Offer?

The Admissions Tests

Most medical schools require you to sit some form of admissions test as a graduate. There is the Graduate Medical Schools Admissions Test (GAMSAT), University Clinical Aptitude Test (UCAT) and, finally, BioMedical Admissions Test (BMAT). Different universities use different exams so make sure you check way ahead of time so you can prepare. I'll write more about those later on in the chapter, but these exams are the schools' way of standardising your academic ability. It depends on the exam and the provider, but you must book and sit an exam before your UCAS application is even submitted. For example, I started researching the GAMSAT in June, sat it in September and sent my UCAS off in October. Make a good note of your test scores and make several copies. This first stage needs to be a reflection—hopefully your scores are good enough, but are they suitable for your chosen medical schools? The schools all set committee-chosen thresholds. The GAMSAT cut off for interview in my year was 59 out of 100.

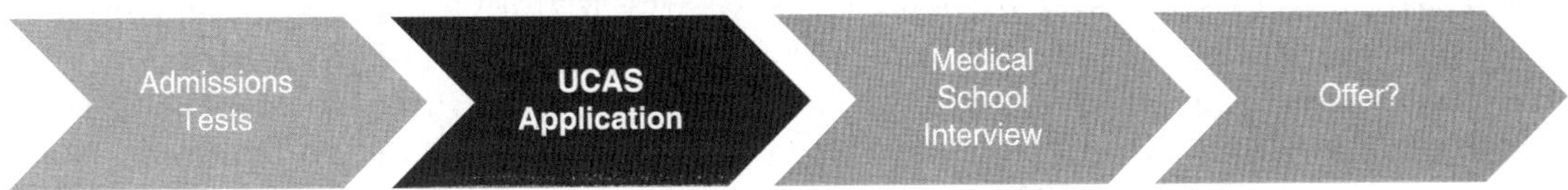

Your UCAS

Hopefully you've already been through this process as a graduate, but if you sat your degree in the days before UCAS, it's an online service through which all UK university applications are submitted (UCAS). I'll write about good personal statements shortly, but the sooner you get your UCAS application ready to send off, the better. Trust me! Filling in the personal details is the easy part. Don't forget to include your admissions test score(s). Medicine UCAS applications also have earlier submission deadlines in October, so don't delay!

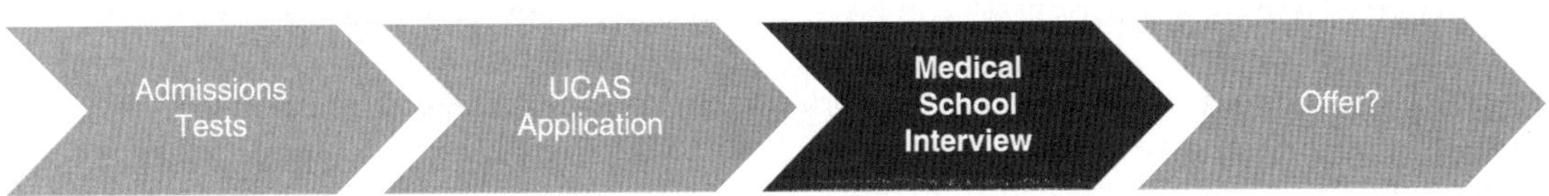

Your Interview

It's becoming a theme, but again, it varies by school. There are two main types of medical school interviews: traditional panel and multiple mini-interviews (MMIs).

A traditional interview is when you sit in front of a panel of medical and lay interviewers and answer all kinds of questions and scenarios. They probe several facets of your character, alongside your motivations for studying medicine. They won't ask you to outline the steps involved in a percutaneous nephrolithotomy; that fun starts AFTER you've been accepted!

An MMI is sort of like a selection centre. You attend with a clutch of candidates, and you are given a briefing on how the day will run. After that, it does exactly what it says on the tin. You rotate between several stations, and each station lasts a few minutes. You meet a different assessor at each one, and you perform different tasks or answer different questions in each station. I'll elaborate in a bit.

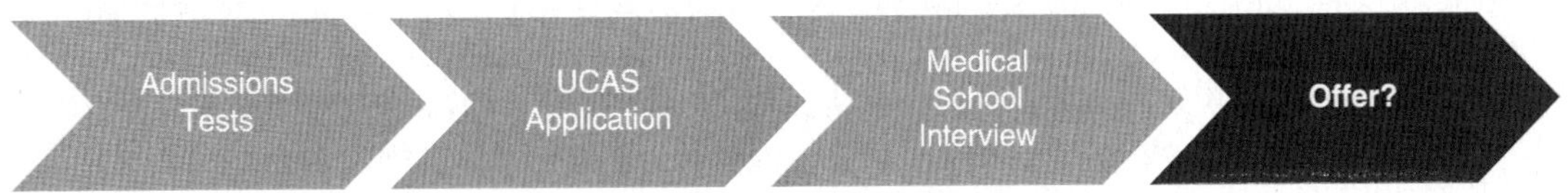

Your Offer?

Just remember, someone has to fill all those places, so it might as well be you.

> Get your UCAS application ready as soon as possible. The longer you leave it the less time you have to prepare it to an excellent standard.

The application timeline can differ, but you're looking at about a year from start to end.

WHAT OTHER ROUTES ARE THERE INTO MEDICINE?

Don't feel as a graduate that you are confined to a GEM course—you are equally valid if you apply for a normal undergraduate course with your degree. The only difference is you will have to present your admission test score rather than your A-Level grades if you're applying as an undergraduate (although some schools still want those too). There are the traditional 5-year courses on offer, and in some cases even 6-year courses available, with the year-long 'access' course added, although these access courses are only available to those who have never taken any science A-Levels, and having a degree precludes some access courses. What about international universities? In some countries, you don't even have to pay tuition fees. Maybe they have better food too?

Loyalty also counts. If you have a degree from a particular university, see if there are any special dispensations for its medical school. Exeter grants a guaranteed interview for their medical sciences alumni and so do several other universities, which can act as an advantage.

Applying for a GEM course can be very competitive, even more competitive than the undergraduate one. Most people think that because you're a graduate, fewer people will be applying. That is not true. A lot of the GEM programs have about 40 spaces for thousands of applicants, so you really have to stand out. The A100 (undergraduate) course is equally competitive if not more competitive. That's because not only do you have school-leavers, but you also have graduates applying too. The thing about graduates is that they're older and have committed 3 years to a degree already. This means their newly acquired skills and commitment can act as real competition for fresh school-leavers applying for their first degree.

GAINING WORK EXPERIENCE AND EXTRACURRICULAR ACTIVITIES

Everyone has their preconceptions about what doctors do and what their job is like, but you absolutely must have some exposure to the medical world before you decide to apply to medicine. There are two main reasons for this. First, medical schools want to know that they won't be investing hundreds of thousands of pounds in your training to decide it isn't for you and pull the plug in your first year of practice.

The second reason is that you need to see for yourself what the working life of a doctor is *really* like. Some doctors may have nice cars and country club holidays, but what you don't see are the long hours, emotional stress, social pressures and other stresses of the vocation. Being a doctor is immensely rewarding, but it takes a certain type of person. The biggest thing I took away from my work experience wasn't necessarily the medical knowledge but the first-hand interaction with patients and staff. It didn't dissuade me from pursuing the medical dream, but some patients had a profound effect on me, and I will never forget them or their cases.

Of course, it isn't just work experience that counts; they are just as interested in what you choose to do outside your studies. If you are amazing at your studies but don't do anything outside them at all, then you're a bit boring, aren't you? It may sound blunt, but assessors are looking for motivation and the constant drive to better yourself as a person. Doctors are required to not only constantly learn, but also be a well-rounded person, and have an escape from work in the form of a worthwhile hobby or sport. Extracurricular pursuits take effort, dedication, diligence, time management, enthusiasm… ticking all the boxes essentially! You'll find that assessors get particularly excited about roles to do with teamwork and leadership. You don't necessarily have to have created and run a Fortune 500 company, but do you have any leadership experiences you can draw on? Were you captain of a sports team or a team leader for an important event? If not, think of something you could get involved in. It could really be anything; it doesn't have to be medical. Just something you enjoy, preferably with a teamwork element to it. A running club or competitive swimming perhaps?

Arguably one of the more difficult parts of preparing to go to medical school is securing work experience. If, like me, you shudder at the thought of your letter requesting work experience getting laughed at and shredded, I am happy to be living proof of the contrary. Just ask. Doctors and medical staff are busy people, but most would be happy to take you for a day of shadowing or to answer some questions. There are other forms of work experience that get you patient contact: voluntary ambulance services, charity work, youth leaders and hospital volunteering. Have a look on the internet for inspiration, and give them a call or, better yet, send them a letter. Explain who you are, what you intend to do and how you will benefit from the experience. There's quite a lot going on out there. When I got my letter telling me I had a week watching surgery, it felt like I'd won the lottery.

Of course, COVID-19 has changed the world significantly and now you may even have more hoops to jump through to get some form of work experience. Now luckily, we live in the 21st century, where the existence of technology has made our lives super easy. You can now join virtual work experience, complete online courses, the list is endless, but I guess the real question is, will it be enough? Ultimately, what are admissions tutors looking for? They want to see that you have the skills and the experience and know enough to want to pursue a career in medicine. If you have the opportunity to do in-person work experience, we wholeheartedly recommend it as you get to see and understand more in the real world than through the lens of a computer camera. Both in-person and virtual work experience opportunities are equally valuable as long as you are able to reflect on your experiences in your personal statement or during your medical school interview.

Now comes the question of how much work experience are they looking for? There is no set limit. Some schools *suggest* about a week's worth, but this is only a guide, and it is cumulative. They are looking for what you learned from your experience, as that is what they will ask about in the interview. They won't care if you witnessed open-heart surgery in Zanzibar or only got a day shadowing hospital porters; it's all about reflection and what you learned. An example I can relate to you—I spent 3 days teaching a bunch of Girl Guides first aid. What good is that? Well, dissect it. I had to take my knowledge of the subject and tailor my communications style to impart the same knowledge in a way that the girls could understand, but also in a fun way so that they could enjoy and retain it better. This is a good skill for a physician, as you will have to explain complicated terminology and medical advice to the patient and their families in a way that they understand. I guarantee most of your experiences can in some way give you a skill you can bring to medical school. The best thing to do is to write them all down and have examples ready for each skill the interviewers want.

By the same token, any work experience is good experience. Don't be put off by people saying they spent 3 months in Nepal saving lives in hospital before their first cup of Earl Grey. If they can't relate what they took from it, then it was a waste of time anyway. When it comes to work experience, think outside the box. It's not just doctors you can shadow; you can write to clerical staff, porters, social workers and academics. Even if they can't help you, they can probably refer you to someone who can. Also, do any of your friends or colleagues have acquaintances in that field? Ask to be put in touch.

Now we have covered making the most of work experiences from a general perspective. If you always wanted to do medicine but were unable to get into medical school the first time, the logical second choice will be to pursue a science-related degree such as Biomedical Sciences, Biological Sciences, Pharmacy or anything similar. What we may consider 'traditional' work experience may not immediately be obvious when you're doing these degrees, as you may not get direct patient contact or be involved in healthcare.

But, and this is a big BUT, you are spending 3 to 4 years studying the core principles of medical sciences and most likely conducting medical research as well. The GMC Tomorrow's Doctors publication states that one of the outcomes for medical graduates is *'Doctor as a scientist'* and therefore you will automatically be more qualified than a graduate of any other discipline. The key is to make the most of experiences and see how it can be applied to the medical school application.

The major points that you must get across are the appreciation that doctors need to be aware of medical research and many doctors get involved extensively in clinical trials, laboratory research and publishing in peer-reviewed journals. As a science graduate, you have experience in the methodology of research, conducted research in your final year project and, if applicable, presented your research at conferences, and if you're very lucky published in journals as well. It is crucial that you get these points across in your personal statement in at least one paragraph and be well read in your own research so that you're ready to talk about it at the interview.

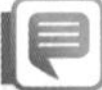

If you're still studying for your science undergraduate degree, start reflecting on your research activities and how they could be clinically applicable. This will help you remember what you did when it comes to apply. If you have the time, start preparing a portfolio with evidence of your scientific achievements, be it giving a presentation, attending a conference or completing extra courses. This will allow you to have the competitive edge.

Dr Navin Nagesh, Academic Doctor, Oxford University

Lastly, work experience is extra important for graduates because it gives you a window into what you're getting into. What's their working life like? How will it affect your living arrangements, finances and family? Don't forget to cover these questions too.

Work Experience?

Work experience is definitely something all too commonly asked about in your interview. It's vital for boosting your application and for you as an individual. Medicine is a long slog, particularly after getting a degree already, and you really need to be sure. Getting a part-time job in a hospital is really helpful. I've worked in my local trust since I was 18 years old and it's such a good way to see the hospital, how it's run and what a doctor actually does every day. Alongside this, I have gained numerous placements with consultants, and have volunteered with both elderly and disabled adults too. Experiencing different areas of healthcare gives you a more holistic background for your decision as to why you chose medicine over other career options. Also, it might actually make you realise you prefer something else.

Chloe, Graduate Medical Student, King's College London

In summary, there are loads of things you can do to gain work experience. Network constantly, make new contacts and write to everyone you can. For every no there'll be a yes somewhere. Work experience is precious—take notes and keep a diary, and constantly think, how will this help you in a medical interview?

PERSONAL STATEMENT

Unfortunately, 47 lines isn't much to convince someone why you deserve a place in medical school. It's even less when you have to include a mini-biography, your experiences and your motivations. Hopefully you've written a personal statement before—and there are guides that go into far more detail than I can in this chapter, but what I will include is whether your personal statement is any different from an undergraduate application, and on what the emphasis should be placed.

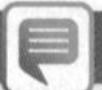

Personal Statement?

My top tip is: Get it done early and show it to people. You will most likely have advisors at university that can help. Your personal or academic tutor is also a really good person to go to. However, it is not the be-all and end-all. For example, Warwick University does not even consider it, whereas Kings College London looks at it alongside your reference and your UCAT score.

For the personal statement I think it's very important to make sure you show how and what you've learnt from your experiences, and how this educates you and motivates you for a career in medicine.

Chloe G., Graduate Medical Student, Kings College London

You are at least 3 years ahead of a school-leaver. During that time, you have accomplished a degree and hopefully some life experience in the interim. Your studies have granted you access to higher education facilities and you may have produced several pieces of research-grade coursework to be granted your degree, alongside juggling work and extracurricular events and activities. Sell yourself! Don't apologise for anything. Any degree involves writing skills alongside quantitative fluency, presentation and computer skills.

We already extensively covered the structure of the medical school personal statement in Chapter 8. But as a graduate, there are a few things you should definitely consider that the average school-leaver might not have. So let's recap the basic personal statement structure and how as a graduate you can add further value.

In the first paragraph, it should be clear that you are a graduate, as it's not ideal for the reader to find out by chance later on in the statement. There are many ways of making this clear. It's ultimately your personal statement and you should take full ownership of the first paragraph, as it's usually the most personal.

Examples of good introductions are addressing the elephant in the room, which is, why are you a graduate applicant? If you studied a nonscience subject, you should be very honest about why you chose it. Having a clear passion in life is very admirable, and the more honest you are about this the better you'll score. Also mention, if applicable, that you were not aware of medicine as a career when you were a school-leaver, and after studying the degree that you were passionate about, you looked at medicine more seriously and found that it was the profession with which you want to continue your life.

If you are a science graduate, you can still be passionate about your chosen subject, but there are greater opportunities to make links to medicine. This can be in the form of enjoying the clinical application of the content that you're learning, getting involved in clinical research or being more honest and saying that laboratory research is not for you. Nobody can judge you for your passion for medicine, and the more open and honest you are, the better. Don't worry about sounding cliché; if something is cliché, it's because it's very common for applicants to consider.

As we progress to the second and third paragraphs, the school-leavers will be talking about their clinical work experiences. 'But my clinical work experiences are from 3 to 4 years ago when I first applied?' There is no time limit on a life experience; if you did it and you learnt from it, don't be embarrassed to use it. Of course you can mention that you had this experience before your degree and then reflect on other work experiences you may have had that have given you a worldview of medicine. 'What if I didn't do any clinical work experience during my undergraduate?' This is also fine; as previously mentioned, you can relate any life experience to how it will make you a more compassionate, safer and more competent doctor. If you did a science degree, then write about your research activity and passion for advancing medical care; if you did a nonscience degree, then write about your transferable skills. In summary, the bulk of the personal statement will be focused on how your life experiences have guided your decision towards medicine. If that is clear to the reader then you've done a good job.

The final paragraph is very important. The reader needs to understand that you appreciate the longevity of your chosen path, know the social and financial implications of a medical degree as a graduate, but have made a mature and realistic decision. You can also use this opportunity to discuss your aspirations for after medical school. This is harder for school-leavers, as all they've seen is A-Levels/IB, but you've lived out in the real world; some of you may have even had careers. The most impressive graduate applicants have a view of what they would like to pursue after medical school in terms of specialities, whether they want to split clinical work with research, or they would just like to do clinical work, as that's why they have left the science world. It is important that you are most honest in the first and last paragraphs of your personal statement. The middle section is a given, as most applicants will describe impressive activities, but for us to understand what kind of person you've become and wish to be is the most valuable aspect of the personal statement for graduates.

- Be careful with sweeping statements.

A sentence as innocent as, 'My passion for science will be an asset in medical school' can potentially be ripped apart. If you like science, why not be a scientist instead? How will it be an asset, we've got lots of scientists here? They'll (hopefully) not be as nasty as that, but you need to think about each assertion. If you frame the same statement like this, 'My scientific training and curiosity equips me with logical reasoning, which would be vital in patient care and diagnoses', you've narrowed down the statement and made it more relevant.

- Examine properly your motivations for applying to medicine.
  If you want to join a select community of like-minded individuals who use knowledge and skill to better the lives of patients and their families while continually aiming to improve themselves and the vocation, then you're along the right lines. You want to help people, but everyone says that, and there are other ways you can help people. Why do you want to help people by specifically practicing medicine? Get through the superficial layers and to the core of why you want to do this.
- Assessors don't need to be impressed by overly long words or terminology.
- Just be honest.
  You're effectively writing an advert of yourself. If you have strong convictions that you are ready to be a doctor, this should come across in your writing.
- Self-confidence is important, but don't be cocky!

Dr Ollie Rupar, A&E, Royal Devon and Exeter Hospital

Take your time with your personal statement, let it be scrutinised by friends and family, and do your research. You deserve this place—show them why!

Make sure that you have properly examined and understand your reasoning for wanting to become a doctor. Medical schools want to know that you have a firm conviction to enter medicine for the right reasons, so be prepared for 'Why do you want to be a doctor?'

Jamie, Graduate Entry Medical School Applicant, UK

MAKE USE OF YOUR FORMER DEGREE AND ITS MODULES

As you'll recall from your former undergraduate degree, you get the blessing of picking most of your university modules, and this means you get to learn what you want. How cool is that?! Unlike in A-Level or school in general, where you must do whatever is specified in the curriculum, a degree allows flexibility. Of course, you can pick modules that would help you with your medicine degree, but the truth is it won't make a huge difference since you will cover all essentials during your time as a medical student. This should motivate you to choose modules you truly enjoy during your undergraduate degree as this will make you happier and will make you more likely to score well when it comes to exams. You can however make the most of your undergraduate modules by discussing some of your favourite ones in your personal statement or during the interview.

Now then, let's talk about the one thing all students hate: The dreaded dissertation. Most graduate students (including myself) hate writing their dissertation. It is the longest essay of your life and it feels pointless, but once it's done you soon realise it can be more useful to your medical school application than you can imagine. Remember, as a doctor, you won't just be working in the clinical environment; you can also do research, which is something that A-Level and school students don't have. The skills you gain from a lab are still used in medicine. Have you been synthesising drugs, working with cells and testing samples of blood? These are all examples that can make you stand out from the crowd. Another thing you can do is volunteer in a research lab at your university. This will enable you to develop key skills you can mention in your personal statement and discuss during your interview while volunteering and supporting university staff and your supervisor. Alternatively, you can speak to a researcher in your university and apply for a summer studentship. All of these things will show your passion and commitment and hopefully bring you one step closer to studying medicine.

Prior to applying to graduate entry medicine, I studied a degree in chemistry (a BSc). I didn't have as many modules linked to medicine due to the nature of my degree. I tried to think of ways to stand out, so I decided to speak to my lecturer about doing a project with one of her collaborators with the School of Medicine and Dentistry. The next thing I knew, I had a project linked to pharmacology. I was designing drugs and then synthesising them and testing them on my receptor. I had an amazing experience, and I completely enjoyed the project. All it took was courage and confidence to ask! In fact, my supervisor enjoyed working with me so much that he offered me a master's degree (an MSc), but of course, I wanted to study medicine, so instead, he helped me get funding so I could work in his lab for the summer. I also had the opportunity to talk about my project in my medical school interviews, and they loved it. It showed my understanding of various medical issues and how my research will deepen my understanding.

Aisha, Graduate Entry Medical School Applicant, UK

ENTRANCE EXAMINATIONS

I mentioned earlier that graduates are expected to sit an admissions test or entrance examination. They all follow different formulae, but they are all designed to give a fair assessment of your intelligence to the medical schools. They are extremely important and should be taken seriously, as they determine if you even get an interview or not. I'll talk briefly about the main triad of admissions tests before sharing some useful tips. BMAT and UCAT are covered in Chapter 7.

The Graduate Medical Schools Admissions Test (GAMSAT)

The GAMSAT is similar in structure to the BMAT, but it is much longer and there is more emphasis on science. It is another pen-to-paper exam, and lasts 5½ hours. There are three separate exams: Section I, **Reasoning in Social Sciences and Humanities** (100 minutes, probes your understanding of people and how they tick); Section II, **Written Communication** (two 30-minute essays, each on a one or two word random theme); and Section III, **Reasoning in Biological and Physical Sciences** (170 minutes, the really hard paper testing biology, chemistry and physics at around A2 level).

Cardiff, Exeter, Keele, Liverpool, Nottingham, Plymouth, St Andrew's, St. George's and Swansea use GAMSAT. It is a more widely used exam and the one with the meanest reputation. I recommend at least 4 months preparation but it can be done in a month (stressfully!).

These exams are very difficult, and apart from maybe the science sections, you can't study for them. They test intelligence rather than knowledge retention. Don't be put off by how hard you've heard a particular exam is; they are all hideous, but remember that if your score is good enough for medical school, then you've aced probably one of the hardest exams around! With decent research and a lot of preparation, you shouldn't have any surprises, and you'll know which test is best suited for your needs. You should consider the admissions test as the first action in applying for medical school before anything else, as they take many months of hard work and more than a few coffee-fuelled chemistry binges, but any hurdle can be overcome with the right amount of dedication.

HOW EARLY SHOULD I PREPARE AS A GRADUATE?

You don't necessarily have to apply in the same year you decide you want to go for medicine—there's no rush. People in their forties and fifties get in after a lifetime of doing something else! When you do go for it, the whole process from researching admissions tests to (hopefully) receiving an offer takes around a year, and it's quite stop-start with periods of study followed by long periods of waiting. Patience is key here. Everyone has their own comfortable preparation time, so the timetable I'll present here is only a guide, but the timings here should give you some indication of how much time you need to allot to each stage, assuming around 1 to 5 hours of work a day.

Admissions Tests

UCAT—Around a **month** of preparation.

BMAT and **GAMSAT**—At least **2 months** but preferably longer. Five months is a bit excessive, you need to have a life too!

UCAS Application and Personal Statement

Leave a good **month** to go over it and submit early if possible, so you don't have to worry about it later. The personal statement should take a **week** at least.

Interview

A **month** of good, solid prep and mock interviews should suffice. There's only so much they can ask you! YouTube has some great channels for interview questions and how MMI works, so check it out.

> I started preparing for this process probably at the beginning of my second year. This in all honesty was probably a bit premature but different programmes require different things, for example work experience requirements and their respective entrance exams. For example, Warwick requires 70 hours from a minimum of two placements in the past 2 years and sometimes these can be difficult to obtain at the last minute. Additionally, some exams take longer to prepare for than others, so this needs to be taken into consideration.
>
> **Chloe, Graduate Medical Student, Kings College London**

FINANCE—HOW TO COPE AS A GRADUATE STUDENT (DOMESTIC AND INTERNATIONAL)

Ah...how are you going to fund the little venture of medical school? Finance is a major concern of undergraduate and graduate medical students alike, especially with the restriction of bursaries and the shrinking amount of financial help available. Further complications are added for GEM students, because the financial help you will receive depends on the type of medical course you enrol in, your sources of expenditure and what funding options you choose, whether you are a domestic or international student and whether you can get any help from student-funding bodies. This section will be broken down into two parts: what you will be spending money on as a GEM student and where your income is going to come from.

WHAT DO MEDICAL STUDENTS SPEND MONEY ON?

Chances are, as a graduate already, you have a fair understanding of just how expensive and sometimes frugal a student's life is. There's no other way to put it—becoming a doctor will be an investment, not only emotionally and academically, but also financially. I write this section exclusively from the view of a prospective graduate student, assuming you have a degree and probably some form of paid employment. This section will be illuminating and depressing in equal measure, but it is vital you consider how a potential medical degree will affect your piggy bank.

Admissions Tests

Your expenditure will probably begin before you even apply to medical school! If you recall, the first stage of any graduate medical application is the admissions tests. Because external companies administer the tests, they all set fees for sitting the test and any study materials you may require. If you choose, you may also need to budget for attending prep courses for the exams, and they aren't cheap! It is always worthwhile doing your research into what schools you want to apply to and what admissions test they require. If they do require different tests and you have already shortlisted your chosen medical schools, then by all means sit whatever admissions tests are required. However, if you can narrow down your choices to schools that only require one type of test, then you are already being shrewd with your expenditure. As a guide for what to expect, I will list some rough prices for you to consider:

GAMSAT 2023 fees:

- £271 (roughly equivalent in international test centres)
- +£60 late registration fee (check the dates!)
- +£40–80 admin fees (deferral, remarking and cancellation charges)
- +£10–28 per GAMSAT revision item (practice tests and booklets)

BMAT 2022 fees:

- £46 EU and UK entry fee
- £78 International entry fee
- +£33–34 admin fees (late entry, results enquiries and appeals)

With the BMAT, test centres may charge a small additional fee to cover administration costs. However, the BMAT has several means by which you can apply for financial support. See http://www.admissionstestingservice.org/for-test-takers/bmat/dates-and-costs/ for more details. Please note, UK medical schools have decided to remove BMAT from their selection criteria as of 2024. However, there are several medical schools around the world who are still using the BMAT. For a full list, please visit their official website.

UCAT 2023 fees:

- Test taken in the UK: £70
- Test taken outside the UK: £115

UCAS Applications

UCAS is probably the cheapest thing you'll have to pay for on this list. It's £13 for a single choice, or £24 for multiple choices or late applications.

Travel and Accommodation

When preparing for graduate medicine, networking and studying, these costs will soon add up. Medicine has moved with the times and is now a very interconnected but spread out vocation, so you will have to travel between lectures, sites and hospitals to all kinds of conferences and events. Great for the travel, sad for the wallet! On top of this, of course, you will have to consider relocation or student accommodation costs. There may be means to help you with this such as scholarships or grants, but this is where your research is key.

Tuition Fees, Living Costs and Course Resources

Again, make sure you do your research thoroughly. Most, if not all, universities now charge the maximum £9250 a year fees with the recent Teaching Excellence Framework (TEF) policies, and this increases markedly for international students. What you will find, however, is that your tuition fees actually cover very little. You will probably still have to pay for textbooks, stethoscopes, lab wear, printing, food and society memberships. There are more details on how to cover tuition fees in the following section.

HOW CAN I FUND ALL THIS?!

Before we begin this section, it is important to make a distinction between what sort of 'graduate' medicine you're applying for. Four-year graduate GEM courses generally have more funding options than a 5- or 6-year undergraduate course, because it is not considered equivalent to doing a second undergraduate degree. Due to budget constraints, student finance services will currently not give a tuition fee loan to undergraduate medicine degree if you already possess a degree in any subject. With any problem though, there are solutions. There are several means for both domestic and international students to fund their studies, some harder than others. The following section will only outline suggestions to get you started; it is up to you to research and decide the most appropriate methods for your situation.

Student Finance

Even if you're applying for a 4-year GEM course, you are still expected to make a contribution to the course fees in at least year one. According to 2022 information, your contribution will be £3465 with a non-means-tested Student Finance Loan covering the rest of the year's fees. On top of this, you may be eligible for a living costs loan of up to £12,000, depending on your circumstances, which is partly means tested. 'Circumstances' in this respect means the assessment criteria by which the student loans companies determine how much they should pay you. They account for current income, whether you have any dependents, your parental income and other indicators.

To reiterate, if you are applying for an undergraduate medicine course, as a graduate student, you will not be eligible for the tuition fee loan from Student Finance. However, since medicine is considered a part-time 'Equivalent or lower qualification (ELQ)' exception, you will be eligible to get the minimum maintenance loan of £6780. You could only get this loan if you are a domestic student or an EU student holding a pre-settled or settled status under the EU Settlement Scheme. The application requires the students to physically fill out the PN1 form with a pen and either post it to the Student Finance Company (SFC) or scan the completed pages of the PN1 form and upload it to your Student Finance account online. If you want to get more maintenance loan due to your household income being below a certain threshold outlined by the SFC, you can then fill out the PN1 form, which allows you to get a maximum loan of £12,667 on the condition that your household income is £25,000 or less and that you live in London, away from your parents. Along with the PN1 form, you are also asked to provide evidence of your parents' gross income in the tax year during which you are applying. This could be a P60 form or a statement letter from your parents' employer. If your household income has dropped by 15% or more and, thereby, you want the income that your parents will earn in the following tax year to be assessed, you will need to fill out the Current Year Income Assessment Form, along with providing evidence of the predicted gross income of your parents. It is recommended that you start your maintenance loan application by the 31st of May, so that you could receive the money before your course term starts, as the application process takes around 3 to 4 months. Please note, this information is subject to change from year to year so please double check on the official website to avoid disappointment.

In addition, personal factors may also make you eligible for certain grants, like childcare and adult dependents grants. Check out all the details and how to apply for student finance on www.gov.uk/studentfinance.

There are several different things that may make you eligible for some financial help. Are you from a disadvantaged background? Do you have any children or are you married? Are you an international student? Universities try very hard indeed to attract as many applicants as possible, so research what they can do for you. What help can they or will they offer you to get your application? It's worth an ask!

NHS Bursary

If you intend on being a physician in the National Health Service (NHS), then they can provide some funding in the final 3 years of a 4-year GEM course. In years 2, 3 and 4 (providing you meet their eligibility criteria), the NHS will pay the first £3715 of your annual tuition fee, and the rest can be covered by student finance. The NHS can also contribute towards living costs, travel expenses and personal circumstances. More details are on the NHS Business Services Authority website (https://www.nhsbsa.nhs.uk/nhs-bursary-students). For those in an undergraduate course, the NHS bursary is not accessible until the final year of your course.

Paid Work

This is probably the solution favoured by old-schoolers and parents. You can always fund your studies through your own finances, particularly if you have been working for several years prior to your medical school application. Using money earned from work cuts out the formalities and stress of numerous funding applications, but of course it also means you will be out of pocket. It is highly inadvisable to have a job while at medical school. Unless you're extremely savvy at time management, it probably won't work very well. However, there's nothing stopping you working during the holidays for a few extra pennies or even working for a few years before applying. There are many ways you can earn cash, and some more bizarre than others—you can be a private tutor, a translator, which can be a good opportunity for international students, as you are more likely to speak several languages, or ironically volunteer yourself for paid medical trails! Hey, money is money, right?

University Support

Whether you are enrolled in a graduate or undergraduate medical course, universities will probably have some mechanism of financial support for exceptional or disadvantaged students. It is a good idea to contact your universities of choice regarding this. If you have particular problems that may affect your studies, there are bursaries and grants available from the institutions or from other bodies—always check the available information for more details.

The Military

The armed forces are in great need of trained medical officers, and as a result the UK armed forces offer generous funding packages to support you. If you decide that being a medical officer in the military is for you, then go into your local Armed Forces Careers Office (AFCO) and speak to a representative from your chosen military branch. Explain your situation and ask them what support is available. All branches will cover at least 3 years tuition fees, in addition to paying you a salary and a book allowance. In return, however, you are required to join your chosen armed force as an officer cadet, for example in the University's Air Squadron, Royal Naval Unit, or Officer Training Corps, and sign on for an officer's commission for at least 6 years after you graduate.

Other Loans

You may wish to consider professional development loans or research other methods pertinent to your funding, but be very careful to consider all angles. What is the interest rate? What company will provide it? What are the terms and conditions? Always make sure it is feasible and read the small print.

> While finishing my undergraduate neuroscience degree and preparing to re-apply to medical school, no one talked about the financial aspect of applying to medicine. Due to personal reasons, I couldn't afford to pay for my medical degree out of pocket. At the time, I felt optimistic and wrongly assumed the situation would soon be resolved. I focused on entrance exams and practical steps of the application process only to soon realise that I had missed several deadlines for scholarships and bursaries. Luckily everything worked out in the end, but my top tip is to start researching scholarships, bursaries and loans as early as possible and to apply far in advance to avoid disappointment.
>
> **Polen, Graduate Entry Medical School Applicant, UK**

COPING AS A MATURE STUDENT

Studying for your first undergraduate degree undoubtedly has its difficulties, namely funding, what clothes to wear and how to get rid of the mould from your student flat ceiling, but returning to university as a graduate, particularly if you've had a large gap since you left university, presents many unique considerations.

On the positive side, you already have at least one degree under your belt. You are familiar with all the 'fresher' stuff already—how to critique sources, how to research, how to disseminate information and how to work in groups on projects. Universities always favour a graduate on a medical course because they won't have to 'hold hands' with them and teach them how university works—they've already been there and done that. The student can also act as a mentor for other undergraduates who may struggle to adapt to university life. Graduates also possess more life experience and academic know-how, and this exposure to the world outside academia and the medical sphere will make you a much more well-rounded person, with a variety of transferrable skills and experiences to draw on during your time in medical school.

On the other hand, you may be joining a cohort of very enthusiastic, very young undergraduates. Not many of them will have the same challenges you will be considering, such as a partner, family, housing or even children—being an adult, basically. Rejoining university as a graduate will painfully remind you how fast-paced and relentless university can be, especially when you're ultimately training to save peoples' lives. Inside and outside of medical school, people will look to you for inspiration and leadership, and sometimes you may feel that you are scrutinised just that little bit more than your colleagues. This extra pressure, alongside your financial and personal concerns, can quickly prove overwhelming. There may be times where you question your motivations, whether you've made a mistake, or how you will ever graduate. It's entirely natural to doubt yourself—in fact, it's a good sign that you're not being overconfident. In these situations though, you must remind yourself why you started this in the first place. Remember your burning desire to become a member of one of the most trusted and revered disciplines there is. Medical school, and being a doctor, is hard. Many try and few succeed, but the very fact that you're even in a position to apply to medical school, and become a doctor if you succeed, means that you're one of the very, very slim percentage of people who possess the 'right stuff'. The potential is in you somewhere, the medical school has already seen it, you just need to find it within yourself and unlock it.

There is always support for you if you struggle to cope. Universities have extremely good wellbeing and support services available to their students, and you can always ask any family or friends for a friendly ear or to help you with your studies.

> I already had an undergraduate degree, but when I first started, I was still anxious about starting medicine. Especially being a graduate student, it can seem different or even scary, but it wasn't. You have to remember that you have the experience of those 3 years as an undergraduate student so you can definitely do it, but also, you're all in the same boat. Everyone will feel the same as you and will want to make friends. My top advice is to enjoy the process as much as you can and remember, you should feel proud that this is what you worked for all those years in preparation for getting accepted.
>
> **Aisha, Graduate Entry Medical School Applicant, UK**

INTERNATIONAL MEDICAL STUDENTS

Welcome to the UK, my fellow overseas student! You may be applying to study in the UK or wishing to apply to the UK. You may have already accepted a place in a UK university and are just wondering what it's like to be a medical student in the UK. In any sense, I'll try my best to convey exactly that from my perspective, as I am one myself. However, I don't want you to take this as official advice, as I am just one international student out of hundreds.

APPLICATION: HOW IS IT DIFFERENT?

If you're reading this, chances are you've already looked up the technical side of this. Luckily for you, the application process is not that much more difficult for an international student than it is for a local student, as it is still done through UCAS. Here are some things to keep in mind.

Grades/Qualifications

Your attained qualifications from your home country may be from a different system than is generally used in the UK. Here, the most recognised qualifications from secondary school or college are the IGCSE/GCSE, A-Levels and the IB. Furthermore, certain subject requirements may hinder your progress in applying to medical school. For example, most universities require Biology and Chemistry A-Levels in order for you to be considered at all. If your qualifications do not match what the universities want, you may run into some trouble. Furthermore, each university's requirements are different, so extra research to help you pick your four choices may prove to be advantageous.

> Originally from Egypt, having lived the majority of my life in Dubai, I found moving to the UK and settling into university a very smooth process, which was partly due to the assistance provided to me during international week. Initially wanting to go to a city-based university, I found myself pleasantly surprised at how much I suited the campus life like that in the University of Nottingham.

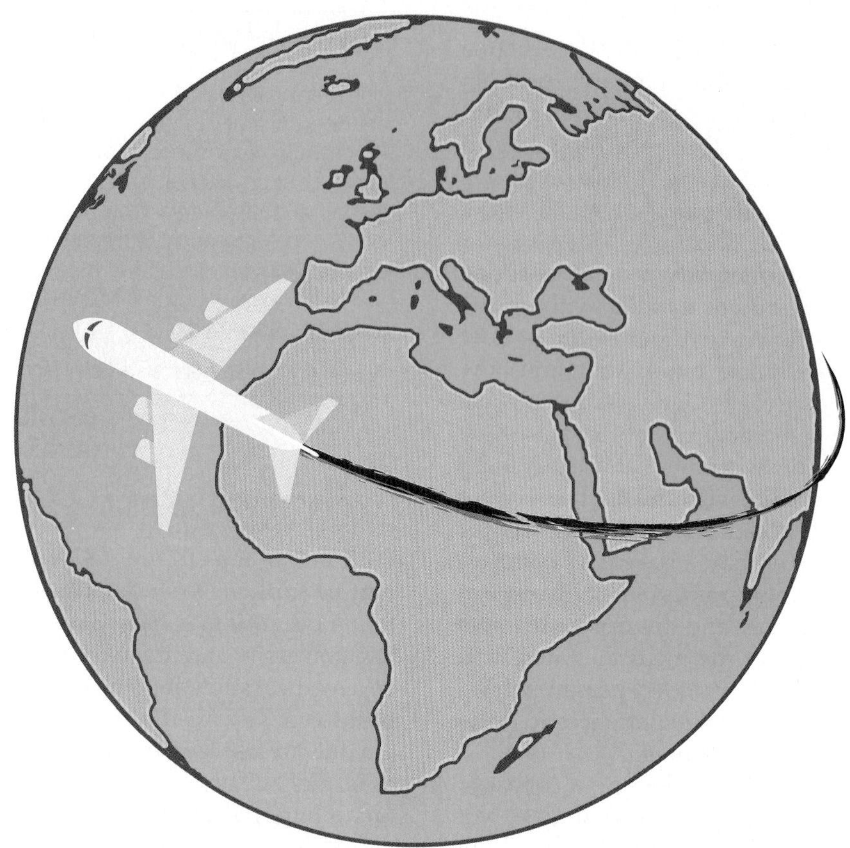

> University is a different type of learning environment, where the success achieved in your course is dependent on how hard you work and the passion you have for the subject. Some personal advice is to throw yourself at all opportunities that come your way—they will always act as a step forward to enhance your CV and will often lead to bigger and better prospects.
>
> **Fady Anis, Medical Student, Nottingham Medical School**

English

If you are an international applicant and have not completed any accepted qualifications to prove your English proficiency (such as an IGCSE in English), universities have every right to doubt your English ability. You may therefore be required to take English proficiency tests such as the International English Language Testing System (IELTS) or Test of English as a Foreign Language (TOEFL). International students who wish to study medicine at undergraduate level are required to achieve an IELTS score of 7.0 overall, with no less than 6.5 in any one component of reading, writing, speaking and listening. The exam operates a pass/fail policy; therefore, getting a higher score than the requirement does not put you at an advantage. Keep in mind that a pass on these tests has a limited period of validity. For example, the IELTS has a 2-year period of validity from the original test date, meaning that if you need to go through more than two rounds of application cycles, you will have to take it again (and I suggest you take it as few times as possible, it's not cheap).

Permit to Study in the UK

If you are not a holder of an UK passport (including EU student from 1 August 2021), then you will be classified as an international student. You are therefore required to obtain a Tier 4 (General) student visa if you're 16 and over in order to study in the UK (check out the UK government website). This is only obtainable after you've received an offer, and you have proven that you have enough money to support yourself and pay for your course. Post-Brexit, this is the case for European students too, unless they are able to apply for settled or presettled status (which applies to students who have been living in the UK for 3 or more years—more on this online on the UK government website directly).

According to the official UCAS website, Irish nationals are able to study within the UK under the Common Travel Area arrangement. Irish students will therefore be eligible for home fee status.

Fees

Before you get too giddy about studying medicine in the UK as an international student, let me remind you that it comes with a premium price tag. While local students pay around £9250 annually, international students pay almost triple that. Taking that into account, imagine what your total payment towards the university will be at the end of your course. Medicine courses are generally 5 to 6 years long, amounting to approximately £135,000—£162,000 by the time you graduate.

International students are embraced at the university, and I found that when I was not treated like everyone else, it was because people were celebrating my culture. With over 340 societies it was easy to find others who shared my interests, and whenever I longed to meet people of similar background, I went to the German society events.

Waseem Hasan, Medical Student, Imperial College London

Education is invaluable, and knowledge is power, but I seriously suggest you spend some time with a calculator and your parents to discuss whether the reality of your situation allows you to spend this sum to become a UK-qualified doctor.

Furthermore, this financial burden may be expected to rise in the coming years, as the government plans to increase medical school by removing a cap of university places to tackle workforce shortages. This does not, however, mean that more international students will necessarily be recruited. If anything, the number of places may stay the same, and the costs required to educate a larger cohort will be put on our shoulders.

Personal Statement and Interview

There may be a certain question that you feel the admissions committee of every university would want to ask you if you're an international student, and that's, 'Why UK?' From personal experience, there is no need to write why you did not pursue a degree in medicine in your home country or other countries. You may choose to write this if you feel that it has a large impact upon how examiners envision you through your personal statement. Otherwise, there is not much that is different regarding the writing of your personal statement.

Regarding the same question in the interview process, in the five medical school interviews that I had, MMI and panel styles included, no one asked me why I decided to study here as opposed to anywhere else. If it turns out to be the case for you, remember that everyone has their own reasons for going to the UK to study medicine. As long as the reason is genuine, no reason is more valid than another. In a way, this question is meant to test your argumentative skills, to see if you can back up your opinion with valid points. Interviewers may challenge you, so be prepared.

Other questions that may pop up and pose a challenge to international students are those pertaining to the NHS. Foreign students not used to the UK healthcare system may struggle with this question due to the fact that they are not exposed to it on a day-to-day basis. You do not need to go to the extent of buying an entire book on how the NHS works, because that will end up just being a waste of your time. It is healthier to your interview practice if you know a general overview of how the NHS functions and the current events surrounding it.

A minor thing that you may find peculiar in the interview process is that you may be grouped with other international students when going for an interview. This seemed to be a trend for me, where four out of the five universities I applied to grouped me with at least 30 other international applicants. Understandably, this is a stressful time where everyone is reciting their answers in their heads, but it's also a good chance to meet other people who may be your future coursemates while you standby in the waiting room.

Additionally, keep in mind that if you apply to universities around the UK, any offers for interviews will require you to prearrange travel (unless able to arrange for the interview to take place online—especially in a post-pandemic world where most universities understand travel restrictions). This includes flights and especially trains. Trains from central London to locations such as Newcastle can take up to 3 hours, so be prepared for these long journeys. Also, take into account interview start times, as some may be in the early morning, which would require you to find a place to stay overnight.

REFLECTIONS OF AN INTERNATIONAL MEDICAL STUDENT IN THE UK

Going abroad for a while can be tough. Luckily for me, transitioning into university was no different for me, as I had studied college in the UK as well, so I understood most things about the UK student lifestyle. However, as home is still thousands of miles away from Britain, I can empathise with a lot of problems that every international student has. Here are some common problems and how I've learned to combat them.

Culture Shock

It is perfectly normal to be surprised by foreign habits and mannerisms when you haven't come into contact with them before. One particular example for me was English sarcasm. The way that my friends and I speak back home is very direct—if we mean something, we'll say it with blatant intent. If sarcasm does come up in conversation, we are generally quite obvious about it and express it in our intonations. In my experience, English sarcasm can be incredibly subtle, so I could never tell if anyone was being serious or not! This is something that you will have to get used to, along with other bits of culture.

Despite the exciting course at my medical school (Aberdeen), I admit that it was difficult to move out of my comfort zone and adjust to the new environment. Coming from hot and humid Singapore, I remember feeling miserable in Scotland's dreary weather. The culture and people were very different, and I was definitely homesick. Over time though, these differences are actually what I have come to love about the place. The slower and more laid back pace of life is refreshing, the cold air invigorating and, of course, the freedom of independence most liberating!

I come from a big family of six and often missed their noise and company, which is why I was so thankful for my flatmates, whose friendship made our little flat feel more like home. The bonding and cultural exchange over food in our kitchen brings back great memories—whether it was watching them cry over my 'spicy' curry, eating helping after helping of Danish rice pudding or discovering what makes a quintessential American breakfast.

Being an international student is not easy, but it is comforting to know there are others in the same boat. Moreover, the opportunity to meet diverse people and experience new cultures is invaluable and worth cherishing.

Sarah Mow, Medical Student, Aberdeen Medical School

Reflect on why you want to be a doctor and enter medicine. How will you benefit from it and how will you benefit others? Do you think your motivations are good or will others disagree? Also, reflect on whether medicine as a second degree is feasible. Think about where you will get your funding, and how it will affect you and your family on a personal level. If you think you can do it then go for it! These are the uncomfortable questions that you will have to ask yourself, however.

Homesickness

When I first started studying abroad, I was lucky to have my parents send me on my way. Moreover, I was lucky to have a large(ish) community of people from the same place as I at my school. This enabled me to adapt to the new environment at a good pace, as I had all these people around me in the same exact position. We learned new things about this domain together and eventually became close friends. This didn't change when I progressed into university, as I sought the same learning experiences with new friends. Indeed, after all of that, I did miss a bit of home. I missed friends, food and the entire buzz of my home city. Something I do not take for granted, however, is the day and age that I live in, to be blessed with revolutionary modes of communication via the internet. Even though I was planted in a country that was quite unlike mine, this advantage helped me get through moments of homesickness. I was, overall, happy with where I was as long as I could confide in close friends and family. Furthermore, getting to talk to them during term time made seeing them in the summer holidays that much sweeter.

Homesickness is something that you must face on a day-to-day basis for the entire length of your course if you are to study medicine in the UK. That is the harsh reality that almost every international medical student will have to face. Remember, however, that hard work pays off, and if you can endure these few years of being away from home, then it will be worth it.

Friends and Colleagues at University

Just because I graduated from college and continued into university did not mean that I lost this sense of community. I was eager to learn more about the culture in which I was immersed, but also eager to stay in touch with my roots. This pushed me to find other like-minded people, which in fact I found through my course. As medicine is typically a close-knit course (depending on your cohort size), if you try, you can get to know many people, a lot of whom will surprise you in how well you can relate to them, even if they aren't from the same background as you. You can also get to know more like-minded people if you just join societies. University societies are there for a reason, and that is to gather people together with similar interests. Do not be afraid that just because you are from another country that chess society will be different—it's not. Chess is chess, and so are many other sports and activities.

As most medical schools within the UK, my university (Bristol) is nothing if not diverse, and as an international student I found it very stimulating meeting students of different ages, ethnicities and backgrounds, and being able to interact and learn from one another's experiences. The friends I made at university have different lifestyles and different goals, but we support and respect one another to the best of our ability.

Kiyara Fernando, Medical Student, Bristol Medical School

To take it one step further, you can get to know other people from other universities as well. Mutual friends go a long way, and especially with the invention of Facebook, you can get to know other medics/international medics and share your experiences with them.

Being an international student studying medicine in the UK represents a challenge that is more than simply tackling the difficult and large expanse of material covered at medical school; rather, it encompasses a diverse range of other challenges ranging from settling into a brand new environment and adapting to an unfamiliar culture (as is the case for those who have moved directly from their home country), meeting and making new friends of differing backgrounds and, most crucially, in most incidences having to support themselves and their wellbeing while being stationed thousands of miles away from their homes and families.

Academically, many internationals like ourselves are coping and performing exceptionally well. There is a very strong sense of unity and cohesion within the international cohort, and they are highly supportive of one another, in particular sharing information and learning resources through social media. My colleague David and I have been involved in a vast amount of activities from being on the committee of the surgical society, to presenting posters at conferences, to competing for the healthcare basketball team! Thus, this is an excellent example of the variety of activities that international students here at Cardiff and throughout the UK in general get up to beyond the classroom, and is a fair reflection of the admirable efforts of international students to make the most of the opportunities available to them.

Timothy Woo & David Li, Medical Students, Cardiff Medical School

On the academic side of things, it may be advantageous for you to get to know lecturers and doctors as well while you're at university. In reality, networking is a good skill to possess. Having a connection with someone may in the future bring up more opportunities for you and give you more chances to speak with professionals at the top of their field. As they have experienced medical school, foundation school and much more medical training, every one of them is a walking textbook that you can ask to learn more about where you want to end up later on. Who knows when the reference letter will come in useful?

Language

If English is not your strongest language, it will be difficult for you to really study medicine in the UK. I would like to say that this depends on what aspect of your English is best, whether it's speaking, writing, listening or reading, but in an English-speaking country you will have to do all of those things, especially when you dedicate yourself to such a subject. Lectures will be in English, notes will be in English, patients and doctors will speak in English, so there really is no escape. However, the entirely immersive experience that you have in an English-speaking society is probably the best way to improve. Simple things to improve all aspects of your English skills, such as writing a diary, reading the newspaper and conversing with others, are small steps towards mastering it. Medicine itself has a lot of Latin terms where one can easily see patterns depending on their usages, so that's already one hurdle cleared.

> Academic-wise, I felt prepared for my course companions; however, communication was the biggest problem for me when I came to the UK because English was not my first language. I struggled with the Scottish accent when I first arrived—it took me a few months to understand their accent and the way they speak. It's frustrating in the beginning, but you get used to it. On a final note, enjoy the sun as much as you can before you come here—the UK weather is definitely not the best in the world.
>
> **Eric Fung, Medical Student, Edinburgh Medical School**

NOT READY YET: COPING WITH REJECTION

Hopefully it won't happen to you, but being rejected from your chosen medical schools the first time you apply is a very real prospect. Medical school vacancies are extremely competitive, and it would be no exaggeration to say that over 20 applicants per place is fairly normal. Believe me, I know because I've been there, and seeing several red cross rejections on UCAS is a crippling blow to your self-esteem. You may doubt your achievements or think of jacking it all in. However, not achieving a place in medical school should be seen as an opportunity, rather than a failure. Let me explain.

ACCEPTANCE

The most important thing you can do in an unsuccessful year is to accept what's happened. It's horrible, it's upsetting, but you were probably still in the better percentage of candidates. It may be a setback, but that's all it is. You can always reapply as many times as you like, and each rejection makes you work on where you were weaker, so you are stronger for next time. Take some time off, have a break. You were probably under a lot of pressure waiting for university decisions to arrive, so you won't do yourself any favours by burning yourself out. Take a few weeks off, go on a short staycation, visit your friends and spend some quality time or just do something else. The time away will help you come to terms with the rejections and refocus.

SEEK FEEDBACK

Once you feel a bit better, email your schools and politely ask for feedback if they haven't provided any. It will probably prove very useful, and you may be pleasantly surprised to find out you did much better than you thought. I received my first rejection because I was only one point off an offer, so it was far from an outright failure!

What was it that contributed most to your failure? Was it your personal statement? Your UCAT, BMAT, A-Level grades, or was it your interview performance? Whatever it might be, find out what your weaknesses are and start REFLECTING on them. A mistake only becomes a mistake if you don't make an effort to learn anything from it.

COME UP WITH A PLAN

Once you know what you have to work on, it is the time to make an action plan. Is there anything you can do during this application cycle? In the following, we talk about a few options that may be available to you. Here's what you need to know.

What About Your Fifth Option on UCAS?

Most medical school applicants usually have a biomedical sciences or medical sciences degree as their fifth option on UCAS. Were you successful in this? If so, is this something you'd like to do and reapply to medical school as a graduate? If you want to go into graduate medicine, have a read through our section on this.

What If You Have Been Rejected From All Five Universities on UCAS? UCAS Extra

If you've been rejected from all five universities on UCAS, you are entitled to use 'UCAS Extra'. This is an extra option on UCAS that you can use for any university of your choice that will still consider your application. The good thing is you can choose any subject (if they still accept applications), and you also have the opportunity to change your personal statement. This means that you can change your personal statement from medicine to biomedical sciences and send your application to a university that will accept you. You can read more about this at https://www.ucas.com/ucas/undergraduate/apply-and-track/track-your-application/extra-choices. This fits in well with transfer schemes (described later) and universities where you may consider applying to medicine as a graduate.

Are There Any Other Ways of Getting Into Medical School Using Your Current Application?

There are a few medical schools in the UK offering a transfer scheme from biomedical science degrees into medicine after the successful completion of Year 1. However, these are VERY competitive, and usually only 5% to 10% of students who are at the top of the cohort after the first year get the chance to transfer. That doesn't mean it's impossible, it just means there is a lot of hard work, but if you're ready to give it a go, there's nothing that can stop you from achieving it. In fact, one of this book's authors did a year of medical sciences at Exeter Medical School, ended up in the top 10% of the class, and successfully transferred into medicine. There is hope, but there's also hard work.

Here are a couple of the universities currently offering transfer schemes. To find out more, research online and email the admissions team, as this information is likely to change from year to year and varies depending on cohort numbers. You would also benefit from speaking to a student who transferred in the past, so do your best to get in touch with one.

Transfer from Biomedical Sciences into Medicine Schemes:

- **Bradford University**. Transfer into **Leeds Medical School** (two chances to transfer, once at the end of the Foundation Year, and again at the end of Year 1 of Clinical Sciences)
- **Exeter Medical School**. Top 10 students only out of a cohort of 200+ from Medical Sciences)
- **Leicester University**. From Biomedical Sciences, very competitive.
- **Newcastle University**. Top seven students only, from Biomedical Sciences.

There may be other schemes that we are not aware of yet. Have a thorough look online and email admission tutors from individual medical schools where you may want to reapply.

Students rejected in the past often try to secure an offer at one of the previously mentioned universities for biomedical sciences through either UCAS Extra or UCAS Clearing (https://www.ucas.com/ucas/undergraduate/apply-and-track/results/no-offers-learn-how-clearing-works), because if they couldn't transfer after the first year, they would then apply to Graduate Medicine after spending 3 years at the aforementioned institutions.

Make a Decision and Have Faith in the Path You Have Chosen

Which journey are you going to take? Are you going to try transferring? Reapplying? What about Graduate Medicine?

It simply doesn't matter, to be honest with you. All journeys lead to the same destination. Be it Graduate Medicine, a transfer scheme or reapplying after a gap year, if you are persistent and determined enough, you will make it in the end.

People often cry about losing 1 year of their lives, but what's a year of your life if you don't do what you truly love? What's 1 year if you won't be pursuing a job that truly makes you happy? You will be a medical student. You deserve a place at medical school. Keep pushing, keep working, and you will succeed. We hope the following stories from students who did not make it into medicine the first time they applied will inspire you.

> Realising that you won't start studying medicine next autumn can bring out emotions, 'what ifs', and lots of confusion. Then you realise that acting like everything is over is not helpful in any way and you're not actually a failure at all. Then you have another realisation, and that's realising all the opportunities out there that will help you find a way into medicine and help you grow as a person. As long as you have the determination, you will find a way to reach your goal and nothing will be able to stop you.
>
> **Beatrice Golban, Medical Student, University of Bristol**

> Disappointment. That word resonates with students, scientists and practically anyone who has envisioned a goal that they failed to meet. That word particularly stung 2 years ago when I realised my final option was to study biomedical sciences—not medicine. Not because my grades didn't make the cut—in fact, I scored as the top 1% in the world for the Diploma Programme in 2016. Instead, I let myself down on the admission test. After realising I'd be a life sciences student instead, I chose not to regret the path that I am on today. As Warren stated, 'We are products of our past, but we do not have to be prisoners of it'. My drive to study medicine has never been more intense than it is now. Rather than feeling inadequate, I've gained a more profound appreciation for the science at work propelling the clinical aspect of medicine.
>
> Currently at UCL, my stream concentrates on human anatomy and physiology, which has encouraged me to increase my knowledge of the biological principles that define the human body. Everything I am learning inspires me to become a better scientist and doctor. I believe that through this alternative journey, I've thoroughly developed my capabilities to become the best possible human I can be, in order to serve our society and contribute to restoring human health.
>
> **Evita Müller, Medical Student, University College London**

> Being rejected from medical school the first time around cannot be described in words. Frustration, anger, tears and confusion—these overwhelmed me for a few days, weeks, even months. I felt stupid, incapable of achieving what was perhaps my biggest dream. What was even more frustrating was that I didn't receive any interview invitations. I never had the chance to prove who I am. I was simply rejected due to my

background and international examinations, which the admission teams could not translate because they never had an applicant with my background before then.

My frustration, anger and feelings of uselessness transformed into motivation and determination, fuelling my passion to keep going until I eventually made it. They say there's always a rainbow behind the clouds, and you only get to see it if you make it through the storm. In my case, there was certainly a hell of a storm, but here I am, in my fourth year as a medical student, only 1 year away from becoming a doctor.

As a medical student, inspired by the frustration of not making it into medicine on the first try, I put a team together and we created what has become Medefine Education—a network of hundreds of passionate medical students from all over the UK, ready to share their best tips to help new applicants, like yourself. This is why today, I am writing this book to give you the best advice I would have given myself 5 years ago.

There definitely is a rainbow behind the clouds, and I am grateful to be here, sharing my story with you. I hope that you too will stay motivated and determined, and one day reach your goal of studying medicine in the UK. It doesn't matter how many times you try and fail. What matters is how many times you get up and try again. I wish you all the best, and don't ever forget: If you want to become a doctor, if you're willing to put in the hard work, then your wish will one day come true.

Dr Bogdan Chiva Giurca, Medical Doctor

TAKING A GAP YEAR AND REAPPLYING

TAKING A GAP YEAR

Over the years, we have received several questions from students who are willing to take a gap year before they start medical school. Whether it's because they didn't make it on the first try or because they want to explore other areas before committing to medicine, taking a gap year is a reasonable thing to do.

Here are some of the most frequently encountered questions about gap years.

DO I GET MARKED DOWN ON MY APPLICATION FOR TAKING A GAP YEAR?

Taking a gap year is completely your choice, and universities do not mark you down as long as you can explain your decision. In fact, if you do the 'right stuff', it will increase your chances of getting in. We will talk more about the 'right stuff' soon, but here's a simple example. If you were an admission tutor, would you choose a student who has some work experience or a student who has some work experience and a whole year of volunteering in an underdeveloped country during their gap year?

If this is your first application to medical school, you have two options. First, you can apply using **deferred entry** in October during your final year of school. This means you'll go on your gap year knowing whether you have been accepted or not. You can read more about this on each medical school's information page under 'deferred entry'. Second, you can apply in October after your final year of school (during your gap year). This gives you the opportunity to add your plans for your gap year in your personal statement, which may give you an advantage over other applicants.

If you are reapplying to medical school, please read the final section of this chapter, as you may want to check which universities accept applicants who are reapplying and which don't.

CAN I TRAVEL DURING MY GAP YEAR?

What you do during your work experience is completely up to you, as long as it can be considered a 'learning experience' that will make you a better applicant and perhaps a better doctor someday.

To answer the previous question, the answer is yes and no. By that we mean yes you can travel, but not if you're just travelling to have fun. If you travel to gain work experience and explore different cultures, that's a good enough reason. If you're planning a trip to Ibiza with your mates, you may want to avoid mentioning that in your personal statement, although I suppose your first aid skills may improve by looking after your mate who's had a few too many drinks.

SHOULD I MENTION MY GAP YEAR IN MY PERSONAL STATEMENT AND DURING MY INTERVIEW?

Absolutely, it is a MUST. You must put to good use all these new experiences and shine bright in front of the admission tutors and interviewing panel. You have something extra; why not talk about it? If you do not mention it, however, the gap in your studies will pose certain questions and you will most definitely be asked about this during your interview.

THE 'RIGHT STUFF' FOR YOUR GAP YEAR

Here are some of our top tips for a well-spent gap year.

Come Up with a Plan

We've mentioned this already, but sitting down and creating a list of the things you want to achieve during this year is crucial. Don't let the year start and blindly choose random activities that are thrown at you. Design your own year and make it worth it.

Reflect on the Following

- Where would I like to go? (Be it home or in a different country, it makes no difference)
- What would I like to do?
  - Work experience?
  - Exam preparation? (AS/A Level grades, UCAT, BMAT)
  - Travelling?
  - Volunteering?
  - Sports and other activities?
- If I imagined the perfect gap year, what would it look like and why?

Take Part in Work Experience, Volunteering or Other Extracurricular Activities

Be it in a general practice (GP) surgery or a remote, low-income country, what matters is what you learn during your work experience. Stay organised and use the advice in our Work Experience chapter as well as the reflective templates to log and reflect upon your experiences.

Our previous chapter covered what counts as work experience. In short, it can be part of a hospital, GP setting, care homes, charities, hospices or any other area of your choice, as long as you can reason that what you learnt can be applied in a clinical setting.

You can also join several international volunteer projects or extracurricular activities that can be found online. There may even be paid positions such as teaching children in various countries how to speak English. Explore all your options before making a decision.

Get Involved in Some Research

Some of you may have done a bit of research as part of A-Levels or your Extended Project Qualification (EPQ) projects. If you haven't experienced research firsthand, joining a lab for a couple of weeks or months may be a useful experience if you correlate it with the role of a doctor as a researcher.

Find Time to Reflect on Your Previous Application (If Applicable)

- What went wrong?
- How can I use this year to improve?
- Are there any preparatory courses that I can join?
- Can I get a better letter of recommendation?

Find Time to Relax

It is important to remember that universities look for well-rounded individuals. You may want to allocate time to sports or hobbies that you truly love. Remember, at the end of the day, medical schools are looking for humans, not robots. Medical school can be very stressful, and admission tutors appreciate when you convey an understanding of this and then go on to demonstrate productive techniques you've developed in your gap year that will allow you to cope with stress.

> Following my unsuccessful first attempt of getting into medical school, I decided to take a gap year and apply again.
>
> My top tip for you is to invest in yourself during this year. I used my year to repair everything that went wrong in my previous application. I learnt how to write better personal statements, I worked harder on entrance exams including the UCAT and BMAT, and I did more preparation for interviews.
>
> I ended up working in a clinic in Malaysia alongside doctors and nurses. I found it highly rewarding and when I reflected on my work experience, I realised how unprepared I was when I first applied to medical school. In any case, I felt like now I deserved a place at medical school and it eventually happened.
>
> **Akash, Medical Student, Leicester Medical School**

REAPPLYING TO MEDICAL SCHOOL

First, you need to make sure that the universities you are reapplying to allow you to do so. There are a few medical schools that only allow you to apply once. Using one of your UCAS choices on such a medical school would simply be a waste of your resources.

Here's a list of the medical schools that only allow you to apply once. We strongly recommend that you get in touch with each of the four medical schools you are about to reapply to and ask whether they are okay with you doing so. It's always best to make sure especially as this information changes from year to year.

Universities that will not consider your application if you reapply:

- Birmingham Medical School
- Keele Medical School
- Lancaster Medical School
- University College London

When the time comes to reapply, be honest in your personal statement. Medical schools won't judge you at all for being rejected; they know how hard it is to be accepted. State how you have bettered yourself since your rejection, how you understand why you failed, how you sought feedback and how you changed in light of the feedback received. The very fact that you are reapplying looks good and shows real determination, something that makes a very good doctor. *Someone* has to gain that place in medical school, so why shouldn't it be you?

Similarly, adopt the same attitude during your medical school interviews. Be grateful for being there once again, and demonstrate how you used your previous failure as a learning experience that made you more determined and motivated to pursue a career in medicine.

However, you may find that medicine is indeed not for you, and that's absolutely fair! There are hundreds of other roles in the healthcare sector that may align more closely with your interests and skills than you think. Have a look around and see what's out there, you may be surprised!

FINAL THOUGHTS

I truly wish all of you every success. Unfortunately, not everyone makes the cut first time round, but that is just the nature of medicine as a profession. By accepting the best, that's what makes it such a revered and trusted discipline. With positivity and tenacity, there's no reason why you shouldn't succeed. Best of luck to you all.

SUMMARY, TEST YOURSELF AND REFLECTION

If You Want to Succeed

- **You can never start preparing too early.** Doing a little bit here and there is far more effective than cramming in a couple of weeks.
- **Be reflective.** Question your motivations—is medicine truly what you want to do? List your reasons.
- **Don't be fazed by adversity.** Many outstanding professionals failed their application at least once. Don't be fazed by that C grade at A-level or how difficult you've heard the GAMSAT is—just go in there and do your absolute best; that's all you can do!
- Remember, some people might try to psych you out or talk down your achievements, not always maliciously, but **have faith in yourself**. The very fact that you are in a position to apply to medical school, sit an admissions test or get an interview is an achievement in itself. You ARE capable, and don't let naysayers tell you otherwise.
- Don't do what I did and leave yourself only a month to study for the GAMSAT—it's not worth the stress.
- **Networking** is so useful—even if it's just swapping numbers or emails, every contact is potentially someone who can really help you later.

Test Yourself

- What exams do you need to consider, and which universities can you apply to?
- When is your UCAS application deadline?
- How much time do you need to prepare for your exams?

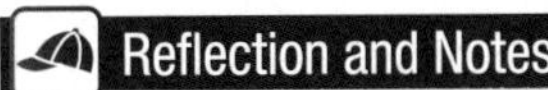

Reflection and Notes

RESOURCES

ACER. (2017). Graduate medical school admissions test – Information booklet. Australian Council for Educational Research.

The Medic Portal. (2017). Which UK medical schools offer the graduate entry medicine courses? Available at https://www.themedicportal.com/application-guide/graduate-entry-medicine.

UCAS. (2017). Filling in your UCAS undergraduate application. Available at https://www.ucas.com/ucas/undergraduate/apply-and-track/filling-your-ucas-undergraduate-application.

University of Nottingham. (2017). Funding for GEM (graduate entry medicine) students. Available at http://www.nottingham.ac.uk/studentservices/support/financialsupport/studentfunding/fundingforgemstudents.aspx.

The Geeky Corner

Bogdan Chiva Giurca

One of the most common questions we get from medical school applicants is 'What should I read/watch/do to expand my knowledge in preparation for the application process?' Hundreds of you wrote back to us asking for a list of suggestions, so we came up with a 'geeky corner' for you all. This is a place where you can find recommendations and suggestions for some of the best medically related films, books, museums and other places to visit.

Well, here it is – an area full of resources, put together by medical students all over the UK, your own geeky corner. Enjoy!

BOOKS

- 'When Breath Becomes Air'—Paul Kalanithi (our personal favourite!)
- 'Trust me, I'm a (Junior) Doctor'—Max Pemberton
- 'Being Mortal'—Atul Gawande
- 'The Checklist Manifesto'—Atul Gawande
- 'This Is Going to Hurt'—Adam Key
- 'Do No Harm'—Henry Marsh
- 'Your Life in My Hands'—Rachel Clarke
- 'Complications'—Atul Gawande
- 'The Gene: An Intimate History'—Siddhartha Mukherjee
- 'How We Do Harm'—Otis Brawley
- 'The Man Who Mistook His Wife for a Hat'—Oliver Sacks
- 'Medical Ethics: A Very Short Introduction'—Tony Hope
- 'The Health Gap'—Michael Marmot
- 'The Emperor of All Maladies'—Siddhartha Mukherjee
- 'How Doctors Think'—Jerome Groopman
- 'Bad Pharma'—Ben Goldacre
- 'I Think You'll Find It's a Bit More Complicated Than That'—Ben Goldacre
- 'The Intern Blues'—Robert Marion
- 'The Anatomy of Home'—Jerome Groopman
- 'A Not Entirely Benign Procedure: Four Years as a Medical Student'—Perri Klass
- 'How We Live'—Sherwin Nuland
- 'The Lives of a Cell: Notes of a Biology Watcher'—Lewis Thomas
- 'Snowball in a Blizzard: The Tricky Problem of Uncertainty in Medicine'—Steve Hatch
- 'Medicine's Strangest Cases'—Michael O'Donnell
- 'Adventures in Human Being'—Gavin Francis
- 'Fragile Lives: A Heart Surgeon's Stories of Life and Death on the Operating Table'—Stephen Westaby
- 'Trauma: My Life as an Emergency Surgeon'—James Cole
- 'A Cabinet of Medical Curiosities'—Jan Bondeson
- 'Better: A Surgeon's Notes on Performance'—Atul Gawande
- 'It's All in Your Head: Stories from the Frontline of Psychosomatic Illness'—Suzanne O'Sullivan
- 'The Healing of America: A Global Quest for Better, Cheaper, and Fairer Health Care'—T.R. Reid
- 'How Not to Die: Discover the Foods Scientifically Proven to Prevent and Reverse Disease' —Michael Greger
- 'Awakenings'—Oliver Sacks

FILMS, PODCASTS, TV SERIES, ONLINE VIDEOS, LECTURE SERIES

- Patch Adams (Film, 1998)—Directed by Tom Shadyac, Universal Pictures. Patch Adams (Film, 1998)—Directed by Tom Shadyac, Universal Pictures.
- Wit (Film, 2001)—Directed by Mike Nichols, HBO Films.
- The Doctor (Film, 1991)—Directed by Randa Haines, Touchstone Pictures.
- Science and Medicine Playlist: TED videos (Video playlist, ongoing)—TED.com.
- Trust Me I'm a Doctor (TV series, 2014–present)—BBC Two.
- The English Surgeon (Documentary, 2007)—Directed by Geoffrey Smith, BBC Storyville.
- House MD (TV series, 2004–12)—Created by David Shore, Fox Broadcasting Company.
- Scrubs (TV series, 2001–10)—Created by Bill Lawrence, NBC/ABC.
- One Flew Over the Cuckoo's Nest (Film, 1975)—Directed by Miloš Forman, United Artists.
- Madame Curie (Film, 1943)—Directed by Mervyn LeRoy, Metro-Goldwyn-Mayer.

- The 'Hospital' (TV series, 1971)—Directed by Frederick Wiseman, Zipporah Films.
- Grey's Anatomy (TV series, 2005-present)—Created by Shonda Rhimes, ABC.
- The Doctor Who Gave Up Drugs (Documentary, 2016)—BBC One.
- Atul Gawande's 2014 Reith Lecture Series (Podcast, 2014)—BBC Radio 4.
- Hospital (BBC Documentary, 2017–present)—BBC Two.
- Emergency Room (American medical drama, 1994–2009)—Created by Michael Crichton, NBC.
- Big Think (Online forum, ongoing)—BigThink.com.
- Gattaca (Film, 1997)—Directed by Andrew Niccol, Columbia Pictures.
- The Elephant Man (Film, 1980)—Directed by David Lynch, Paramount Pictures.
- Something the Lord Made (Film, 2004)—Directed by Joseph Sargent, HBO Films.
- Our healthcare systems are making doctors mentally ill (TEDx Talk, 2017)—by Zeshan Qureshi, TEDx.

MUSEUMS AND SCIENCE GALLERIES (LONDON)

- The Wellcome Collection
- The Old Operating Theatre
- Alexander Fleming's Laboratory
- Hunterian Museum, Royal College of Surgeons
- Barts Pathology Museum
- Florence Nightingale Museum
- Royal College of Physicians Museum
- Science Museum

Hopefully, these lists will keep you busy in those moments of heavy-duty procrastination. If you have any further suggestions, or if there's a book that had a big impact on your learning and decision to choose medicine, we'd love to hear from you.

Finally, as we were compiling this list, several medical students suggested that you listen to and read other things outside medicine. Being well rounded is very important, and so is finding enough time to relax and recharge your batteries during periods of intense stress.

Index

Note: Page numbers followed by *b* indicate boxes, *f* indicate figures and *t* indicate tables.

M

N

O

P

V

W